A Dictionary of Neurological Signs

A.J. Larner

A Dictionary of Neurological Signs

Fourth Edition

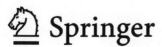 Springer

A.J. Larner, MA, MD, MRCP(UK),
DHMSA, PhD
Walton Centre for Neurology and
Neurosurgery
Liverpool
UK

ISBN 978-3-319-29819-1   ISBN 978-3-319-29821-4   (eBook)
DOI 10.1007/978-3-319-29821-4

Library of Congress Control Number: 2016938226

Printed on acid-free paper

This Springer imprint is published by Springer Nature
The registered company is Springer International Publishing AG Switzerland

To Sue
Nil satis nisi optimum

The dictionary is the only place where success comes before work

Arthur Brisbane

Foreword to the First Edition (2001)

Neurology has always been a discipline in which careful physical examination is paramount. The rich vocabulary of neurology replete with eponyms attests to this historically. The decline in the importance of the examination has long been predicted with the advent of more detailed neuroimaging. However, neuroimaging has often provided a surfeit of information from which salient features have to be identified, dependent upon the neurological examination. A dictionary of neurological signs has a secure future.

A dictionary should be informative but unless it is unwieldy, it cannot be comprehensive, nor is that claimed here. Andrew Larner has decided sensibly to include key features of the history as well as the examination. There is no doubt that some features of the history can strike one with the force of a physical sign. There are entries for "palinopsia" and "environmental tilt" both of which can only be elicited from the history and yet which have considerable significance. There is also an entry for the "head turning sign" observed during the history taking itself as well as the majority of entries relating to details of the physical examination.

This book is directed to students and will be valuable to medical students, trainee neurologists, and professions allied to medicine. Neurologists often speak in shorthand and so entries such as "absence" and "freezing" are sensible and helpful. For the more mature student, there are the less usual as well as common eponyms to entice one to read further than the entry which took you first to the dictionary.

Queen Square, London, UK   Martin N. Rossor

Preface to the Fourth Edition

Those who have read Linda Mugglestone's engaging book on the subject of dictionaries [1] might rightly object (and vehemently so) to this volume calling itself a dictionary. It is not, by any stretch of the imagination, an example of modern systematic corpus lexicography. Rather, it is based on "individual and *ad hoc* reading" (page 56) to gather evidence which, in a generous mood, might be termed "fieldwork" (59), or perhaps more accurately "armchair lexicography" (59), the finished work thus representing the author's "fallibility of aspiration" (80). Such accusations cannot justly be rebutted, but in my defence I might state that this all too human product *is* like other dictionaries in that it is a highly mutable text, bound to change and not stasis (15) – this is the 4th edition in 15 years! – which seeks to probe the nature of words (19). The hope is that this endeavour to produce a lexicon of neurology will remain relevant to those engaged in the assessment and examination of individuals with neurological symptoms.

Should dictionaries be simply descriptive, and neither prescriptive (a recommendation for what should be used) nor proscriptive (a recommendation for what should not be used)? [1]. A scientific vocabulary should surely err on the side of exactness. Possibly for this reason, I have been afflicted with an increasing sense of dissatisfaction with the largely descriptive nature of this book (one might almost say it is akin to flower arranging), perhaps prompted by experience with the use of diagnostic and screening tests where a more rigorous quantitative evaluation is required [2]. The same methodology based around conditional probabilities is certainly applicable to the assessment of neurological signs [3] and it is good to see this being applied to more of the signs described in this book (see, for example, Babinksi's sign, Kernig's sign), as well as evaluations of inter-rater agreement [4]. An attempt has been made to evaluate some of the signs used in cognitive neurology in this way ("attended alone" sign, "head turning" sign, applause sign) [5]. Nevertheless, a Pubmed search using terms such as "sign", "sensitivity and specificity", "diagnostic accuracy", etc., will afford few hits (<50 at time of writing, and even fewer specifically for neurological signs).

Debate continues between those neurologists who appear to advocate less [6] or more [7] neurological examination in clinical practice, but the dichotomy is probably illusory, since most would agree that focused examination which aims to test the diagnostic hypotheses generated from the clinical history taking is the ideal. I'm sure that I examine far less than I used to, presumably because with increasing experience the likely differential diagnosis is pretty clear based on the history alone. Clinical examination never takes place in a vacuum. Thus Martin Rossor was (hopefully) prescient in his Foreword to the first edition (2001) when he opined that "A dictionary of neurological signs has a secure future".

Liverpool, UK   A.J. Larner

References

1. Mugglestone L. Dictionaries: a very short introduction. Oxford: Oxford University Press; 2011.
2. Larner AJ, editor. Cognitive screening instruments. A practical approach. London: Springer; 2013.
3. Larner AJ. Diagnostic test accuracy studies in dementia. A pragmatic approach. London: Springer; 2015.
4. Thaller M, Hughes T. Inter-rater agreement of observable and elicitable neurological signs. Clin Med. 2014;14:264–7.
5. Larner AJ. Neurological signs of possible diagnostic value in the cognitive disorders clinic. Pract Neurol. 2014;14:332–5.
6. Hawkes CH. I've stopped examining patients. Pract Neurol. 2009;9:192–4.
7. Warlow CP. Why I have not stopped examining patients. Pract Neurol. 2010;10:126–8.

Acknowledgements

In preparing this fourth edition, particular thanks are due to friends and colleagues who have commented on the earlier editions, namely (in alphabetical order) Alasdair Coles, Anu Jacob, Alex Leff, Miratul Muqit, Parashkev Nachev, and Sivakumar Sathasivam. At Springer, I am grateful for support and encouragement received from Joanna Bolesworth. All errors and shortcomings which remain are entirely my own work.

Contents

A

Abadie's Sign

Abadie's sign is the absence or diminution of subjective pain sensation when exerting deep pressure on the Achilles tendon by squeezing. This is a frequent finding in the tabes dorsalis variant of neurosyphilis, *i.e.* with dorsal column disease, but now is more usually encountered in the context of diabetes mellitus as a consequence of intratendinous changes which might predispose to tendon rupture. The sign has also been reported in adrenomyeloneuropathy.

References

Abate M, Schiavone C, Salini V, Andia I. Revisiting physical examination: Abadie's sign and Achilles intratendinous changes in subjects with diabetes. *Med Princ Pract.* 2014; **23**: 186–8.

Ohtomo R, Matsukawa T, Tsuji S, Iwata A. Abadie's sign in adrenomyeloneuropathy. *J Neurol Sci.* 2014; **340**: 245–6.

Cross Reference

Argyll Robertson pupil

Abdominal Paradox

- see PARADOXICAL BREATHING

Abdominal Reflexes

Both superficial and deep abdominal reflexes are described, of which the superficial (cutaneous) reflexes are the more commonly tested in clinical practice. A wooden stick or pin is used to scratch the abdominal wall, from the flank to the midline, parallel to the line of the dermatomal strips, in upper (supraumbilical), middle (umbilical), and lower (infraumbilical) areas. The manoeuvre is best performed at the end of expiration when the abdominal muscles are relaxed, since the reflexes may be lost with muscle tensing; to avoid this, patients should lie supine with their arms by their sides. Superficial abdominal reflexes are lost in a number of circumstances:

- Normal ageing.
- Obesity.
- Following abdominal surgery.
- Following multiple pregnancies.
- In acute abdominal disorders (Rosenbach's sign).

However, absence of all superficial abdominal reflexes may be of localising value for corticospinal pathway damage (upper motor neurone lesions) above T6. Lesions at or below T10 lead to selective loss of the lower reflexes with the upper and middle reflexes intact, in which case Beevor's sign may also be present. All abdominal reflexes are preserved with lesions below T12.

Abdominal reflexes are said to be lost early in multiple sclerosis, but late in motor neurone disease, an observation of possible clinical use, particularly when differentiating the progressive lateral sclerosis variant of motor neurone disease from multiple sclerosis. However, no prospective study of abdominal reflexes in multiple sclerosis has been reported.

Reference

Dick JPR. The deep tendon and the abdominal reflexes. *J Neurol Neurosurg Psychiatry.* 2003; **74**: 150–3.

© Springer International Publishing Switzerland 2016
A.J. Larner, *A Dictionary of Neurological Signs*,
DOI 10.1007/978-3-319-29821-4_1

Cross References
Beevor's sign; Upper motor neurone (UMN) syndrome

Abducens (VI) Nerve Palsy
Abducens, abducent, or sixth, cranial nerve palsy causes a selective weakness of the lateral rectus muscle resulting in impaired abduction of the affected eye, manifest clinically as diplopia on lateral gaze, or on shifting gaze from a near to a distant object.

Abducens nerve palsy may occur anywhere along its nuclear, fascicular, subarachnoid, petrous apex, cavernous sinus, and orbital course. It may be an isolated finding or be associated with accompanying neurological features which may assist with topographical diagnosis, for example with ipsilateral postganglionic Horner syndrome (posterior cavernous sinus: Parkinson syndrome) or twelfth nerve palsy (clivus).

Many causes of abducens nerve palsy have been described, but the most common include:

- Microinfarction in the nerve, due to hypertension, diabetes mellitus.
- Raised intracranial pressure: a "false-localising sign", possibly caused by stretching of the nerve in its long intracranial course over the ridge of the petrous temporal bone.
- Nuclear pontine lesions: congenital, *e.g.* Duane retraction syndrome, Möbius syndrome.
- Mass lesions anywhere along the course.

Bilateral abducens palsy is more often seen with tumours, subarachnoid haemorrhage, meningitis, Wernicke's encephalopathy, and raised intracranial pressure.

Isolated weakness of the lateral rectus muscle causing impaired abduction may also occur in myasthenia gravis. In order not to overlook this fact, and miss a potentially treatable condition, it is probably better to label isolated abduction failure of the eye initially as "lateral rectus palsy", rather than abducens nerve palsy, until the aetiological diagnosis is established.

Excessive or sustained convergence associated with a midbrain lesion (at the diencephalic-mesencephalic junction) may also result in slow or restricted abduction, so called pseudo-abducens palsy or "midbrain pseudo-sixth".

Reference
Leigh RJ, Zee DS. The neurology of eye movements. 4th ed. Oxford: Oxford University Press; 2006. p. 416–23.
Cross References
Diplopia; "False-localising signs"

Abductor Sign
The abductor sign is tested by asking the patient to abduct each leg whilst the examiner opposes movement with hands placed on the lateral surfaces of the patient's legs: the leg contralateral to the abducted leg shows opposite actions dependent upon whether paresis is organic or non-organic. Abduction of a paretic leg is associated with the sound leg remaining fixed in organic paresis, but in non-organic paresis there is hyperadduction. Hence the abductor sign is suggested to be useful to detect non-organic paresis.
Reference
Sonoo M. Abductor sign: a reliable new sign to detect unilateral non-organic paresis of the lower limb. *J Neurol Neurosurg Psychiatry*. 2004; **75**: 121–5.
Cross Reference
Functional weakness and sensory disturbance

Absence
An absence, or absence attack, is a brief interruption of awareness of epileptic origin. This may be a barely noticeable suspension of speech or attentiveness, without postictal confusion or any awareness that an attack has occurred, as in idiopathic generalized epilepsy of absence type (absence epilepsy; petit mal), a disorder exclusive to childhood and associated with 3 Hz spike and slow wave EEG abnormalities.

Absence epilepsy may be confused with a more obvious distancing, staring, "trance-like" state, or "glazing over", unresponsive to question or command, possibly with associated automatisms such as lip smacking, due to a complex partial seizure of temporal lobe origin ("atypical absence").

Ethosuximide and/or sodium valproate are the treatments of choice for idiopathic generalized absence epilepsy, whereas carbamazepine, sodium valproate, or lamotrigine are first-line agents for localisation-related complex partial seizures.

Cross References
Automatism; Seizures

Abulia

Abulia (or aboulia) is a "syndrome of hypofunction", characterized by lack of initiative, spontaneity and drive (aspontaneity), apathy, slowness of thought (bradyphrenia), and blunting of emotional responses and response to external stimuli. It may be confused with the psychomotor retardation of depression and is sometimes labelled as "pseudodepression". More plausibly, abulia has been thought of as a minor or partial form of akinetic mutism. A distinction may be drawn between abulia major (= akinetic mutism) and abulia minor, a lesser degree of abulia associated particularly with bilateral caudate nucleus stroke and thalamic infarcts in the territory of the polar artery and infratentorial stroke. There may also be some clinical overlap with catatonia and athymhormia.

Abulia may result from frontal lobe damage, most particularly that involving the frontal convexity, and has also been reported with focal lesions of the caudate nucleus, thalamus and midbrain. As with akinetic mutism, it is likely that lesions anywhere in the "centromedial core" of brain frontal-subcortical circuitry, from frontal lobes to brainstem, may produce this picture.

Pathologically, abulia may be observed in:

- Infarcts in anterior cerebral artery territory and ruptured anterior communicating artery aneurysms, causing basal forebrain damage.
- Closed head injury.
- Parkinson's disease; sometimes as a forerunner of a frontal type dementia.
- Other causes of frontal lobe disease: tumour, abscess.
- Metabolic, electrolyte disorders: hypoxia, hypoglycaemia, hepatic encephalopathy.

Treatment is of the underlying cause where possible. There is anecdotal evidence that dopaminergic therapy such as bromocriptine and levodopa may sometimes help.

References
Fisher CM. Abulia. In: Bogousslavsky J, Caplan L, editors. Stroke syndromes. Cambridge: Cambridge University Press; 1995. p. 182–7.
Ghoshal S, Gokhale S, Rebovich G, Caplan LR. The neurology of decreased activity: abulia. *Rev Neurol Dis*. 2011; **8**: e55–67.
Vijayaraghavan L, Krishnamoorthy ES, Brown RG, Trimble MR. Abulia: a Delphi survey of British neurologists and psychiatrists. *Mov Disord*. 2002; **17**: 1052–7.

Cross References
Akinetic mutism; Apathy; Athymhormia; Bradyphrenia; Catatonia; Frontal lobe syndromes; Psychomotor retardation

Acalculia

First named and described by Henschen in 1919, acalculia or dyscalculia is difficulty or inability in performing simple mental arithmetic. This depends on two processes: number processing and calculation. A deficit confined to the latter process is termed anarithmetia. Acalculia may be classified as:

- *Primary*:
  A specific deficit in arithmetical tasks, more severe than any other co-existing cognitive dysfunction.

- *Secondary*:
  In the context of other cognitive impairments, for example of language (aphasia, alexia or agraphia for numbers), attention, memory, or space perception (*e.g.* neglect). Acalculia may occur in association with alexia, agraphia, finger agnosia, right-left disorientation and difficulty spelling words as one part of the Gerstmann syndrome associated with lesions of the dominant parietal lobe.

Secondary acalculia is the more common variety.

Isolated acalculia may be seen with lesions of:
- Dominant (left) parietal/temporal/occipital cortex, especially involving the angular gyrus (Brodmann areas 39 and 40).
- Medial frontal lobe (perhaps as a consequence of impaired problem solving ability).
- Subcortical structures (caudate nucleus, putamen, internal capsule).

Impairments may be remarkably focal, for example one operation (*e.g.* subtraction) may be preserved whilst all others are impaired.

In patients with mild to moderate Alzheimer's disease with acalculia but no attentional or language impairments, cerebral glucose metabolism was found to be impaired in the left inferior parietal lobule and inferior temporal gyrus. Preservation of calculation skills in the face of total language dissolution (production and comprehension) has been reported with focal left temporal lobe atrophy.

References
Boller F, Grafman J. Acalculia: historical development and current significance. *Brain Cogn.* 1983; **2**: 205–23.
Denburg N, Tranel D. Acalculia and disturbances of body schema. In: Heilman KM, Valenstein E, editors. Clinical neuropsychology. 4th ed. Oxford: Oxford University Press; 2003. p. 161–84.
Gitelman DR. Acalculia: a disorder of numerical cognition. In: D'Esposito M, editor. Neurological foundations of cognitive neuroscience. Cambridge: MIT Press; 2003. p. 129–63.

Cross References
Agraphia; Alexia; Aphasia; Gerstmann syndrome; Neglect

Accommodation Reflex
- see PUPILLARY REFLEXES

Achilles Reflex
- see ANKLE JERK, ANKLE REFLEX

Achromatopsia
Achromatopsia, or dyschromatopsia, is an inability or impaired ability to perceive colours. This may be ophthalmological or neurological in origin, and congenital or acquired; only in the latter case does the patient complain of impaired colour vision.

Achromatopsia is most conveniently tested for clinically by using pseudoisochromatic figures (*e.g.* Ishihara plates), although these were specifically designed for detecting congenital colour blindness and test the red-green channel more than blue-yellow. Sorting colours according to hue, for example with the Farnsworth-Munsell 100 Hue test, is more quantitative, but more time consuming. Difficulty performing these tests does not always reflect achromatopsia (see Pseudoachromatopsia).

Probably the most common cause of achromatopsia is inherited "colour blindness", of which several types are recognized: in monochromats only one of the three cone photoreceptor classes is affected, in dichromats two; anomalous sensitivity to specific wavelengths of light may also occur (anomalous trichromat). These inherited dyschromatopsias are binocular, symmetrical, and do not change with time. There are also a number of retinal dystrophies characterised by achromatopsia, photophobia, nystagmus, and severely reduced visual acuity for which a number of mutant genes have been characterised (CNGA3, CNBG3, GNAT2, PDE6C, PDE6H, ATF6).

Acquired achromatopsia may result from damage to the optic nerve or the cerebral cortex. Unlike inherited conditions, these deficits are noticeable (patients describe the world as looking "grey" or "washed out"; *grisaille* is the technical, artistic, term) and may be confined to only part of the visual field (*e.g.* hemiachromatopsia). Optic neuritis typically impairs colour vision (red-green > blue-yellow) and this defect may persist even when other features of the acute inflammation (impaired visual acuity, central scotoma) remit.

Cerebral achromatopsia results from cortical damage to the inferior occipitotemporal area, most usually as a result of infarction. Area V4 of the visual cortex, which is devoted to colour processing, is located in the occipitotemporal (fusiform) and lingual gyri. There is also a loss of colour imagery. Unilateral lesions may produce a homonymous hemiachromatopsia. Lesions in this region may also produce prosopagnosia, alexia, and visual field defects, either a peripheral scotoma which is always in the upper visual field, or a superior quadrantanopia, reflecting damage to the inferior limb of the calcarine sulcus in addition to the adjacent fusiform gyrus. Transient achromatopsia in the context of vertebrobasilar ischaemia has been reported.

The differential diagnosis of achromatopsia encompasses colour agnosia, a loss of colour knowledge despite intact perception; and colour anomia, an inability to name colours despite intact perception.

References
Bartolomeo P, Bachoud-Lévi AC, Thiebault de Schotten M. The anatomy of cerebral achromatopsia: a reappraisal and comparison of two case reports. *Cortex*. 2014; **56**: 138–44.
Zeki S. A century of cerebral achromatopsia. *Brain*. 1990; **113**: 1721–77.

Cross References
Agnosia; Alexia; Anomia; Prosopagnosia; Pseudoachromatopsia; Quadrantanopia; Scotoma; Xanthopsia

Acoasm
- see HALLUCINATION

Acousticopalpebral Reflex
- see BLINK REFLEX

Acroparaesthesia
- see PARAESTHESIA

Action Dystonia
- see DYSTONIA

Action Myoclonus
- see MYOCLONUS

Adiadochokinesia
- see DYSDIADOCHOKINESIA

Adie's Syndrome, Adie's Tonic Pupil
- see HOLMES-ADIE PUPIL, HOLMES-ADIE SYNDROME

Adson's Test
Adson's test may be helpful in the diagnosis of vascular thoracic outlet syndrome, along with Roos test. The arm is extended at the elbow, abducted, then rotated posteriorly; following deep inspiration, the patient's head is turned from one side to the other. Loss of the radial pulse may occur in normals but a bruit over the brachial artery is thought to suggest the

presence of entrapment. A Doppler Adson's test over the subclavian artery may predict successful outcome from thoracic outlet decompression surgery.

Reference
Lee AD, Agarwal S, Sadhu D. Doppler Adson's test: predictor of outcome of surgery in non-specific thoracic outlet syndrome. *World J Surg.* 2006; **30**: 291–2.

Cross Reference
Roos test

Adventitious Movements
- see STEREOTYPY

Affective Agnosia
- see AGNOSIA; APROSODIA, APROSODY

Afferent Pupillary Defect (APD)
- see RELATIVE AFFERENT PUPILLARY DEFECT (RAPD)

Age-Related Signs
A number of neurological signs are reported to be more prevalent with increasing age, and related to ageing *per se* rather than any underlying age-related disease. Hence these signs are not necessarily of pathological significance when assessing the neurological status of older individuals, although there are methodological difficulties in reaching such conclusions.

A brief topographical overview of age-related signs includes:

- *Cognitive function*:
    Loss of processing speed, cognitive flexibility, efficiency of working memory (sustained attention).
    Preservation of vocabulary, remotely learned information including semantic networks, and well-encoded new information.
- *Cranial nerves*:
    I: olfactory sense diminished.
    II, III, IV, VI: presbyopia; reduced visual acuity, depth perception, contrast sensitivity, motion perception; "senile miosis"; restricted upward conjugate gaze.
    VIII: presbycusis; impaired vestibulospinal reflexes.
- *Motor system*:
    Appearance: loss of muscle bulk; "senile" tremor.
    Tone: rigidity; *gegenhalten*/paratonia.
    Power: decline in muscle strength.
    Co-ordination: impaired speed of movement (bradykinesia).
    Reflexes:
        Phasic muscle stretch reflexes: depressed or absent, especially ankle (Achilles tendon) jerk; jaw jerk.
        Cutaneous (superficial) reflexes: abdominal reflexes may be depressed with ageing.
        Primitive/developmental reflexes: glabellar, snout, palmomental, grasp reflexes may be more common with ageing.
    Impairments of gait; parkinsonism.
- *Sensory system*:
    Decreased sensitivity to vibratory perception; ± pain, temperature, proprioception, two-point discrimination.

Neuroanatomical correlates of some of these signs have been defined. There does seem to be an age-related loss of distal sensory axons and of spinal cord ventral horn motor neurones accounting for sensory loss, loss of muscle bulk and strength, and reflex diminution.

References

Franssen EH. Neurologic signs in ageing and dementia. In: Burns A, editor. Ageing and dementia: a methodological approach. London: Edward Arnold; 1993. p. 144–74.

Larner AJ. Neurological signs of ageing. In: Sinclair A, Morley JE, Vellas B, editors. Pathy's principles and practice of geriatric medicine. 5th ed. Chichester: Wiley; 2012. p. 609–16.

McGeer PL, McGeer EG, Suzuki JS. Aging and extrapyramidal function. *Arch Neurol.* 1977; **34**: 33–5.

Vrancken AFJE, Kalmijn S, Brugman F, Rinkel GJE, Notermans NC. The meaning of distal sensory loss and absent ankle reflexes in relation to age. A meta-analysis. *J Neurol.* 2006; **253**: 578–89.

Cross References

Frontal release signs; Parkinsonism; Reflexes

Ageusia

Ageusia or hypogeusia is a loss or impairment of the sense of taste (gustation). This may be tested by application to each half of the protruded tongue the four classical tastes (sweet, sour, bitter, salt).

Isolated ageusia is most commonly encountered as a transient feature associated with coryzal illnesses of the upper respiratory tract, as with anosmia. Indeed, many complaints of loss of taste are in fact due to anosmia, since olfactory sense is responsible for the discrimination of many flavours. Ageusia as an adverse drug effect is described (*e.g.* with clopidogrel).

Neurological disorders may also account for ageusia. Afferent taste fibres run in the facial (VII) and glossopharyngeal (IX) cranial nerves, from taste buds in the anterior two-thirds and posterior one-third of the tongue respectively. Central neuronal processes run in the solitary tract in the brainstem and terminate in its nucleus (nucleus tractus solitarius), the rostral part of which is sometimes called the gustatory nucleus. Fibres then run to the ventral posterior nucleus of the thalamus, hence to the cortical area for taste adjacent to the general sensory area for the tongue (insular region).

Lesions of the facial nerve proximal to the departure of the chorda tympani branch in the mastoid (vertical) segment of the nerve (*i.e.* proximal to the emergence of the facial nerve from the stylomastoid foramen), can lead to ipsilateral impairment of taste sensation over the anterior two-thirds of the tongue, along with ipsilateral lower motor neurone facial weakness (*e.g.* in Bell's palsy), with or without hyperacusis.

Lesions of the glossopharyngeal nerve causing impaired taste over the posterior one-third of the tongue usually occur in association with ipsilateral lesions of the other lower cranial nerves (X, XI, XII; jugular foramen syndrome) and hence may be associated with dysphonia, dysphagia, depressed gag reflex, vocal cord paresis, anaesthesia of the soft palate, uvula, pharynx and larynx, and weakness of trapezius and sternocleidomastoid.

Ageusia as an isolated symptom of neurological disease is extremely rare, but has been described with focal central nervous system lesions (infarct, tumour, demyelination) affecting the nucleus of the tractus solitarius (gustatory nucleus) and/or thalamus, and with bilateral insular lesions. Anosmia and dysgeusia have also been reported following acute zinc loss.

Reference

Finelli PF, Mair RG. Disturbances of smell and taste. In: Bradley WG, Daroff RB, Fenichel GM, Jankovic J, editors. Neurology in clinical practice. 5th ed. Philadelphia: Butterworth Heinemann Elsevier; 2008. p. 255–62.

Cross References

Anosmia; Bell's palsy; Cacogeusia; Dysgeusia; Facial paresis, Facial weakness; Hyperacusis; Jugular foramen syndrome

Agnosopsia

This term has been suggested to describe the retention of accurate visual perceptual judgements despite lacking conscious visual perception, in other words knowing without seeing. Anopsognosia has also been used to describe this phenomenon. Unlike blindight, patients have some residual awareness of the presentation of stimuli.

Reference

Carota A, Calabrese P. The achromatic "philosophical zombie", a syndrome of cerebral achromatopsia with color anopsognosia. *Case Rep Neurol.* 2013; **5**: 98–103.

Cross Reference

Blindsight

Agnosia

Agnosia is a deficit of higher sensory (most often visual) processing causing impaired recognition. The term, coined by Freud in 1891, means literally "absence of knowledge", but its precise clinical definition continues to be a subject of debate. Lissauer (1890) originally conceived of two kinds of agnosia:

- *Apperceptive*:
    in which there is a defect of complex (higher order) perceptual processes.

- *Associative*:
    in which perception is thought to be intact but there is a defect in giving meaning to the percept by linking its content with previously encoded percepts (the semantic system); this has been described as "a normal percept that has somehow been stripped of its meaning", or "perception without knowledge".

These deficits should not be explicable by a concurrent intellectual impairment, disorder of attention, or by an inability to name or describe the stimulus verbally (anomia). As a corollary of this last point, some argue that there should be no language disorder (aphasia) to permit a diagnosis of agnosia.

Intact perception is sometimes used as a *sine qua non* for the diagnosis of agnosia, in which case it may be questioned whether apperceptive agnosia is truly agnosia. However, others retain this category, not least because the supposition that perception is normal in associative visual agnosia is probably not true. Moreover, the possibility that some agnosias are in fact higher order perceptual deficits remains: examples include some types of visual and tactile recognition of form or shape (*e.g.* agraphognosia; astereognosis; dysmorphopsia); some authorities label these phenomena "pseudoagnosias". The difficulty with definition perhaps reflects the continuing problem of defining perception at the physiological level. Other terms which might replace agnosia have been suggested, such as non-committal terms like "disorder of perception" or "perceptual defect", or as suggested by Hughlings Jackson "imperception".

Theoretically, agnosias can occur in any sensory modality, but some authorities believe that the only unequivocal examples are in the visual and auditory domains (*e.g.* prosopagnosia, and pure word deafness, respectively). Nonetheless, many other "agnosias" have been described, although their clinical definition may lie outwith some operational criteria for agnosia. With the passage of time, acquired agnosic defects merge into anterograde amnesia (failure to learn new information).

Anatomically, agnosias generally reflect dysfunction at the level of the association cortex, although they can on occasion result from thalamic pathology. Some may be of localizing value. The neuropsychological mechanisms underpinning these phenomena are often ill understood.

References

Bauer RM, Demery JA. Agnosia. In: Heilman KM, Valenstein E, editors. Clinical neuropsychology. 4th ed. Oxford: Oxford University Press; 2003. p. 236–95.

Critchley M. The citadel of the senses and other essays. New York: Raven Press; 1986. p. 239.

Farah MJ. Visual agnosia: disorders of object recognition and what they tell us about normal vision. Cambridge: MIT Press; 1995.
Ghadiali E. Agnosia. *Adv Clin Neurosci Rehabil.* 2004; **4**(5): 18–20.
Cross References
Agraphognosia; Alexia; Amnesia; Anosognosia; Aprosodia, Aprosody; Asomatognosia; Astereognosis; Auditory agnosia; Autotopagnosia; Dysmorphopsia; Finger agnosia; Phonagnosia; Prosopagnosia; Pure word deafness; Simultanagnosia; Tactile agnosia; Topographagnosia; Visual agnosia; Visual form agnosia

Agrammatism

Agrammatism is a reduction in, or loss of, the production or comprehension of the syntactic elements of language, for example articles, prepositions, conjunctions, verb endings (*i.e.* the non-substantive components of language), whereas nouns and verbs are relatively spared. Despite this impoverishment of language, or "telegraphic speech", meaning is often still conveyed to auditors because of the high information content of verbs and nouns.

Agrammatism is encountered in Broca's type of non-fluent aphasia, associated with lesions of the posterior inferior part of the frontal lobe of the dominant hemisphere (Broca's area), and also in progressive non-fluent aphasia (the agrammatic variant of primary progressive aphasia) in which there may also be speech apraxia. Agrammatic speech may also be dysprosodic.
Cross References
Aphasia; Aprosodia, Aprosody; Speech apraxia

Agraphaesthesia

Agraphaesthesia, dysgraphaesthesia, or graphanaesthesia, is a loss or impairment of the ability to recognize letters or numbers written or traced on the skin, *i.e.* of graphaesthesia. This ability was first described by Henry Head in 1920. Whether this is a perceptual deficit or a tactile agnosia ("agraphognosia") has been debated.

It has been observed with defects at all levels of the nervous system from periphery, to spinal cord, to parietal cortex, and is usually if not invariably associated with other sensory deficits (*e.g.* two-point discrimination). Hence it would seem to have little value as a localizing sign. By contrast, stereognosis and Braille reading are complex motion-dependent derived functions, so their concurrence with agraphaesthesia would point to a cortical lesion (*e.g.* as seen in corticobasal degeneration).
Reference
Bender MB, Stacy C, Cohen J. Agraphesthesia. A disorder of directional cutaneous kinesthesia or a disorientation in cutaneous space. *J Neurol Sci.* 1982; **53**: 531–55.
Cross References
Agnosia; Astereognosis; Tactile agnosia; Two-point discrimination

Agraphia

Agraphia, or dysgraphia, is a loss or disturbance of the ability to write or spell. Since writing depends not only on language function but also on motor, visuospatial and kinaesthetic function, many factors may lead to dysfunction. Agraphias may be classified as follows:

- *Central, aphasic, or linguistic dysgraphias*:
    These are usually associated with aphasia and alexia, and the deficits mirror those seen in the Broca/anterior/motor and Wernicke/posterior/sensory types of aphasia. Oral spelling is impaired. From the linguistic viewpoint, two types of paragraphia may be distinguished, *viz.*:
    Surface/lexical/semantic dysgraphia: misspelling of irregular words, producing phonologically plausible errors (*e.g.* simtums for symptoms); this is seen with left temporoparietal lesions, *e.g.* Alzheimer's disease, Pick's disease;
    Deep/phonological dysgraphia: inability to spell unfamiliar words and non-words; semantic errors; seen with extensive left hemisphere damage.

- *Mechanical agraphia*:

  Impaired motor control, due to paresis (as in dominant parietal damage), apraxia (may be accompanied by ideomotor limb apraxia), dyskinesia (hypokinetic or hyperkinetic), or dystonia; oral spelling may be spared.

- *Neglect* (*spatial*) *dysgraphia*:

  Associated with other neglect phenomena consequent upon a non-dominant hemisphere lesion; there may be missing out or misspelling of the left side of words (paragraphia); oral spelling may be spared.

- *Pure agraphia*:

  A rare syndrome in which oral language, reading and praxis are normal.

A syndrome of agraphia, alexia, acalculia, finger agnosia, right-left disorientation and difficulty spelling words (Gerstmann syndrome) may be seen with dominant parietal lobe pathologies.

Writing disturbance due to abnormal mechanics of writing is the most sensitive language abnormality in delirium, possibly because of its dependence on multiple functions.

References

Benson DF, Ardila A. Aphasia: a clinical perspective. New York: Oxford University Press; 1996. p. 212–34

Roeltgen DP. Agraphia. In: Heilman KM, Valenstein E, editors. Clinical neuropsychology. 4th ed. Oxford: Oxford University Press; 2003. p. 126–45.

Cross References

Alexia; Allographia; Aphasia; Apraxia; Broca's aphasia; Fast micrographia; Gerstmann syndrome; Hypergraphia; Macrographia; Micrographia; Neglect; Wernicke's aphasia

Agraphognosia
- see AGRAPHAESTHESIA

Agrypnia (Excitata)

Agrypnia (from the Greek, to chase sleep), or agrypnia excitata, is characterised by severe, total insomnia of long duration, sometimes with persistent motor and autonomic hyperactivation (hence agrypnia excitata).

Recognised causes of agrypnia include trauma to the brainstem and/or thalamus, von Economo's disease, and trypanosomiasis.

Agrypnia excitata (AE) has been used to describe three particular disorders: fatal familial insomnia, a prion disease associated with thalamic degeneration; Morvan's syndrome, an autoimmune encephalitis often associated with autoantibodies directed against voltage-gated potassium channels; and delirium tremens, an alcohol withdrawal syndrome. The pathophysiology of AE in these various conditions is thought to be loss of cortico-limbic inhibitory control of the hypothalamus and ascending brainstem reticular formation.

Reference

Provini F. Agrypnia excitata. *Curr Neurol Neurosci Rep*. 2013; **13**: 341.

Akathisia

Akathisia is a feeling of inner restlessness, often associated with restless movements of a continuous and often purposeless nature, such as rocking to and fro, repeatedly crossing and uncrossing the legs, standing up and sitting down, pacing up and down (forced walking, tasikinesia). Moaning, humming, and groaning may also be features. Voluntary suppression of the movements may exacerbate inner tension or anxiety. The Barnes Akathisia Rating Scale is the standard assessment scale.

Recognized associations of akathisia include Parkinson's disease and neuroleptic medication use (acute or tardive side effect), suggesting that dopamine depletion may contribute to the pathophysiology. Dopamine depleting agents (*e.g.* tetrabenazine, reserpine) may also cause akathisia. Acute akathisia following pontine infarction is reported.

Treatment of akathisia by reduction or cessation of neuroleptic therapy may help, but may exacerbate coexistent psychosis. Centrally acting β-blockers such as propranolol may also be helpful, as may anticholinergic agents, amantadine, clonazepam, and clonidine.

References

Barnes TR. A rating scale for drug-induced akathisia. *Br J Psychiatry*. 1989; **154**: 672–6.
Sachdev P. Akathisia and restless legs. Cambridge: Cambridge University Press; 1995.

Cross References

Parkinsonism; Tasikinesia; Tic

Akinesia

Akinesia is a lack of, or an inability to initiate, voluntary movements. More usually in clinical practice there is a difficulty (reduction, delay), rather than complete inability, in the initiation of voluntary movement, perhaps better termed bradykinesia, or reduced amplitude of movement or hypokinesia. These difficulties cannot be attributed to motor unit or pyramidal system dysfunction. Reflexive motor activity may be preserved (*kinesis paradoxica*). There may be concurrent slowness of movement, also termed bradykinesia.

Akinesia may co-exist with any of the other clinical features of extrapyramidal system disease, particularly rigidity, but the presence of akinesia is regarded as an absolute requirement for the diagnosis of parkinsonism.

Hemiakinesia may be a feature of motor neglect of one side of the body (possibly a motor equivalent of sensory extinction). Bilateral akinesia with mutism (akinetic mutism) may occur if pathology is bilateral. Pure akinesia, without rigidity or tremor, may occur: if levodopa-responsive, this is usually due to Parkinson's disease; if levodopa-unresponsive, it may be the harbinger of progressive supranuclear palsy. A few patients with PSP have "pure akinesia" without other features until late in the disease course; freezing of gait may also be a feature.

Neuroanatomically, akinesia is a feature of disorders affecting:

- Frontal-subcortical structures, *e.g.* the medial convexity subtype of frontal lobe syndrome.
- Basal ganglia.
- Ventral thalamus.
- Limbic system (anterior cingulate gyrus).

Neurophysiologically, akinesia is associated with loss of dopamine projections from the substantia nigra to the putamen.

Pathological processes underpinning akinesia include:
- Neurodegeneration, *e.g.* Parkinson's disease, progressive supranuclear palsy (Steele-Richardson-Olszewski syndrome), multiple system atrophy (striatonigral degeneration); akinesia may occur in some frontotemporal lobar degeneration syndromes, Alzheimer's disease, and some prion diseases.
- Hydrocephalus.
- Neoplasia, *e.g.* butterfly glioma of the frontal lobes.
- Cerebrovascular disease.

Akinesia resulting from nigrostriatal dopamine depletion (*i.e.* idiopathic Parkinson's disease) may respond to treatment with levodopa or dopamine agonists. However, many parkinsonian/akinetic-rigid syndromes show no or only partial response to these agents.

References

Imai H. Clinicophysiological features of akinesia. *Eur Neurol*. 1996; **36**(Suppl 1): 9–12.
Riley DE, Fogt N, Leigh RJ. The syndrome of "pure akinesia" and its relationship to PSP. *Neurology*. 1994; **44**: 1025–9.

Cross References
Akinetic mutism; Bradykinesia; Extinction; Freezing of gait; Frontal lobe syndromes; Hemiakinesia; Hypokinesia; Hypometria; *Kinesis paradoxica*; Neglect; Parkinsonism

Akinetic Mutism
Akinetic mutism is a "syndrome of negatives", characterized by lack of voluntary movement (akinesia), absence of speech (mutism), lack of response to question and command, but with normal alertness and sleep-wake cycles (*cf.* coma). Blinking (spontaneous and to threat) is preserved. Frontal release signs, such as grasping and sucking, may be present, as may double incontinence, but there is a relative paucity of upper motor neurone signs affecting either side of the body, suggesting relatively preserved descending pathways. Akinetic mutism represents an extreme form of abulia, hence sometimes referred to as abulia major.
    Pathologically, akinetic mutism is associated with bilateral lesions of the "centromedial core" of the brain interrupting reticular-cortical or limbic-cortical pathways but which spare corticospinal pathways; this may occur at any point from frontal lobes to brainstem.
    Different forms of akinetic mutism are sometimes distinguished, *e.g.* according to lesion location:

- Fronto-diencephalic: associated with bilateral occlusion of the anterior cerebral arteries or with haemorrhage and vasospasm from anterior communicating artery aneurysms; damage to the cingulate gyri appears crucial but not sufficient for this syndrome.
- Akinetic mutism with disturbances of vertical eye movements and hypersomnia: associated with paramedian thalamic and thalamo-mesencephalic strokes.

Or according to lesion location and clinical phenotype:

- Mesencephalic-diencephalic region, also called apathetic akinetic mutism or somnolent mutism;
- Anterior cingulate gyrus and adjacent frontal lobes, also called hyperpathic akinetic mutism, a more severe presentation.

Other structures (*e.g.* globus pallidus) have sometimes been implicated. Pathology may be vascular, neoplastic, or structural (subacute communicating hydrocephalus), and evident on structural brain imaging. Akinetic mutism may be the final state common to the end-stages of a number of neurodegenerative pathologies. EEG may show slowing with lack of desynchronization following external stimuli.
    Occasionally, treatment of the cause may improve akinetic mutism (*e.g.* relieving hydrocephalus). Agents such as dopamine agonists (*e.g.* bromocriptine), ephedrine and methylphenidate have also been tried.

References
Cairns H. Disturbances of consciousness with lesions of the brain stem and diencephalon. *Brain*. 1952; **75**: 109–46.
Nagaratnam N, Nagaratnam K, Ng K, Diu P. Akinetic mutism following stroke. *J Clin Neurosci*. 2004; **11**: 25–30.
Ross ED, Stewart RM. Akinetic mutism from hypothalamic damage: successful treatment with dopamine agonists. *Neurology*. 1981; **31**: 1435–9.
Shetty AC, Morris J, O'Mahony P. Akinetic mutism – not coma. *Age Ageing*. 2009; **38**: 350–1.
Cross References
Abulia; Akinesia; Athymhormia; Blink reflex; Catatonia; Coma; Frontal lobe syndromes; Frontal release signs; Grasp reflex; Locked-in syndrome; Mutism

Akinetic Rigid Syndrome
- see PARKINSONISM

Akinetopsia
Akinetopsia is a specific inability to see objects in motion, the perception of other visual attributes such as colour, form, and depth, remaining intact. This statokinetic dissociation may be known as Riddoch's phenomenon; the syndrome may also be called cerebral visual motion blindness. Such cases, although exceptionally rare, suggest a distinct neuroanatomical substrate for movement vision, as do cases in which motion vision is selectively spared in a scotomatous area (Riddoch's syndrome).

Akinetopsia reflects a lesion selective to area V5 of the visual cortex. Clinically there may be associated acalculia and aphasia.

References
Zeki S. Cerebral akinetopsia (cerebral visual motion blindness). *Brain.* 1991; **114**: 811–24.
Zihl J, Von Cramon D, Mai N. Selective disturbance of movement vision after bilateral brain damage. *Brain.* 1983; **106**: 313–40.

Cross References
Acalculia; Aphasia; Riddoch's phenomenon; *Zeitraffer* phenomenon

Alalia
Alalia is now an obsolete term, once used to describe a disorder of the material transformation of ideas into sounds. Lordat used it to describe the aphasia following a stroke.

Reference
Bogousslavsky J, Assal G. Stendhal's aphasic spells: the first report of transient ischemic attacks followed by stroke. In: Bogousslavsky J, Hennerici MG, Bäzner H, Bassetti C, editors. Neurological disorders in famous artists – part 3. Basel: Karger; 2010. p. 130–42. [at 139].

Cross References
Aphasia; Aphemia

Alexia
Alexia is an acquired disorder of reading. The word dyslexia, though in some ways equivalent, is often used to denote a range of disorders in people who fail to develop normal reading skills in childhood. Alexia, in contrast, may be described as an acquired dyslexia. Alexia may be categorised as:

- *Peripheral*:
    A defect of perception or decoding the visual stimulus (written script); other language functions are often intact.
- *Central*:
    A breakdown in deriving meaning; other language functions are often also affected.

Peripheral alexias include:

- *Alexia without agraphia*:
    Also known as pure alexia or pure word blindness. This is the archetypal peripheral alexia. Patients lose the ability to recognise written words quickly and easily; they seem unable to process all the elements of a written word in parallel. They can still access meaning but adopt a laborious letter-by-letter strategy for reading, with a marked word-length effect (*i.e.* greater difficulty reading longer words). Patients with pure alexia may be able to identify and name individual letters, but some cannot manage even this ("global alexia"). Tracing letters with a finger may speed up recognition ("Wilbrand's sign"). Strikingly, the patient can write at normal speed (*i.e.* no agraphia) but is then unable to read what they have just written. Alexia without agraphia often coexists with a right homonymous hemianopia, and colour anomia or impaired colour perception (achromatopsia); this latter may be restricted

to one hemifield, classically right-sided (hemiachromatopsia). Pure alexia has been characterized by some authors as a limited form of associative visual agnosia or ventral simultanagnosia. The term word blindness was first used by Henry Charlton Bastian in 1869; Sir William Broadbent (1872) and James Hinshelwood (1895) were also early writers on the subject.

- *Hemianopic alexia*:

    This occurs when a right homonymous hemianopia encroaches into central vision. Patients tend to be slower with text than single words as they cannot plan rightward reading saccades.

- *Neglect alexia*:

    Or hemiparalexia, results from failure to read either the beginning or end of a word (more commonly the former) in the absence of a hemianopia, due to hemispatial neglect.

The various forms of peripheral alexia may coexist; following a stroke, patients may present with global alexia which evolves to a pure alexia over the following weeks.

Pure alexia is caused by damage to the left occipito-temporal junction or its afferent inputs from early mesial visual areas or its efferent outputs to the medial temporal lobe. Global alexia usually occurs when there is additional damage to the splenium or white matter above the occipital horn of the lateral ventricle. Hemianopic alexia is usually associated with infarction in the territory of the posterior cerebral artery damaging geniculostriate fibres or area V1 itself, but can be caused by any lesion outside the occipital lobe that causes a macular splitting homonymous field defect. Neglect alexia is usually caused by occipito-parietal lesions, right-sided lesions causing left neglect alexia.

Central (linguistic) alexias include:

- *Alexia with aphasia*:

    Patients with aphasia often have coexistent difficulties with reading (reading aloud and/or comprehending written text) and writing (alexia with agraphia, such patients may have a complete or partial Gerstmann syndrome, the so-called "third alexia" of Benson). The reading problem parallels the language problem; thus in Broca's aphasia reading is laboured with particular problems reading function words (of, at) and verb inflections (-ing, -ed); in Wernicke's aphasia numerous paraphasic errors are made.

From the linguistic viewpoint, different types of paralexia (substitution in reading) may be distinguished:

- *Surface dyslexia*:

    Reading by sound: there are regularization errors with exception words (*e.g.* pint pronounced to rhyme with mint), but non-words can be read; this may be seen with left medial ± lateral temporal lobe pathology, *e.g.* infarction, semantic dementia, late Alzheimer's disease.

- *Phonological dyslexia*:

    Reading by sight: difficulties with suffixes, unable to read non-words; left temporo-parietal lobe pathology.

- *Deep dyslexia*:

    The inability to translate orthography to phonology, manifesting as an inability to read plausible non-words (as in phonological dyslexia), plus semantic errors related to word meaning rather than sound (*e.g.* sister read as uncle); visual errors are also common (*e.g.* sacred read as scared). Deep dyslexia is seen with extensive left hemisphere temporo-parietal damage.

The term transcortical alexia has been used to describe patients with Alzheimer's disease with severe comprehension deficits who nonetheless are able to read aloud virtually without error all regular and exception words.

References
Coslett HB. Acquired dyslexia. In: D'Esposito M, editor. Neurological foundations of cognitive neuroscience. Cambridge: MIT Press; 2003. p. 109–27.
Farah MJ. Visual agnosia: disorders of object recognition and what they tell us about normal vision. Cambridge: MIT Press; 1995.
Leff A, Starrfelt R. Alexia, Diagnosis, treatment and theory. London: Springer; 2014.
Cross References
Acalculia; Achromatopsia; Agnosia; Agraphia; Aphasia; Broca's aphasia; Gerstmann syndrome; Hemianopia; Macula sparing, Macula splitting; Neglect; Prosopagnosia; Saccades; Simultanagnosia; Visual agnosia; Visual field defects; Wernicke's aphasia; Wilbrand's sign

Alexithymia
Alexithymia is a reduced ability to identify and express ones feelings. This may contribute to various physical and behavioural disorders. It may be measured using the Toronto Alexithymia Score. There is evidence from functional imaging studies that alexithymics process facial expressions differently from normals, leading to the suggestion that this contributes to disordered affect regulation. Alexithymia is a common finding in split-brain patients, perhaps resulting from disconnection of the hemispheres.

References
Kano M, Fukudo S, Gyoba J, et al. Specific brain processing of facial expressions in people with alexithymia: an $H_2^{15}O$-PET study. *Brain*. 2003; **126**: 1474–84.
TenHouten WD, Hoppe KD, Bogen JE, Walter DO. Alexithymia: an experimental study of cerebral commissurotomy patients and normal control subjects. *Am J Psychiatry*. 1986; **143**: 312–6.

"Alice in Wonderland" Syndrome
The name "Alice in Wonderland" syndrome was coined by Todd in 1955 to describe the phenomena of micro- or macrosomatognosia, altered perceptions of body image, although these had first been described by Lippman in the context of migraine some years earlier. It has subsequently been suggested that Charles Lutwidge Dodgson's own experience of migraine, recorded in his diaries, may have given rise to Lewis Carroll's descriptions of Alice's changes in body form, graphically illustrated in *Alice's Adventures in Wonderland* (1865) by Sir John Tenniel. Some authors have subsequently interpreted these as somesthetic migrainous auras whereas others challenge this on chronological grounds, finding no evidence in Dodgson's diaries for the onset of migraine until after he had written the Alice books. Moreover, migraine with somesthetic auras is rare, and Dodgson's diaries have no report of migraine-associated body image hallucinations.

Other conditions may also give rise to the phenomena of micro- or macrosomatognosia, including epilepsy, encephalitis, cerebral mass lesions, schizophrenia, and drug intoxication.

References
Fine EJ. The Alice in Wonderland syndrome. *Prog Brain Res*. 2013; **206**: 143–56.
Larner AJ. The neurology of "Alice". *Adv Clin Neurosci Rehabil*. 2005; **4**(6): 35–6.
Todd J. The syndrome of Alice in Wonderland. *CMAJ*. 1955; **73**: 701–4.
Cross References
Aura; Metamorphopsia

Alien Grasp Reflex
The term alien grasp reflex has been used to describe a grasp reflex occurring in full consciousness, which the patient could anticipate but perceived as alien (*i.e.* not modified by will), occurring in the absence of other abnormal movements. These phenomena were associated with an intrinsic tumour of the right (non-dominant) frontal lobe. It was suggested that the grasp reflex and alien hand syndromes are not separate entities but part of the spectrum of frontal lobe dysfunction, the term "alien grasp reflex" attempting to emphasize the overlap.

Reference
Silva MT, Howard RS, Kartsounis LD, Ross Russell RW. The alien grasp reflex. *Eur Neurol.*
1996; **36**: 55–6.

Cross References
Alien hand, Alien limb; Grasp reflex

Alien Hand, Alien Limb
An alien limb, most usually the arm but occasionally the leg, is one which manifests slow,
involuntary, wandering (levitating), quasi-purposive movements. An arm so affected may
show apraxic difficulties in performing even the simplest tasks, and may be described by the
patient as uncooperative or "having a mind of its own" (hence alternative names such as
anarchic hand sign, *le main étranger*, and "Dr Strangelove syndrome"). These phenomena
may be associated with a prominent grasp reflex, forced groping, intermanual conflict, magnetic movements of the hand, and levitation of the limb.

Different types of alien hand/limb have been described, reflecting the differing anatomical locations of underlying lesions:

- Anterior or motor types:
    Callosal type: characterized primarily by intermanual conflict.
    Frontal type: shows features of environmental dependency, such as forced grasping
    and groping, and utilization behaviour.

- Sensory or posterior variant:
    Resulting from a combination of cerebellar, optic, and sensory ataxia; rare.

A paroxysmal alien hand has been described, probably related to seizures of frontomedial
origin.

Recognized pathological associations of alien limb include:

- Corticobasal (ganglionic) degeneration.
- Corpus callosum tumours, haemorrhage.
- Medial frontal cortex infarction (territory of the anterior cerebral artery).
- Trauma and haemorrhage affecting both corpus callosum and medial frontal area.
- Alzheimer's disease, familial Creutzfeldt-Jakob disease (very rare).
- Posterior cerebral artery occlusion (sensory variant).
- Following commissurotomy (corpus callosotomy alone insufficient).

Disconnection of parietal cortex (especially right side) from other cortical areas may underpin alien limb phenomenon.

References
Brion S, Jedynak CP. Troubles du transfer interhemisphérique. A propos de trois observations de
tumeurs du corps calleux. Le signe de la main étrangère. *Rev Neurol (Paris)*. 1972; **126**: 257–66.
Fisher CM. Alien hand phenomena: a review with the addition of six personal cases. *Can J
Neurol Sci.* 2000; **27**: 192–203.
Graff-Radford J, Rubin MN, Jones DT, et al. The alien limb phenomenon. *J Neurol.* 2013;
260: 1880–8.

Cross References
Alien grasp reflex; Apraxia; Ataxia; "Compulsive grasping hand"; Forced groping; Grasp
reflex; Intermanual conflict; Levitation; Magnetic movements; Utilization behaviour

Alienation Du Mot
This has been used to describe a loss of the feeling of familiarity with a word, part of the
comprehension deficit seen in semantic dementia.

Reference
Poeck K, Luzzatti C. Slowly progressive aphasia in three patients: the problem of accompanying neuropsychological deficit. *Brain*. 1988; **111**: 151–68.

Alloacousia
Alloacousia describes a form of auditory neglect seen in patients with unilateral spatial neglect, characterised by spontaneous ignoring of people addressing the patient from the contralesional side, failing to respond to questions, or answering as if the speaker were on the ipsilesional side.
Reference
Heilman K, Valenstein E. Auditory neglect in man. *Arch Neurol*. 1972; **26**: 32–5.
Cross Reference
Neglect

Alloaesthesia
Alloaesthesia (allesthesia, alloesthesia) is the condition in which a sensory stimulus given to one side of the body is perceived at the corresponding area on the other side of the body after a delay of about half a second. The trunk and proximal limbs are affected more often than the face or distal limbs. Early reports were those of Allen (1928) and Bender et al. (1949); in the former, when an object was placed in the patient's left hand following the removal of a large meningioma from the posterior Rolandic area of the left cortex, another similar object was felt spontaneously in the right hand; this disappeared 1 week after operation.

Tactile alloaesthesia may be seen in the acute stage of right putaminal haemorrhage (but seldom in right thalamic haemorrhage) and occasionally with anterolateral spinal cord lesions. The author has seen a patient report sensation below the stump of an amputated leg following stimulation of the contralateral remaining leg, a phenomenon which might be termed "phantom alloaesthesia". "Mirror pain", which has been reported after percutaneous cordotomy interrupting spinothalamic tracts to alleviate refractory pain syndromes (ML Sharma, personal communication), may share a similar neurobiological substrate. The mechanism of alloaesthesia is uncertain: some consider it a disturbance within sensory pathways, others that it is a sensory response to neglect.

Visual alloaesthesia, the illusory transposition of an object seen in one visual field to the contralateral visual field, is also described, for example in "top of the basilar" syndrome or with occipital lobe tumours.
References
Allison RS. The senile brain. A clinical study. London: Edward Arnold; 1962. p. 24,57,65.
Kasten E, Poggel DA. A mirror in the mind: a case of visual allaesthesia in homonymous hemianopia. *Neurocase*. 2006; **12**: 98–106.
Kawamura M, Hirayama K, Shinohara Y, Watanabe Y, Sugishita M. Alloaesthesia. *Brain*. 1987; **110**: 225–36.
Cross References
Allochiria; Allokinesia, Allokinesis; Neglect

Allochiria
Allochiria is the mislocation of sensory stimuli to the corresponding half of the body or space, a term coined by Obersteiner in 1882. There is overlap with alloaesthesia, a term originally used by Stewart (1894) to describe stimuli displaced to a different point on the same extremity.

Transposition of objects may occur in patients with neglect, *e.g.* from the neglected side (usually left) to the opposite side (usually right): for example in a patient with left visuospatial neglect from a right frontoparietal haemorrhage, a figure was copied with objects from the left side transposed to the right.

Allochiria, understood to mean "right-left confusion", is reported in synaesthetes.

References
Halligan PW, Marshall JC, Wade DT. Left on the right: allochiria in a case of left visuospatial neglect. *J Neurol Neurosurg Psychiatry*. 1992; **55**: 717–9.
Meador KJ, Allen ME, Adams RJ, Loring DW. Allochiria vs allesthesia. Is there a misperception? *Arch Neurol*. 1991; **48**: 546–9.
Walsh RD, Floyd JP, Eidelman BH, Barrett KM. Balint syndrome and visual allochiria in a patient with reversible cerebral vasoconstriction syndrome. *J Neuroophthalmol*. 2012; **32**: 302–6.
Cross References
Alloaesthesia; Allokinesia, Allokinesis; Neglect; Right-left disorientation; Synaesthesia

Allodynia
Allodynia is the elicitation of pain by light mechanical stimuli (such as touch or light pressure) which do not normally provoke pain (*cf*. hyperalgesia), *i.e.* this is a positive sensory phenomenon. Examples of allodynia include the trigger points of trigeminal neuralgia, the affected skin in areas of causalgia, and some peripheral neuropathies; it may also be provoked, paradoxically, by prolonged morphine use.

Various pathogenetic mechanisms are considered possible, including sensitization (lower threshold, hyperexcitability) of peripheral cutaneous nociceptive fibres (in which neurotrophins may play a role); ephaptic transmission ("cross-talk") between large and small (nociceptive) afferent fibres; and abnormal central processing.

The treatment of neuropathic pain is typically with agents such as amitriptyline, duloxetine, gabapentin and pregabalin, or carbamazepine in the case of trigeminal neuralgia. Interruption of sympathetic outflow, for example with regional guanethidine blocks, may sometimes help, but relapse may occur.
Cross References
Hyperalgesia; Hyperpathia

Allographia
This term has been used to describe a peripheral agraphia syndrome characterized by problems spelling both words and nonwords, with case change errors such that upper and lower case letters are mixed when writing, with upper and lower case versions of the same letter sometimes superimposed on one another. Such errors may increase in frequency with word length. Sometimes cursive script is retained whilst writing the same material in upper case is impaired. These defects have been interpreted as a disturbance in selection of allographic forms in response to graphemic information outputted from the graphemic response buffer.
References
De Bastiani P, Barry C. A model of writing performance: evidence from a dysgraphic patient with an "allographic" writing disorder. *Boll Soc Ital Biol Sper*. 1985; **61**: 577–82.
Menichelli A, Rapp B, Semenza C. Allographic agraphia: a case study. *Cortex*. 2008; **44**: 861–8.
Cross Reference
Agraphia

Allokinesia, Allokinesis
Allokinesis has been used to denote a motor response in the wrong limb (*e.g.* movement of the left leg when attempting to move a paretic left arm), or transposition of the intended movement to the contralateral side; the movement may also be in the wrong direction. Others have used the term to denote a form of motor neglect, akin to alloaesthesia and allochiria in the sensory domain, relating to incorrect responses in the limb ipsilateral to a frontal lesion, also labelled disinhibition hyperkinesia.
References
Fisher CM. Neurologic fragments. I. Clinical observations in demented patients. *Neurology*. 1988; **38**: 1868–73. [at 1873].

Heilman KM, Valenstein E, Day A, Watson R. Frontal lobe neglect in monkeys. *Neurology*. 1995; **45**: 1205–10.
Cross References
Alloaesthesia; Allochiria; Neglect

Alternate Cover Test
- see COVER TESTS

Alternating Fist Closure Test
In the alternating fist closure test, patients are asked to open and close the fists alternating (*i.e.* open left, close right, and vice versa) at a comfortable rate. Patients with limb-kinetic apraxia cannot keep pace and lose track.
Cross References
Apraxia; Frontal lobe syndromes

Alternating Sequences Test
- see APRAXIA; FRONTAL LOBE SYNDROMES

Altitudinal Field Defect
Altitudinal visual field defects are horizontal hemianopias, in that they respect the horizontal meridian; they may be superior or inferior. Altitudinal field defects are characteristic of (but not exclusive to) disease in the distribution of the central retinal artery. Central vision may be preserved (macula sparing) because the blood supply of the macula often comes from the cilioretinal arteries. Recognised causes of altitudinal visual field defects include:

- *Monocular*:
    Central retinal artery occlusion (CRAO).
    Acute ischaemic optic neuropathy (AION).
    Retinal detachment.
    Choroiditis.
    Glaucoma.
    Chronic atrophic papilloedema.

- *Bilateral*:
    Sequential CRAO, AION.
    Bilateral occipital (inferior or superior calcarine cortices) lesions.

Cross References
Hemianopia; Macula sparing, Macula splitting; Quadrantanopia; Visual field defects

Amaurosis
Amaurosis describes visual loss, with the implication that this is not due to refractive error or intrinsic ocular disease. The term is most often used in the context of "amaurosis fugax", a transient monocular blindness, which is most often due to embolism from a stenotic ipsilateral internal carotid artery (ocular transient ischaemic attack). Giant cell arteritis, systemic lupus erythematosus and the anti-phospholipid antibody syndrome are also recognised causes. Gaze-evoked amaurosis has been associated with a variety of mass lesions and is thought to result from decreased blood flow to the retina from compression of the central retinal artery on eye movement.

Amblyopia
Amblyopia refers to poor visual acuity, most usually in the context of a "lazy eye", in which the poor acuity results from the failure of the eye to establish normal cortical representation of visual input during the critical period of visual maturation (between the ages of 6 months and 3 years). This may result from:

- Strabismus.
- Uncorrected refractive error.
- Stimulus deprivation.

Amblyopic eyes may demonstrate a relative afferent pupillary defect, and sometimes latent nystagmus.

Amblyopia may not become apparent until adulthood, when the patient suddenly becomes aware of unilateral poor vision. The finding of a latent strabismus (heterophoria) may be a clue to the fact that such visual loss is long-standing.

The word amblyopia has also been used in other contexts: bilateral simultaneous development of central or centrocaecal scotomas in chronic alcoholics has often been referred to as tobacco-alcohol amblyopia, although nutritional optic neuropathy is perhaps a better term.

Cross References
Esotropia; Heterophoria; Nystagmus; Relative afferent pupillary defect (RAPD); Scotoma

Amimia
- see HYPOMIMIA

Amnesia
Amnesia is an impairment of episodic memory, or memory for personally experienced events (autobiographical memory). This is a component of long-term (as opposed to working) memory which is distinct from memory for facts (semantic memory), in that episodic memory is unique to the individual whereas semantic memory encompasses knowledge held in common by members of a cultural or linguistic group. Episodic memory generally accords with the lay perception of memory, although many complaints of "poor memory" represent faulty attentional mechanisms rather than true amnesia. A precise clinical definition for amnesia has not been demarcated, perhaps reflecting the heterogeneity of the syndrome.

Amnesia may be retrograde (for events already experienced) or anterograde (for newly experienced events). Retrograde amnesia may show a temporal gradient, with distant events being better recalled than more recent ones, relating to the duration of anterograde amnesia.

Amnesia may be acute and transient or chronic and persistent. In a pure amnesic syndrome, intelligence and attention are normal and skill acquisition (procedural memory) is preserved. Amnesia may occur as one feature of more widespread cognitive impairments, *e.g.* in Alzheimer's disease.

Various psychometric tests of episodic memory are available. These include the Wechsler Memory Score (WMS-R), the Recognition Memory Test which has both verbal (words) and visual (faces) subdivisions, the Rey Auditory Verbal Learning Test (immediate and delayed free recall of a random word list), and the Rey-Osterrieth Complex Figure (non-verbal memory). Retrograde memory may be assessed with a structured Autobiographical Memory Interview, and with the Famous Faces Test. Poor spontaneous recall, for example of a word list, despite an adequate learning curve, may be due to a defect in either storage or retrieval. This may be further probed with cues: if this improves recall, then a disorder of retrieval is responsible; if cueing leads to no improvement, or false-positive responses to foils (as in the Hopkins Verbal Learning Test) are equal or greater than true positives, then a learning defect (true amnesia) is the cause.

The neuroanatomical substrate of episodic memory is a distributed system in the medial temporal lobe and diencephalon surrounding the third ventricle (the circuit of Papez) comprising the entorhinal area of the parahippocampal gyrus, perforant and alvear pathways, hippocampus, fimbria and fornix, mammillary bodies, mammillothalamic tract, anterior thalamic nuclei, internal capsule, cingulate gyrus, and cingulum. Basal forebrain structures (septal nucleus, diagonal band nucleus of Broca, nucleus basalis of Meynert) are also involved.

Classification of amnesic syndromes into subtypes has been proposed, since lesions in different areas produce different deficits reflecting functional subdivision within the system; thus left temporal lesions produce problems in the verbal domain, right sided lesions affect non-verbal/visual memory. A distinction between medial temporal pathology (*e.g.* hippocampus), leading to difficulty encoding new memories (anterograde amnesia and temporally limited retrograde amnesia), and diencephalic pathology (*e.g.* Korsakoff's syndrome), which causes difficulty retrieving previously acquired memories (extensive retrograde amnesia) with diminished insight and a tendency to confabulation, has been suggested, but overlap may occur. A frontal amnesia has also been suggested, although impaired attentional mechanisms may contribute. Functional imaging studies suggest medial temporal lobe activation is required for encoding with additional prefrontal activation with "deep" processing; medial temporal and prefrontal activation are also seen with retrieval.

Many causes of amnesia are recognised, including:

- Acute/transient:
    Closed head injury.
    Drugs.
    Transient global amnesia.
    Transient epileptic amnesia.
    Transient semantic amnesia (very rare).
- Chronic/persistent:
    Alzheimer's disease (may show isolated amnesia in early disease).
    Sequela of herpes simplex encephalitis.
    Limbic encephalitis (paraneoplastic or non-paraneoplastic).
    Hypoxic brain injury.
    Temporal lobectomy (bilateral; or unilateral with previous contralateral injury, usually birth asphyxia).
    Bilateral posterior cerebral artery occlusion.
    Korsakoff's syndrome.
    Bilateral thalamic infarction.
    Third ventricle tumour, cyst.
    Focal retrograde amnesia (rare).

Few of the chronic persistent causes of amnesia are amenable to specific treatment. Plasma exchange or intravenous immunoglobulin therapy may be helpful in autoimmune limbic encephalitides, for example associated with autoantibodies directed against voltage-gated potassium channels.

Functional or psychogenic or dissociative amnesia may involve failure to recall basic autobiographical details such as name and address. Reversal of the usual temporal gradient of memory loss may be observed (but this may also be the case in the syndrome of focal retrograde amnesia).

References
Bauer RM, Grande L, Valenstein E. Amnesic disorders. In: Heilman KM, Valenstein E. editors. Clinical neuropsychology. 4th ed. Oxford: Oxford University Press; 2003. p. 495–573.
Brandt J, Van Gorp WG. Functional ("psychogenic") amnesia. *Semin Neurol.* 2006; **26**: 331–40.
Kopelman MD. Disorders of memory. *Brain.* 2002; **125**: 2152–90.
Papanicolaou AC, editor. The amnesias. A clinical textbook of memory disorders. New York: Oxford University Press; 2006.
Cross References
Confabulation; Dementia; Dissociation

Amphigory
Miller Fisher used this term to describe nonsense speech.
References
Fisher CM. Nonsense speech – amphigory. *Trans Am Neurol Assoc*. 1970; **95**: 238–40.
Fisher CM. Neurologic fragments. I. Clinical observations in demented patients. *Neurology*. 1988; **38**: 1868–73. [at 1872].
Cross Reference
Aphasia

Amusia
Amusia is a loss of the ability to appreciate music despite normal intelligence, memory and language function. Subtypes have been described: receptive or sensory amusia is loss of the ability to appreciate music; and expressive or motor amusia is loss of ability to sing, whistle, etc. Clearly a premorbid appreciation of music is a *sine qua non* for the diagnosis (particularly of the former), and most reported cases of amusia have occurred in trained musicians. Others have estimated that amusia affects up to 4% of the population (presumably expressive; = "tone deafness"). Tests for the evaluation of amusia have been described.

Amusia may occur in the context of more widespread cognitive dysfunction, such as aphasia and agnosia, although aphasia without amusia has been reported. Amusia has been reported in association with pure word deafness, presumably as part of a global auditory agnosia. Isolated amusia has been reported in the context of focal cerebral atrophy affecting the non-dominant temporal lobe. However, functional studies have failed to show strong hemispheric specificity for music perception, but suggest a cross-hemispheric distributed neural substrate. An impairment of pitch processing with preserved awareness of musical rhythm changes has been described in amusics.
Reference
Clark CN, Golden HL, Warren JD. Acquired amusia. *Handb Clin Neurol*. 2015; **129**: 607–31.
Fisher CA, Larner AJ. Jean Langlais (1907–91): an historical case of a blind organist with stroke-induced aphasia and Braille alexia but without amusia. *J Med Biogr*. 2008; **16**: 232–4.
Cross References
Agnosia; Auditory agnosia; Pure word deafness

Amyotrophy
Amyotrophy is a term used to describe thinning or wasting (atrophy) of musculature with attendant weakness. This may result from involvement of:

- Lower motor neurones (in which case fasciculations may also be present):
  Motor neurone disease/Amyotrophic lateral sclerosis.
  Benign focal amyotrophy/monomelic amyotrophy.
  Disinhibition-dementia-parkinsonism-amyotrophy complex (DDPAC).
  Amyotrophic Creutzfeldt-Jakob disease (obsolete term).
  "Asthmatic amyotrophy" (Hopkins' syndrome).

- Nerve roots:
  Diabetic amyotrophy (polyradiculopathy, especially L2-L4).
- Plexus
  Neuralgic amyotrophy (Parsonage-Turner syndrome).

Hence although the term implies neurogenic (as opposed to myogenic) muscle wasting, its use is non-specific with respect to neuroanatomical substrate.
Cross References
Atrophy; Fasciculation; Neuropathy; Plexopathy; Radiculopathy; Wasting

Anaesthesia
Anaesthesia (anesthesia) is a complete loss of sensation; hypoaesthesia (hypaesthesia, hypesthesia) is a diminution of sensation. Hence in Jacksonian terms, these are negative sensory phenomena. Anaesthesia may involve all sensory modalities (global anaesthesia, as in general surgical anaesthesia) or be selective (*e.g.* thermoanaesthesia, analgesia). Regional patterns of anaesthesia are described, *e.g.* "glove-and-stocking anaesthesia" in peripheral neuropathies, "saddle anaesthesia" involving S3-5 dermatomes resulting from a cauda equina syndrome.

Anaesthesia is most often encountered after resection or lysis of a peripheral nerve segment, whereas paraesthesia or dysaesthesia (positive sensory phenomena) reflect damage to a nerve which is still in contact with the cell body.

Anaesthesia dolorosa, or painful anaesthesia, is a persistent unpleasant pain (*i.e.* a positive sensory phenomenon) which may be experienced in the distribution of a resected nerve, *e.g.* following neurolytic treatment for trigeminal neuralgia, usually with delayed onset. This deafferentation pain may respond to various medications, including tricyclic antidepressants, carbamazepine, gabapentin, pregabalin, and selective serotonin reuptake inhibitors.
Cross References
Analgesia; Dysaesthesia; Neuropathy; Paraesthesia

Analgesia
Analgesia or hypoalgesia refers to a complete loss or diminution, respectively, of pain sensation, or the absence of a pain response to a normally painful stimulus. These negative sensory phenomena may occur as one component of total sensory loss (anaesthesia) or in isolation. Consequences of analgesia include the development of neuropathic ulcers, burns, Charcot joints, even painless mutilation or amputation. Analgesia may occur in:

- Peripheral nerve lesions, *e.g.* hereditary sensory and autonomic neuropathies (HSAN), leprosy.
- Central spinal cord lesions which pick off the decussating fibres of the spinothalamic pathway in the ventral funiculus (with corresponding thermoanaesthesia), *e.g.* syringomyelia.
- Cortical lesions, *e.g.* medial frontal lobe syndrome (akinetic type).

Congenital syndromes of insensitivity to pain were once regarded as a central pain asymbolia (*e.g.* Osuntokun's syndrome), but on further follow-up some have turned out to be variants of HSAN.
Reference
Larner AJ, Moss J, Rossi ML, Anderson M. Congenital insensitivity to pain: a 20 year follow up. *J Neurol Neurosurg Psychiatry*. 1994; **57**: 973–4.
Cross References
Anaesthesia; Frontal lobe syndromes

Anal Reflex
Contraction of the external sphincter ani muscle in response to a scratch stimulus in the perianal region, testing the integrity of the S4/S5 roots, forms the anal or wink reflex. This reflex may be absent in some normal elderly individuals, and absence does not necessarily correlate with urinary incontinence. External anal responses to coughing and sniffing are part of a highly consistent and easily elicited polysynaptic reflex, whose characteristics resemble those of the conventional scratch-induced anal reflex.
Reference
Chan CLH, Ponsford S, Swash M. The anal reflex elicited by cough and sniff: validation of a neglected clinical sign. *J Neurol Neurosurg Psychiatry*. 2004; **75**: 1449–51.
Cross References
Reflexes; Urinary incontinence

Anarchic Hand
- see ALIEN HAND, ALIEN LIMB

Anarithmetia
- see ACALCULIA

Anarthria
Anarthria is the complete inability to articulate words (*cf.* dysarthria). This is most commonly seen as a feature of the bulbar palsy of motor neurone disease.

A motor disorder of speech production with preserved comprehension of spoken and written language has been termed pure anarthria; this syndrome has also been labelled at various times and by various authors as aphemia, phonetic disintegration, apraxic dysarthria, cortical dysarthria, verbal apraxia, subcortical motor aphasia, pure motor aphasia, and small or mini Broca's aphasia. It reflects damage in the left frontal operculum, but with sparing of Broca's area. A pure progressive anarthria or slowly progressive anarthria may result from focal degeneration affecting the frontal operculum bilaterally (so-called Foix-Chavany-Marie syndrome).
References
Broussolle E, Bakchine S, Tommasi M, et al. Slowly progressive anarthria with late anterior opercular syndrome: a variant form of frontal cortical atrophy syndromes. *J Neurol Sci.* 1996; **144**: 44–58.
Lecours AR, Lhermitte F. The "pure" form of the phonetic disintegration syndrome (pure anarthria): anatomo-clinical report of a single case. *Brain Lang.* 1976; **3**: 88–113.
Cross References
Aphemia; Bulbar palsy; Dysarthria

Angioscotoma
Angioscotomata are shadow images of the superficial retinal vessels on the underlying retina, a physiological scotoma.
Cross Reference
Scotoma

Angor Animi
Angor animi describes the sense of dying or the feeling of impending death. It may be experienced on awakening from sleep, or as a somesthetic aura of migraine.
Reference
Ryle JA. Angor animi, or the sense of dying. *Guys Hosp Rep.* 1950; **99**: 230–5.
Cross Reference
Aura

Anhidrosis
Anhidrosis, or hypohidrosis, is a loss or lack of sweating. This may be due to primary autonomic failure, or to pathology within the posterior hypothalamus ("sympathetic area").

Anhidrosis may occur in various neurological disorders, including multiple system atrophy, Parkinson's disease, multiple sclerosis, caudal to a spinal cord lesion, and in some hereditary sensory and autonomic neuropathies. Localised or generalised anhidrosis may be seen in Holmes-Adie syndrome, and unilateral anhidrosis may be seen in Horner's syndrome if the symptomatic lesion is distal to the superior cervical ganglion.
Cross References
Dysautonomia; Holmes-Adie pupil, Holmes-Adie syndrome; Horner's syndrome; Hyperhidrosis

Anismus
Anismus, also known as puborectalis syndrome, is paradoxical contraction of the external anal sphincter during attempted defaecation, leading to faecal retention and a complaint of constipation. This may occur as an idiopathic condition in isolation, or as a feature of the off

periods of idiopathic Parkinson's disease. It is thought to represent a focal dystonia, and may be helped temporarily by local injections of botulinum toxin.

Reference
Ron Y, Avni Y, Lukovetski A, et al. Botulinum toxin type-A in therapy of patients with anismus. *Dis Colon Rectum*. 2001; **44**: 1821–6.

Cross References
Dystonia; Parkinsonism

Anisocoria

Anisocoria describes an inequality of pupil size. This may be physiological (said to occur in up to 15% of the population), in which case the inequality is usually mild and does not vary with degree of ambient illumination; or pathological, with many possible causes.

- Structural:
    Ocular infection, trauma, inflammation, surgery.
- Neurological:
    Anisocoria greater in dim light or darkness suggests a sympathetic innervation defect (darkness stimulates dilatation of the normal pupil). The affected pupil is constricted (miosis; oculosympathetic paresis), as in:
    Horner's syndrome.
    Argyll Robertson pupil.
    Cluster headache.
    Anisocoria greater in bright light/less in dim light suggests a defect in parasympathetic innervation to the pupil. The affected pupil is dilated (mydriasis; oculoparasympathetic paresis), as in:
    Holmes-Adie pupil (vermiform movements of the pupil margin may be visible with a slit-lamp).
    Oculomotor (III) nerve palsy (efferent path from Edinger-Westphal nucleus).
    Mydriatic agents (phenylephrine, tropicamide).
    Anticholinergic agents (*e.g.* asthma inhaler accidentally puffed into one eye).

Clinical characteristics and pharmacological testing may help to establish the underlying diagnosis in anisocoria.

Reference
Bremner FD, Smith SE. Pupil abnormality in autonomic disorders. In: Mathias CJ, Bannister R, editors. Autonomic failure. A textbook of clinical disorders of the autonomic nervous system. 5th ed. Oxford: Oxford University Press; 2013. p. 445–53.

Cross References
Argyll Robertson pupil; Holmes-Adie pupil, Holmes-Adie syndrome; Horner's syndrome; Miosis; Mydriasis

Ankle Jerk, Ankle Reflex

Plantar flexion at the ankle following phasic stretch of the Achilles tendon constitutes the ankle jerk or Achilles (tendon) reflex, mediated through sacral segments S1 and S2 and the sciatic and posterior tibial nerves.

This reflex may be elicited in several ways: by a blow with a tendon hammer directly upon the Achilles tendon (patient supine, or prone with knees flexed, or kneeling) or with a direct plantar strike. The latter, though convenient and quick, is probably the least sensitive method, since absence of an observed muscle contraction does not mean that the reflex is absent; the latter methods are more sensitive, although intra- and interobserver agreement may be better with the plantar strike.

The ankle jerk is typically lost in polyneuropathies and in S1 radiculopathy. Loss of the ankle jerk is increasingly prevalent with normal healthy ageing, beyond the age of 60 years, although more than 65% of patients are said to retain their ankle jerks; this observation may depend in part on the method of assessment used.

References

O'Keeffe ST, Smith T, Valacio R, Jack CI, Playfer JR, Lye M. A comparison of two techniques for ankle jerk assessment in elderly subjects. *Lancet*. 1994; **344**: 1619–20.

Ross RT. How to examine the nervous system. 4th ed. Totawa: Humana Press; 2006. p. 169–71.

Vrancken AFJE, Kalmijn S, Brugman F, Rinkel GJE, Notermans NC. The meaning of distal sensory loss and absent ankle reflexes in relation to age. A meta-analysis. *J Neurol*. 2006; **253**: 578–89.

Cross References

Age-related signs; Neuropathy; Reflexes

Annular Scotoma

An annular or ring scotoma suggests retinal disease, as in retinitis pigmentosa or cancer-associated retinopathy (paraneoplastic retinal degeneration).

Cross References

Retinopathy; Scotoma; Visual field defects

Anomia

Anomia, or dysnomia, is a deficit in naming or word-finding. This may be detected as abrupt cut-offs in spontaneous speech with circumlocutions and/or paraphasic substitutions. Formal tests of naming are also available (*e.g.* Graded Naming Test). Patients may be able to point to named objects despite being unable to name them, suggesting a problem in word retrieval but with preserved comprehension. They may also be able to say something about the objects they cannot name (*e.g.* "flies in the sky" for kite) suggesting preserved access to the semantic system.

Category-specific anomias have been described, *e.g.* for colour (*cf.* achromatopsia).

Anomia occurs with pathologies affecting the left temporoparietal area, but since it occurs in all varieties of aphasia is of little precise localizing or diagnostic value. The term anomic aphasia is reserved for unusual cases in which a naming problem overshadows all other deficits. Anomia may often be seen as a residual deficit following recovery from other types of aphasia. Anomia may occur with any dominant hemisphere space-occupying lesion, and as a feature of semantic dementia, being more prominent in this condition than in Alzheimer's disease.

References

Benson DF, Ardila A. Aphasia: a clinical perspective. New York: Oxford University Press; 1996. p. 252–61.

Woollams AM, Cooper-Pye E, Hodges JR, Patterson K. Anomia: a doubly typical signature of semantic dementia. *Neuropsychologia*. 2008; **46**: 2503–14.

Cross References

Aphasia; Circumlocution; Paraphasia

Anopsognosia

- see AGNOSOPSIA

Anosmia

Anosmia is the inability to perceive smells due to damage to the olfactory pathways (olfactory neuroepithelium, olfactory nerves, rhinencephalon). Olfaction may be tested with kits containing specific odours (*e.g.* clove, turpentine); each nostril should be separately tested. Unilateral anosmia may be due to pressure on the olfactory bulb or tract, *e.g.* from a subfrontal meningioma.

Anosmia may be congenital (*e.g.* Kallman's syndrome, hypogonadotrophic hypogonadism, a disorder of neuronal migration) or, much more commonly, acquired. Rhinological disease (allergic rhinitis, coryza) is by far the most common cause; this may also account for the impaired sense of smell in smokers. Head trauma is the most common neurological cause, due to shearing off of the olfactory fibres as they pass through the cribriform plate. Recovery is possible in this situation due to the capacity for neuronal and axonal regeneration within the olfactory pathways. Olfactory dysfunction is also described in Alzheimer's disease and Parkinson's disease, possibly as an early phenomenon, due to pathological involvement of olfactory pathways. Patients with depression may also complain of impaired sense of smell. Loss of olfactory acuity may be a feature of normal ageing.

Reference
Hawkes CH, Doty RL. The neurology of olfaction. Cambridge: Cambridge University Press; 2009.

Cross References
Age-related signs; Ageusia; Cacosmia; Dysgeusia; Mirror movements; Parosmia

Anosodiaphoria
Babinski (1914) used the term anosodiaphoria to describe a disorder of body schema in which patients verbally acknowledge a clinical problem (*e.g.* hemiparesis) but fail to be concerned by it. Anosodiaphoria usually follows a stage of anosognosia.

La belle indifférence describes a similar lack of concern for acknowledged disabilities which are psychogenic.

References
Babinski JM. Contribution à l'étude des troubles mentaux dans l'hémiplégie organique céré-brale (anosognosie). *Rev Neurol.* 1914; **27**: 845–8.
Critchley M. Observations on anosodiaphoria. *L'Encéphalie.* 1957; **46**: 540–6.

Cross References
Anosognosia; *Belle indifférence*; Personification of paralysed limbs

Anosognosia
Anosognosia refers to a patient's unawareness or denial of their illness. The term was first used by von Monakow (1885) and has been used to describe denial of blindness (Anton's syndrome), deafness, hemiplegia (by Babinski), hemianopia, aphasia, and amnesia. Some authorities would question whether this unawareness is a true agnosia, or rather a defect of higher level cognitive integration (*i.e.* perception).

Anosognosia with hemiplegia most commonly follows right hemisphere injury (parietal and temporal lobes) and may be associated with left hemineglect and left-sided hemianopia; it is also described with right thalamic and basal ganglia lesions. Many patients with posterior aphasia (Wernicke type) are unaware that their output is incomprehensible or jargon, possibly through a failure to monitor their own output. Cerebrovascular disease is the most common pathology associated with anosognosia, although it may also occur with neurodegenerative disease, for example the cognitive anosognosia in some patients with Alzheimer's disease (often interpreted by relatives as the patient being "in denial").

The neuropsychological mechanisms of anosognosia are unclear: the hypothesis that it might be accounted for by personal neglect (asomatognosia), which is also more frequently observed after right hemisphere lesions, would seem to have been disproved experimentally by studies using selective hemisphere anaesthesia in which the two may be dissociated, a dissociation which may also be observed clinically. In Alzheimer's disease, anosognosia may be related to memory dysfunction and executive dysfunction

At a practical level, anosognosia may lead to profound difficulties with neurorehabilitation. Temporary resolution of anosognosia has been reported following vestibular stimulation (*e.g.* with caloric testing).

References
Adair JC, Schwartz RL, Barrett AM. Anosognosia. In: Heilman KM, Valenstein E, editors. Clinical neuropsychology. 4th ed. Oxford: Oxford University Press; 2003. p. 185–214.

Babinski JM. Contribution à l'étude des troubles mentaux dans l'hémiplégie organique céré-brale (anosognosie). _Rev Neurol._ 1914; **27**: 845–8.
Prigatano GP, editor. The study of anosognosia. Oxford: Oxford University Press; 2010.
Rosen HJ. Anosognosia in neurodegenerative disease. _Neurocase._ 2011; **17**: 231–41.
Cross References
Agnosia; Anosodiaphoria; Asomatognosia; Cortical blindness; Extinction; Jargon aphasia; Misoplegia; Neglect; Personification of paralysed limbs; Somatoparaphrenia

Anserina
Autonomically mediated piloerection and thermoconstriction may produce "goosebumps", cold and bumpy skin which may be likened to that of a plucked goose. Loss of anserina may be a feature of some autonomic disorders.

Antecollis
Antecollis (or anterocollis) is forward flexion of the neck. It may be a feature of multiple system atrophy (_cf._ retrocollis in progressive supranuclear palsy), a sustained dystonic posture in advanced Parkinson's disease, and, unusually, in spasmodic torticollis.

Forward flexion of the head onto the chest is a feature in the "dropped head syndrome".
Reference
Quinn N. Disproportionate antecollis in multiple system atrophy. _Lancet._ 1989; **1**: 844.
Cross References
Dropped head syndrome; Retrocollis; Torticollis

Anteflexion
Anteflexion is forward flexion of the trunk, as typical of the stooped posture seen in Parkinson's disease.
Cross Reference
Parkinsonism

Anton's Syndrome
Anton's syndrome refers to cortical blindness accompanied by denial of the visual defect (visual anosognosia), with or without confabulation. The syndrome most usually results from bilateral posterior cerebral artery territory lesions causing occipital or occipitoparietal infarctions, but has occasionally been described with anterior visual pathway lesions associated with frontal lobe lesions. It may also occur in the context of dementing disorders or delirium.
References
Abutalebi J, Arcari C, Rocca MA, et al. Anton's syndrome following callosal disconnection. _Behav Neurol._ 2007; **18**: 183–6.
Gassel M, Williams D. Visual function in patients with homonymous hemianopia. III. The completion phenomenon: insight and attitude to the defect: and visual function efficiency. _Brain._ 1963; **86**: 229–60.
Zukic S, Sinanovic O, Zonic L, et al. Anton's syndrome due to bilateral ischemic occipital lobe strokes. _Case Rep Neurol Med._ 2014; **2014**: 474952.
Cross References
Agnosia, Anosognosia, Confabulation, Cortical blindness

Anwesenheit
A vivid sensation of the presence of somebody either somewhere in the room or behind the patient has been labelled as _anwesenheit_ (German: presence), presence hallucination, minor hallucination, or extracampine hallucination. This phenomenon is relatively common in Parkinson's disease, occurring in isolation or associated with formed visual hallucinations.

References
Chan D, Rossor MN. "- but who is that on the other side of you?" Extracampine hallucinations revisited. *Lancet*. 2002; **360**: 2064–6.
Fénélon G, Mahieux F, Huon R, Ziegler M. Hallucinations in Parkinson's disease: prevalence, phenomenology and risk factors. *Brain*. 2000; **123**: 733–45.
Cross References
Hallucination; Parkinsonism

Apallic Syndrome
- see VEGETATIVE STATES

Apathy
Apathy is a common neurobehavioural symptom which may be characterized by lack of motivation relative to the patient's previous level of functioning or the standards of age and culture. This manifests as diminished goal-directed behaviour (lack of effort, dependency on others to structure activity), diminished goal-directed cognition (lack of interest, or of concern about personal problems), and diminished concomitants of goal-directed behaviour (unchanging affect, lack of emotional responsiveness). Various scales and inventories are available to measure apathy.

Listlessness, paucity of spontaneous movement (akinesia) or speech (mutism), and lack of initiative, spontaneity and drive, may all be features of apathy. These are also features of the abulic state, and it has been suggested that apathy and abulia represent different points on a continuum of motivational and emotional deficit, abulia being at the more severe end. The diminished motivation of apathy should not be attributable to impaired level of consciousness, emotional distress, or cognitive impairment although it may coexist with the latter, as in Alzheimer's disease. Apathy is a specific neuropsychiatric syndrome, distinct from depression.

Apathy may be observed in various diseases affecting frontal-subcortical structures, for example in the frontal lobe syndrome affecting the frontal convexity, or following multiple vascular insults to paramedian diencephalic structures (thalamus, subthalamus, posterior lateral hypothalamus, mesencephalon) or the posterior limb of the internal capsule; there may be associated cognitive impairment of the so-called "subcortical" type in these situations (*e.g.* in Huntington's disease). Apathy is also extremely common in Alzheimer's disease. It is also described following amphetamine or cocaine withdrawal, in neuroleptic-induced akinesia, and in psychotic depression and schizophrenia.

Because apathy may reflect reward insensitivity, dopaminergic mechanisms may play a role in the pathophysiology, suggesting that dopaminergic agents may sometimes be helpful. Selective serotonin reuptake inhibitors have also been tried.

References
Bonnelle V, Veromann KR, Burnett Heyes S, et al. Characterization of reward and effort mechanisms in apathy. *J Physiol Paris*. 2015; **109**: 16–26.
Levy ML, Cummings JL, Fairbanks LA, et al. Apathy is not depression. *J Neuropsychiatry Clin Neurosci*. 1998; **10**: 314–9.
Levy R, Dubois B. Apathy and the functional anatomy of the prefrontal cortex-basal ganglia circuits. *Cereb Cortex*. 2006; **16**: 916–28.
Stella F, Radanovic M, Aprahamian I, et al. Neurobiological correlates of apathy in Alzheimer's disease and mild cognitive impairment: a critical review. *J Alzheimers Dis*. 2014; **39**: 633–48.
Thobois S, Lhommee E, Klinger H, et al. Parkinsonian apathy responds to dopaminergic stimulation of D2/D3 receptors with piribedil. *Brain*. 2013; **136**: 1568–77.
Cross References
Abulia; Akinetic mutism; Dementia; Frontal lobe syndromes

Aphantasia
This term has been coined to describe a lack of visual imagery.

Reference
Zeman A, Dewar M, Della Sala S. Lives without imagery – congenital aphantasia. *Cortex*. 2015; **73**: 378–80.

Aphasia
Aphasia, or dysphasia, is an acquired loss or impairment of language function. Language may be defined as the complex system of symbols used for communication (including reading and writing), encompassing various linguistic components (phonetic, phonemic, semantic/lexical, syntactic, pragmatic), all of which are dependent on dominant hemisphere integrity. Non-linguistic components of language (emotion, inflection, cadence), collectively known as prosody, may require contributions from both hemispheres.

Language is distinguished from speech (oral communication), disorders of which are termed dysarthria or anarthria. Dysarthria and aphasia may co-exist but are usually separable.

Clinical assessment of aphasia requires analysis of the following features, through listening to the patient's spontaneous speech, asking questions or giving commands, and asking the patient to repeat, name, read and write:

- *Fluency*: is output effortful, laboured, with agrammatism and dysprosody (non-fluent); or flowing, with paraphasias and neologisms (fluent)?
- *Comprehension*: spared or impaired?
- *Repetition*: preserved or impaired?
- *Naming*: preserved or impaired?
- *Reading*: evidence of alexia?
- *Writing*: evidence of agraphia?

These features allow definition of various types of aphasia (see Table and specific entries; although it should be noted that some distinguished neurologists, such as Macdonald Critchley, have taken the view that no satisfactory classification of the aphasias exists). For example, motor ("expressive") aphasias are characterized by non-fluent verbal output, with intact or largely unimpaired comprehension, whereas sensory ("receptive") aphasias demonstrate fluent verbal output, often with paraphasias, sometimes jargon, with impaired comprehension. Conduction aphasia is marked by relatively normal spontaneous speech (perhaps with some paraphasic errors) but a profound deficit of repetition. In transcortical motor aphasia spontaneous output is impaired but repetition is intact.

	Broca	Wernicke	Conduction	Transcortical: motor/sensory
Fluency	↓↓	N	N	↓/N
Comprehension	N	↓↓	N	N/↓
Repetition	↓	↓	↓↓	N/N
Naming	↓	↓	↓	N?/N?
Reading	↓	↓	↓	N?/N?
Writing	↓	↓	↓	N?/N?

Aphasia most commonly follows a cerebrovascular event: the specific type of aphasia may change with time following the event, and discrepancies may be observed between classically defined clinicoanatomical syndromes and the findings of everyday practice.

Aphasia may also occur with space-occupying lesions and in neurodegenerative disorders, often with other cognitive impairments (*e.g.* Alzheimer's disease) but sometimes in isolation. The classification of these primary progressive aphasias (PPA) is still in flux, but broadly they may be divided into primary non-fluent aphasia (agrammatic variant of PPA) and semantic dementia (semantic variant of PPA), both of which usually have a pathological substrate of one of the frontotemporal dementias; and logopenic variant of PPA which most often has the pathological substrate of Alzheimer's disease.

References
Basso A. Aphasia and its therapy. Oxford: Oxford University Press; 2003.
Benson DF, Ardila A. Aphasia: a clinical perspective. New York: Oxford University Press; 1996.
Caplan D. Aphasic syndromes. In: Heilman KM, Valenstein E, editors. Clinical neuropsychology. 4th ed. Oxford: Oxford University Press; 2003. p. 14–34.
Critchley M. The citadel of the senses and other essays. New York: Raven Press; 1986. p. 96.
LaPointe LL. Aphasia and related neurogenic language disorders. 4th ed. New York: Thieme; 2011.
Spreen O, Risser AH. Assessment of aphasia. Oxford: Oxford University Press; 2003.
Willmes K, Poeck K. To what extent can aphasic syndromes be localized?. *Brain*. 1993; **116**: 1527–40.
Cross References
Agrammatism; Agraphia; Alexia; Anomia; Aprosodia, Aprosody; Broca's aphasia; Circumlocution; Conduction aphasia; *Conduit d'approche*; Crossed aphasia; Dynamic aphasia; Dysarthria; Dysphasia; Jargon aphasia; Neologism; Optic aphasia; Paraphasia; Transcortical aphasias; Wernicke's aphasia

Aphemia
Aphemia was the name originally given by Paul Broca to the language disorder which he observed in his celebrated case, prior to Armand Trousseau's suggestion that the term aphasia was preferable on philological grounds (hence the name "Broca's aphasia" for this phenotype).

The term aphemia is now used to describe a motor disorder of speech production with elements including dysarthria, orofacial apraxia, dysprosody, phonetic and phonemic errors but preserved comprehension of spoken and written language and otherwise preserved cognition. This syndrome, or something akin to it, has also been called phonetic disintegration (*cf.* phonemic disintegration), pure anarthria, apraxic dysarthria, cortical dysarthria, verbal apraxia, subcortical motor aphasia, alalia, pure motor aphasia, small or mini Broca's aphasia, and kinetic speech production disorder, reflecting the differing views as to the nature of the underlying disorder (aphasia, dysarthria, apraxia).

Aphemia probably also encompasses at least some cases of the "foreign accent syndrome", in which altered speech production and/or prosody makes speech output sound foreign to the speaker's native tongue. Such conditions may stand between pure disorders of speech (*i.e.* dysarthrias) and of language (*i.e.* aphasias). They usually reflect damage in the left frontal operculum, but sparing Broca's area. Slowly progressive aphemia may be associated with a left frontal lesion, often affecting the opercular region (*cf.* speech apraxia).
References
Fox RJ, Kasner SE, Chatterjee A, Chalela JA. Aphemia: an isolated disorder of articulation. *Clin Neurol Neurosurg*. 2001; **103**: 123–6.
Henderson VW. Alalia, aphemia, and aphasia. *Arch Neurol*. 1990; **47**: 85–8.
Lecours AR, Lhermitte F. The "pure" form of the phonetic disintegration syndrome (pure anarthria): anatomo-clinical report of a single case. *Brain Lang*. 1976; **3**: 88–113.
Schiff HB, Alexander MP, Naeser MA, Galaburda AM. Aphemia: clinical-anatomic correlations. *Arch Neurol*. 1983; **40**: 720–7.
Cross References
Anarthria; Aphasia; Aprosodia, Aprosody; Dysarthria; Foreign accent syndrome; Phonemic disintegration; Speech apraxia

Aphonia
Aphonia is loss or diminution of vocal sound volume, necessitating mouthing or whispering of words. As for dysphonia, this most frequently follows laryngeal inflammation, although it may follow bilateral recurrent laryngeal nerve palsy. Dystonia of the abductor muscles of the larynx can result in aphonic segments of speech (spasmodic aphonia, or abductor laryngeal dystonia); this may be diagnosed by hearing the voice fade away to nothing when asking the

patient to keep talking, and patients may volunteer that they cannot hold any prolonged conversation. Aphonia of functional or hysterical origin is also recognised.

Aphonia should be differentiated from mutism, in which patients make no effort to speak, and anarthria in which there is a failure of articulation.

Cross References
Anarthria; Dysphonia; Mutism

Aposiopesis
Critchely used this term to denote a sentence which is started but not finished, as in the aphasia associated with dementia.

Reference
Critchley M. The divine banquet of the brain and other essays. New York: Raven Press; 1979. p. 48.

Cross Reference
Aphasia

Applause Sign
The applause sign, also known as the *signe d'applause*, clapping test or three clap test, is elicited by instructing the patient to clap the hands rapidly three times (the examiner may demonstrate). The tendency to clap more than three times, even when demonstrated by the examiner, is judged abnormal.

The applause sign was first reported (2005) in patients with progressive supranuclear palsy (PSP) and later in other parkinsonian disorders such as Parkinson's disease, dementia with Lewy bodies (DLB), corticobasal degeneration, and multiple system atrophy, consistent with basal ganglia pathology (striatal dysfunction), but it has also been reported in cortical dementias, namely Alzheimer's disease (AD) and frontotemporal lobar degenerations (FTLD), as well as in PSP. In AD, applause sign correlates with frontal lobe dysfunction, hence this may be a motor perseveration.

In consecutive patients attending a cognitive disorders clinic, the applause sign was found to be specific (0.89) but not sensitive (0.36) for identification of any cognitive impairment, and hence it may be useful as a non-canonical sign of cognitive impairment in high prevalence settings.

References
Bonello M, Larner AJ. Applause sign: screening utility for dementia and cognitive impairment. *Postgrad Med*. 2016; **128**: 250–3.
Dubois B, Slachevsky A, Pillon B, Beato R, Villalponda JM, Litvan I. "Applause sign" helps to discriminate PSP from FTD and PD. *Neurology*. 2005; **64**: 2132–3.
Luzzi S, Fabi K, Pesallaccia M, Silvestrini M, Provinciali L. Applause sign: is it really specific for Parkinsonian disorders? Evidence from cortical dementias. *J Neurol Neurosurg Psychiatry*. 2011; **82**: 830–3.

Cross References
"Attended alone" sign; "Head turning sign"

Apraxia
Apraxia or dyspraxia is a disorder of movement characterized by the inability to perform a voluntary motor act despite an intact motor system (*i.e.* no ataxia, weakness) and without impairment in level of consciousness. Automatic/reflex actions are preserved, hence there is a voluntary-automatic dissociation; some authors see this as critical to the definition of apraxia. Different types of apraxia have been delineated, the standard classification being that of Liepmann (1900):

- *Ideational apraxia, conceptual apraxia*:
    A deficit in the conception of a movement; this frequently interferes with daily motor activities and is not facilitated by the use of objects; there is often an associated aphasia.

- *Ideomotor apraxia (IMA):*

    A disturbance in the selection of elements that constitute a movement (*e.g.* panto-miming the use of tools); in contrast to ideational apraxia, this is a "clinical" disor-der inasmuch as it does not greatly interfere with everyday activities; moreover, use of objects may facilitate movement; it may often be manifest as the phenomenon of using body part as object, *e.g.* in demonstrating how to use a toothbrush or how to hammer a nail, a body part is used to represent the object (finger used as tooth-brush, fist as hammer).

- *Limb-kinetic, or melokinetic, apraxia:*

    Slowness, clumsiness, awkwardness in using a limb, with a temporal decomposition of movement; it usually coexists with ideomotor apraxia but may be differentiated from it as more distal, unilateral, impairing only fine finger movements and hand postures and affecting both transitive and intransitive movements; it may be difficult to disentangle from pure motor deficits associated with corticospinal tract lesions.

Apraxia may also be defined anatomically:

- *Parietal (posterior):*

    Ideational and ideomotor apraxia are seen with unilateral lesions of the inferior parietal lobule (most usually of the left hemisphere), or premotor area of the fron-tal lobe (Brodmann areas 6 and 8).

- *Frontal (anterior):*

    Unilateral lesions of the supplementary motor area are associated with impairment in tasks requiring bimanual co-ordination, leading to difficulties with alternating hand movements, drawing alternating patterns (*e.g.* m n m n in joined up writing: alternating sequences test, Luria figures). This may be associated with the presence of a grasp reflex and alien limb phenomena (limb-kinetic type of apraxia).

Apraxia is more common and severe with left hemisphere lesions.

Difficulties with the clinical definition of apraxia persist, as for the agnosias. For example, "dressing apraxia" and "constructional apraxia" are now considered visuospatial problems rather than true apraxias. Likewise, some cases labelled as eyelid apraxia or as gait apraxia are not true ideational apraxias.

References

Binkofski F, Reetz K. Apraxia. In: Cappa SF, Abutalebi J, Démonet JF, Fletcher PC, Garrard P, editors. Cognitive neurology: a clinical textbook. Oxford: Oxford University Press; 2008. p. 67–88.

Dovern A, Fink GR, Weiss PH. Diagnosis and treatment of upper limb apraxia. *J Neurol.* 2012; **259**: 1269–83.

Leiguarda RC, Marsden CD. Limb apraxias. Higher-order disorders of sensorimotor integra-tion. *Brain.* 2000; **123**: 860–79.

Zadikoff C, Lang AE. Apraxia in movement disorders. *Brain.* 2005; **128**: 1480–97.

Cross References

Alien hand, Alien limb; Body part as object; Crossed apraxia; Dysdiadochokinesia; Eyelid apraxia; Forced groping; Frontal lobe syndromes; Gait apraxia; Grasp reflex; Optic ataxia; Speech apraxia

Aprosexia

Aprosexia is a syndrome of psychomotor inefficiency, characterized by complaints of easy forgetting, for example of conversations as soon as they are finished, material just read or instructions just given. There is difficulty keeping the mind on a specific task, which is forgot-ten if the patient happens to be distracted by another task. These difficulties, which the patient has insight into and often bitterly complains of, are commonly encountered in the memory clinic. They probably represent a disturbance of attention or concentration, rather than being a harbinger of dementia. These patients generally achieve normal scores on cognitive screening instruments and formal psychometric tests (and indeed may complain that these assessments do not test the function they are having difficulty with). Concurrent sleep disturbance, irritability, and low mood are common and may reflect an underlying affective disorder (anxiety, depression) which may merit specific treatment.

Cross References
Attention; Dementia

Aprosodia, Aprosody
Aprosodia or aprosody (dysprosodia, dysprosody) is a defect in or absence of the ability to produce or comprehend speech melody, intonation, cadence, rhythm, and accentuations, in other words the non-linguistic aspects of language which convey or imply emotion and attitude. Aprosodia may be classified, in a manner analogous to the aphasias, as:

- *Sensory (posterior)*:
   Impaired comprehension of the emotional overtones of spoken language or emotional gesturing, also known as affective agnosia; this may be associated with visual extinction and anosognosia, reflecting right posterior temporoparietal region pathology.

- *Expressive/Motor (anterior)*:
   An inability to produce emotional overtones ("emotional dysprosody", sometimes confusingly referred to as speech dyspraxia); this may occur in isolation with right sided anterior lesions, or in association with linguistic aspects of aphasia such as agrammatism with anterior left hemisphere damage.

References
Ghacibeh GA, Heilman KM. Progressive affective aprosodia and prosoplegia. *Neurology*. 2003; **60**: 1192–4.
Monrad-Krohn GH. Dysprosody or altered "melody of language". *Brain*. 1947; **70**: 405–15.
Ross ED. The aprosodias. In: Farah MJ, Feinberg TE, editors. Patient-based approaches to cognitive neuroscience. 2nd ed. Cambridge: MIT Press; 2006. p. 259–69.

Cross References
Agnosia: Agrammatism; Anosognosia; Aphasia; Aphemia; Broca's aphasia; Fisher's sign; Foreign accent syndrome; Visual extinction

Arc De Cercle
- see OPISTHOTONOS

Arcuate Scotoma
An arcuate scotoma suggests retinal or optic nerve disease, such as glaucoma, acute ischaemic optic neuropathy, or the presence of drusen.

Cross References
Retinopathy; Scotoma; Visual field defects

Areflexia
Areflexia is an absence or a loss of tendon reflexes. This may be physiological, in that some individuals never demonstrate tendon reflexes; or pathological, reflecting an anatomical interruption or physiological dysfunction at any point along the monosynaptic reflex pathway which is the neuroanatomical substrate of phasic stretch reflexes. Sudden tendon stretch, as produced by a sharp blow from a tendon hammer, activates muscle spindle Ia afferents which pass to the ventral horn of the spinal cord, there activating α-motor neurones, the efferent limb of the reflex, so completing the monosynaptic arc. Hence, although reflexes are typically regarded as part of the examination of the motor system, reflex loss may also occur in "sensory" disorders, affecting the Ia afferents from the muscle spindle. It is often possible to "hear" that reflexes are absent from the thud of tendon hammer on tendon.

Areflexia is most often encountered in disorders of lower motor neurones, specifically radiculopathies, plexopathies and neuropathies (axonal and demyelinating). Areflexia may also occur in neuromuscular junction disorders, such as the Lambert-Eaton myasthenic syndrome, in which condition the reflexes may be "restored" following forced muscular contraction (facilitation). Transient areflexia may be seen in central nervous system disorders such as cataplexy, and in acute spinal cord syndromes ("spinal shock", *e.g.* acute compression, acute inflammatory myelopathy).

Cross References

Cataplexy; Facilitation; Hyporeflexia; Lower motor neurone (LMN) syndrome; Plexopathy; Radiculopathy; Reflexes

Argyll Robertson Pupil (ARP)

The Argyll Robertson pupil is small (miosis) and irregular. It fails to react to light (reflex iridoplegia), but does constrict to accommodation (when the eyes converge). In other words, there is light-near pupillary dissociation (a useful mnemonic is ARP = *a*ccommodation *r*eaction *p*reserved).

Since the light reflex is lost, testing for the accommodation reaction may be performed with the pupil directly illuminated: this can make it easier to see the response to accommodation, which is often difficult to observe when the pupil is small or in individuals with a dark iris. There may be an incomplete response to mydriatic drugs. Although pupil involvement is usually bilateral, it is often asymmetric, causing anisocoria.

The Argyll Robertson pupil was originally described in the context of neurosyphilis, specifically tabes dorsalis. If this pathological diagnosis is suspected, a helpful clinical concomitant is the associated loss of deep pain sensation, as assessed, for example, by vigorously squeezing the Achilles tendon (Abadie's sign).

There are, however, a number of recognized causes of ARP besides neurosyphilis, including:

- Multiple sclerosis.
- Encephalitis.
- Diabetes mellitus.
- Syringobulbia.
- Sarcoidosis.
- Lyme disease.
- Pinealoma.
- Herpes zoster.
- Hereditary motor and sensory neuropathies (Charcot-Marie Tooth disease; Dejerine-Sottas hypertrophic neuropathy).

Miosis and pupil irregularity are inconstant findings in some of these situations, in which case the term "pseudo-Argyll Robertson pupil" may be preferred.

The neuroanatomical substrate of the Argyll Robertson pupil is uncertain. A lesion in the tectum of the (rostral) midbrain proximal to the oculomotor nuclei has been suggested. In multiple sclerosis and sarcoidosis, magnetic resonance imaging has shown lesions in the periaqueductal grey matter at the level of the Edinger-Westphal nucleus, but these cases lacked miosis and may therefore be classified as pseudo-Argyll Robertson pupil. Some authorities think a partial oculomotor (III) nerve palsy or a lesion of the ciliary ganglion is a more likely cause.

References

Argyll Robertson D. Four cases of spinal myosis [*sic*]: with remarks on the action of light on the pupil. *Edinb Med J*. 1869; **15**: 487–93.

Aziz TA, Holman RP. The Argyll Robertson pupil. *Am J Med*. 2010; **123**: 120–1.

Grzybowski A, Sak J. Douglas Moray Cooper Lamb Argyll Robertson (1837–1909). *J Neurol*. 2016; **263** :in press.

Thompson HS, Kardon RH. The Argyll Robertson pupil. *J Neuroophthalmol*. 2006; **26**: 134–8.
Cross References
Abadie's sign; Anisocoria; Light-near pupillary dissociation; Miosis; Pseudo-Argyll Robertson pupil

"Arm Drop"
"Arm drop", or the "face-hand test", has been suggested as a useful diagnostic test if hemiparesis or upper limb monoparesis is suspected to be psychogenic: the examiner lifts the paretic hand directly over the patient's face and drops it. It is said that in organic weakness the hand will hit the face, whereas patients with functional weakness avoid this consequence. However, the validity and reliability of this "avoidance testing manoeuvre" has never been examined; its clinical value is therefore doubtful.
Reference
Stone J, Zeman A, Sharpe M. Functional weakness and sensory disturbance. *J Neurol Neurosurg Psychiatry*. 2002; **73**: 241–5.
Cross References
Babinski's trunk-thigh test; Functional weakness and sensory disturbance; Hoover's sign

"Around the Clock" Paralysis
- see SEQUENTIAL PARESIS

Arthrogryposis
- see CONTRACTURE

Asemasia
Asemasia is an inability to indicate by signs or spoken language. The term was invented in the nineteenth century (Hamilton) as an alternative to aphasia, since in many cases of the latter there is more than a loss of speech, including impairments in pantomime (apraxia) and in symbolizing the relationships of things. Hughlings Jackson approved of the term but feared it was too late to displace the word aphasia.
Reference
Critchley M, Critchley EA. John Hughlings Jackson. Father of English neurology. New York: Oxford University Press; 1998. p. 106.
Cross References
Aphasia; Apraxia

Asomatognosia
Asomatognosia is a lack of regard for a part, or parts, of the body, most typically failure to acknowledge the existence of a hemiplegic left arm. Asomatognosia may be verbal (denial of limb ownership) or non-verbal (failure to dress or wash a limb). All patients with asomatognosia have hemispatial neglect (usually left), hence this would seem to be a precondition for the development of asomatognosia; indeed, for some authorities asomatognosia is synonymous with personal neglect. Attribution of the neglected limb to another person is known as somatoparaphrenia.

The neuroanatomical correlate of asomatognosia is damage to the right supramarginal gyrus and posterior corona radiata, most commonly due to a cerebrovascular event. Cases with right thalamic lesions have also been reported. The predilection of asomatognosia for the left side of the body may simply be a reflection of the aphasic problems associated with left-sided lesions that might be expected to produce asomatognosia for the right side.

Asomatognosia is related to anosognosia (unawareness or denial of illness) but the two are dissociable on clinical and experimental grounds. Some authorities consider asomatognosia as a form of confabulation. Asomatognosia and phantom limb may be conceptualised as converse phenomena (brain representation lost/present even though limb is present/lost).

References
Feinberg TE, Venneri A, Simone AM, Fan Y, Northoff G. The neuroanatomy of asomatognosia and somatoparaphrenia. *J Neurol Neurosurg Psychiatry*. 2010; **81**: 276–81.
Heilman KM. Matter of mind. A neurologist's view of brain-behavior relationships. Oxford: Oxford University Press; 2002. p. 122.
Cross References
Anosognosia; Confabulation; Neglect; Phantom limb; Somatoparaphrenia

Astasia
- see CATAPLEXY

Astasia-Abasia
Astasia-abasia is a terminology which has sometimes been given to a disorder of gait characterized by impaired balance (disequilibrium), wide base, shortened stride, start/turn hesitation and freezing. The term has no standardized definition and hence may mean different things to different observers; it has also been used to describe a disorder characterised by inability to stand or walk despite normal leg strength when lying or sitting, believed to be psychogenic (although gait apraxia may have similar features).

Modern clinical classifications of gait disorders subsume astasia-abasia under the categories of subcortical disequilibrium and frontal disequilibrium, *i.e.* gait disorders with prominent disequilibrium or impaired postural control. A transient inability to sit or stand despite normal limb strength has been reported after acute infarction of the thalamus (thalamic astasia), caudal cingulate gyrus, or supplementary motor area.

References
Masdeu JC, Gorelick PB. Thalamic astasia: inability to stand after unilateral thalamic lesions. *Ann Neurol*. 1988; **23**: 596–603.
Nutt JG, Marsden CD, Thompson PD. Human walking and higher-level gait disorders, particularly in the elderly. *Neurology*. 1993; **43**: 268–79.
Cross References
Gait apraxia; Presbyastasis

Astereognosis
Astereognosis is the failure to recognize a familiar object, such as a key or a coin, palpated in the hand with the eyes closed, despite intact primary sensory modalities. Description of qualities such as the size, shape and texture of the object may be possible.

Hence, this would seem to be a failure of higher order (*i.e.* cortical) processing and it is most often associated with lesions of the posterior parietal lobe (post central gyrus) association cortex. There may be associated impairments of two-point discrimination and graphaesthesia (cortical sensory syndrome), although the latter can also occur with more peripheral lesions.

Astereognosis was said to be invariably present in the original description of the thalamic syndrome by Dejerine and Roussy. Very occasional cases in which astereognosis has been observed with subcortical lesions, such as cervical meningioma, have been reported, presumably interrupting sensory pathways which ascend to the thalamus.

Some authorities recommend the terms stereoanaesthesia or stereohypaesthesia as more appropriate descriptors of this phenomenon than astereognosis, to emphasize that this may be a disorder of perception rather than a true agnosia (for a similar debate in the visual domain, see Dysmorphopsia).
Cross References
Agnosia; Agraphaesthesia; Dysmorphopsia; Two-point discrimination

Asterixis
Asterixis is a sudden, brief, arrhythmic lapse of sustained posture due to involuntary interruption in muscle contraction. The term was coined by Raymond Adams and Joseph Foley to describe a movement disorder they saw in the context of liver disease.

Asterixis is most easily demonstrated by observing the dorsiflexed hands with arms outstretched (*i.e.* the motion to indicate "stop"), lapses being seen as flicking or flapping movements of the hands ("flapping tremor"). Movement is associated with EMG silence in anti-gravity muscles for 35–200 ms. These features distinguish asterixis from tremor and myoclonus; the phenomenon has been sometimes described as negative myoclonus (a term to which Adams did not object, although it does not help in understanding the movement) or negative tremor. Asterixis may be bilateral or unilateral.

Recognised causes of asterixis include:

- Hepatic encephalopathy ("liver flap").
- Hypercapnia.
- Uraemia.
- Drug-induced, *e.g.* anticonvulsants, levodopa.
- Structural brain lesions: thalamic lesions (haemorrhage, thalamotomy).

Unilateral asterixis has been described in the context of stroke, contralateral to lesions of the midbrain (involving corticospinal fibres, medial lemniscus), thalamus (ventroposterolateral nucleus), primary motor cortex and parietal lobe; and ipsilateral to lesions of the pons or medulla.

References
Laureno R. Raymond Adams. A life of mind and muscle. Oxford: Oxford University Press; 2009: 92–3, 177, 235–237.
Pal G, Lin MM, Laureno R. Asterixis: a study of 103 patients. *Metab Brain Dis*. 2014; **29**: 813–24.

Cross References
Encephalopathy; Myoclonus; Tremor

Asthenopia
Asthenopia, literally "weak vision", is frequently used to describe "eye strain" due to uncorrected or inadequately corrected refractive errors, such as hyperopia (far-sightedness) or overcorrected myopia. Such refractive errors are sometimes blamed for headache.

Asynergia
Asynergia or dyssynergia is lack or impairment of synergy in sequential muscular contractions in the performance of complex or reflex movements, such that they seem to become broken up into their constituent parts, so called decomposition of movement. This may be evident when performing rapid alternating hand movements. Dyssynergy of speech may also occur, a phenomenon sometimes termed scanning speech or scanning dysarthria. This is typically seen in cerebellar syndromes, most often those affecting the cerebellar hemispheres, and may coexist with other signs of cerebellar disease such as ataxia, dysmetria, and dysdiadochokinesia. Detrusor-sphincter dyssynergia may be a cause of urinary symptoms in spinal cord syndromes (injury, demyelination).

Cross References
Ataxia; Cerebellar syndromes; Dysarthria; Dysdiadochokinesia; Dysmetria; Scanning speech

Ataxia
Ataxia (or dystaxia) refers to a lack of co-ordination of voluntary motor acts, impairing their smooth performance. The rate, range, timing, direction, and force of movement may be affected. Ataxia is used most frequently to refer to a cerebellar problem, but sensory ataxia, optic ataxia, and frontal ataxia are also described, so if possible the term should be qualified rather than used in isolation.

- *Cerebellar ataxia*:

  Defective timing of agonist and antagonist muscle contraction (asynergia) produces jerking, staggering, inaccurate movements (decomposition of movement), which may manifest as intention tremor, dysmetria (past pointing), dysdiadochokinesia, ataxic dysarthria (sometimes known as scanning speech, although this also has other connotations), excessive rebound phenomenon, macrographia, head tremor (titubation), gait ataxia, and abnormal eye movements (nystagmus, square-wave jerks, saccadic intrusions). There may be concurrent limb hypotonia. Cerebellar hemisphere lesions cause ipsilateral limb ataxia (hemiataxia; ataxia on finger-to-nose, finger chase, and/or heel-shin testing) whereas midline cerebellar lesions involving the vermis produce selective truncal and gait ataxia. An International Cooperative Ataxia Rating Scale has been developed to assess the efficacy of treatments for cerebellar ataxia.

- *Sensory ataxia*:

  This results from impaired proprioception, and may be seen in disease of the dorsal (posterior) columns of the spinal cord (hence "spinal ataxia"), sensory neuropathies, and neuronopathies affecting the dorsal root ganglia. It is markedly exacerbated by removal of visual cues (*e.g.* as in Romberg's sign), unlike the situation with cerebellar ataxia, and may also lead to pseudoathetosis.

- *Optic ataxia*:

  Misreaching for visually presented targets, with dysmetria, due to a parieto-occipital lesion, as seen in Balint's syndrome.

- *"Frontal ataxia"*:

  Similar to, and sometimes indistinguishable from, cerebellar ataxia, but results from lesions of the contralateral frontal cortex or frontopontine fibres, often from tumours invading the frontal lobe or corpus callosum. These fibres run in the corticopontocerebellar tract, synapsing in the pons before passing through the middle cerebellar peduncle to the contralateral cerebellar hemisphere.

Triple ataxia, the rare concurrence of cerebellar, sensory and optic types of ataxia, may be associated with an alien limb phenomenon (sensory type).

There are many causes of cerebellar ataxia, including:

- *Inherited*:

  Autosomal recessive: Friedreich's ataxia, ataxia with isolated vitamin E deficiency, ataxia with oculomotor apraxia (AOA types 1 and 2).
  Autosomal dominant: clinically ADCA types I, II, and III, now reclassified genetically as spinocerebellar ataxias: many types (>50) now described.
  Episodic ataxias: channelopathies involving potassium (type 1) and calcium (type 2) ion channels.
  Mitochondrial disorders.
  Huntington's disease.
  Dentatorubropallidoluysian atrophy (DRPLA).
  Inherited prion diseases, especially Gerstmann-Straussler-Scheinker (GSS) syndrome.

- *Acquired*:

  Cerebrovascular events (infarct, haemorrhage): usually cause hemiataxia; postanoxic cerebellar ataxia.
  Inflammatory: demyelination: multiple sclerosis, Miller Fisher variant of Guillain-Barré syndrome, central pontine and extrapontine myelinolysis.
  Inflammatory: infection: cerebellitis with Epstein-Barr virus; encephalitis with *Mycoplasma*; HIV.

Neoplasia: tumours, paraneoplastic syndromes.
Neurodegeneration: one variant of multiple system atrophy (MSA-C); prion diseases (Brownell-Oppenheimer variant of sporadic Creutzfeldt-Jakob disease, kuru); idiopathic late-onset cerebellar ataxia.
Drugs/toxins, *e.g.* alcohol, phenytoin.
Metabolic: vitamin E deficiency, thiamine deficiency (Wernicke's encephalopathy), gluten ataxia, hypothyroidism (debatable).

References
Klockgether T. Sporadic ataxia with adult onset: classification and diagnostic criteria. *Lancet Neurol.* 2010; **9**: 94–104.
Trouillas P, Takayanagi T, Hallett M, et al. International Cooperative Ataxia Rating Scale for pharmacological assessment of the cerebellar syndrome. The Ataxia Neuropharmacology Committee of the World Federation of Neurology. *J Neurol Sci.* 1997; **145**: 205–211.
Cross References
Alien hand, Alien limb; Asynergia; Balint's syndrome; Cerebellar syndromes; Dysarthria; Dysdiadochokinesia; Dysmetria; Head tremor; Hemiataxia; Hypotonia, Hypotonus; Macrographia; Nystagmus; Optic ataxia; Proprioception; Pseudoathetosis; Rebound phenomenon; Rombergism, Romberg's sign; Saccadic intrusion, Saccadic pursuit; Scanning speech; Square-wave jerks; Tandem walking; Tremor

Ataxic Hemiparesis
Ataxic hemiparesis is a syndrome of ipsilateral hemiataxia and hemiparesis, the latter affecting the leg more severely than the arm (crural paresis). There may be additional dysarthria, nystagmus, paraesthesia and pain.
   This syndrome is caused by lacunar (small deep) infarcts in the contralateral basal pons at the junction of the upper third and lower two-thirds. It may also be seen with infarcts in the contralateral thalamocapsular region, posterior limb of the internal capsule (anterior choroidal artery syndrome), red nucleus, and the paracentral region (anterior cerebral artery territory). Sensory loss is an indicator of capsular involvement; pain in the absence of other sensory features is an indicator of thalamic involvement.
References
Arboix A. Clinical study of 23 patients with ataxic hemiparesis [in Spanish]. *Med Clin (Barc).* 2004; **122**: 342–4.
Fisher CM. Ataxic hemiparesis. A pathologic study. *Arch Neurol.* 1978; **35**:126–8.
Gorman MJ, Dafer R, Levine SR. Ataxic hemiparesis: critical appraisal of a lacunar syndrome. *Stroke.* 1998; **29** :2549–55.
Cross References
Ataxia; Hemiataxia; Hemiparesis; Pseudochoreoathetosis

Ataxic Nystagmus
- see INTERNUCLEAR OPHTHALMOPLEGIA (INO); NYSTAGMUS

Athetosis
Athetosis is the name sometimes given to an involuntary movement disorder characterized by slow, sinuous, purposeless, writhing movements, often more evident in the distal part of the limbs. Athetosis often co-exists with the more flowing, dance-like movements of chorea, in which case the movement disorder may be described as choreoathetosis. Indeed the term athetosis is now little used except in the context of "athetoid cerebral palsy". Athetoid-like movements of the outstretched hands may also been seen in the presence of sensory ataxia (impaired proprioception) and are known as pseudoathetosis or pseudochoreoathetosis. Choreoathetoid movements result from disorders of the basal ganglia.

References
Morris JG, Jankelowitz SK, Fung VS, Clouston PD, Hayes MW, Grattan-Smith P. Athetosis
I: historical considerations. *Mov Disord*. 2002; **17**: 1278–80.
Turny F, Jedynak P, Agid Y. Athetosis or dystonia? [in French]. *Rev Neurol (Paris)*. 2004; **160**:
759–64.
Cross References
Chorea, Choreoathetosis; Pseudoathetosis; Pseudochoreoathetosis

Athymhormia
Athymhormia, or athymormia, also known as the robot syndrome, is a name given to a form
of abulia or akinetic mutism in which there is loss of self-autoactivation. Clinically there is a
marked discrepancy between heteroactivation, behaviour under the influence of exogenous
stimulation, which is normal or almost normal, and autoactivation. Left alone, patients are
akinetic and mute, a state also known as loss of psychic self-activation or pure psychic akinesia. It is associated with bilateral deep lesions of the frontal white matter or of the basal
ganglia, especially the globus pallidus. It has also been described as a feature of Perry syndrome. Athymhormia is thus environment-dependent, since patients normalize initiation and
cognition when stimulated, an important differentiation from apathy and akinetic mutism.

References
Habib M. Athymhormia and disorders of motivation in basal ganglia disease. *J
Neuropsychiatry Clin Neurosci*. 2004; **16**: 509–24.
Mori E, Yamashita H, Takauchi S, Kondo K. Isolated athymhormia following hypoxic bilat-
eral pallidal lesions. *Behav Neurol*. 1996; **9**: 17–23.
Cross References
Abulia; Akinetic mutism; Apathy

Atrophy
Atrophy refers to a wasting or thinning of tissues. The term is often applied to wasted muscles, usually in the context of lower motor neurone pathology (in which case it may be synonymous with amyotrophy), but also with disuse. Atrophy develops more quickly after lower,
as opposed to upper, motor neurone lesions. It may also be applied to other tissues, such as
subcutaneous tissue (as in hemifacial atrophy). Muscle atrophy may sometimes be remote
from the affected part of the neuraxis, hence a false-localising sign, for example the wasting
of intrinsic hand muscles sometimes seen with foramen magnum lesions.
Cross References
Amyotrophy; "False-localising signs"; Hemifacial atrophy; Lower motor neurone (LMN)
syndrome; Wasting

"Attended Alone" Sign
Collateral history is crucial in assessing cognitive disorders, especially complaints of memory impairment, for which reason individuals referred to memory clinics are usually asked
to bring with them a spouse, relative or friend who knows them well to provide such history.
Failure to attend with an informant, the "attended alone" sign, is a robust (*i.e.* very sensitive,
> 0.95) marker of the absence of dementia and of cognitive health in patients with subjec-
tive memory complaints. This may be categorized as one of the non-canonical signs useful
in the assessment of cognitive impairment, along with the applause sign and the head turning sign.

References
Larner AJ. Screening utility of the "attended alone" sign for subjective memory impairment.
Alzheimer Dis Assoc Disord. 2014; **28**: 364–5.
Larner AJ. Neurological signs of possible diagnostic value in the cognitive disorders clinic.
Pract Neurol. 2014; **14**: 332–335.

Cross References
Applause sign; Dementia; "Head turning sign"

Attention
Attention is a distributed cognitive function, important for the operation of many other cognitive domains; the terms concentration, vigilance, and persistence may sometimes be used synonymously with attention. Attention denotes the preferential allocation of (finite) neuronal resources to relevant events during a specific time period. It is generally accepted that attention is effortful, selective, and closely linked to intention. Distinction may be made between different types of attention, *viz.*:

- Sustained (vigilance): maintenance of behavioural response over a prolonged time period.
- Selective: focus directed to just one source despite competing or distracting stimuli.
- Divided/executive function: processing more than one information source at a time, generally regarded as the highest level of attention.

Impairment of attentional mechanisms may lead to distractability (with a resulting complaint of poor memory, perhaps better termed aprosexia), disorientation in time and place, perceptual problems, and behavioural problems (*e.g.* disinhibition), as in the cardinal disorder of attention, delirium.

The neuroanatomical substrates of attention encompass the ascending reticular activating system of the brainstem, the thalamus, and the prefrontal (multimodal association) cerebral cortex (especially on the right side). Damage to any of these areas of the "attentional matrix" may cause impaired attention.

Attentional mechanisms may be tested in a variety of ways. Those adapted to "bedside" use all essentially look for a defect in selective attention, also known as working memory or short term memory (although this does not necessarily equate with lay use of the term "short term memory"):

- Orientation in time/place.
- Digit span forwards/backwards.
- Reciting months of the year backwards, counting back from 30 to 1.
- Serial sevens (serial subtraction of 7 from 100, = 93, 86, 79, 72, 65).

In the presence of severe attentional disorder (as in delirium) it is difficult to make any meaningful assessment of other cognitive domains (*e.g.* memory).

Besides delirium, attentional impairments may be seen following head injury, and in ostensibly "alert" patients, *e.g.* with Alzheimer's disease (the dysexecutive syndrome of impaired divided attention).

References
Mesulam MM. Attentional and confusional states. *Continuum (Minneap Minn)*. 2010; **16**: 128–39.
Scholey A. Attention. In: Perry E, Ashton H, Young A, editors. Neurochemistry of consciousness: neurotransmitters in mind. Amsterdam: John Benjamins; 2002. p. 43–63.
Cross References
Aprosexia; Delirium; Dementia; Disinhibition; Dysexecutive syndrome; Frontal lobe syndromes; Pseudodementia

Auditory Agnosia
Auditory agnosia refers to an inability to appreciate the meaning of sounds despite normal hearing (perception of pure tones as assessed by audiological examination) and preservation of other cognitive functions such as language. This agnosia may be general (affecting all types

of sound perception) or selective, *e.g.* for verbal material (pure word deafness) or non-verbal material, either sounds (bells, whistles, animal noises) or music (amusia, of receptive or sensory type).

Reference
Robert Slevc L, Shell AR. Auditory agnosia. *Handb Clin Neurol.* 2015; **129**: 573–87.

Cross References
Agnosia; Amusia; Phonagnosia; Pure word deafness

Auditory Perseveration
- see PALINACOUSIS, PALINACUSIS

Auditory-Visual Synaesthesia
This name has been given to the phenomenon of sudden sound-evoked light flashes in patients with optic nerve disorders. This may be equivalent to noise-induced visual phosphenes or sound-induced photisms. Such synaesthetic perceptions might be accounted for by direct cross-modal activation of occipital cortex by auditory stimuli, or by "disinhibited feedback" coupling the inducing stimulus and synaesthetic sensation in a "sensory nexus" area. Evidence from different patients for both possibilities has been reported.

References
Afra P, Anderson J, Funke M, et al. Neurophysiological investigation of idiopathic acquired auditory-visual synesthesia. *Neurocase.* 2012; **18**: 323–9.
Neufeld J, Sinke C, Zedler M, et al. Disinhibited feedback as a cause of synesthesia: evidence from a functional connectivity study on auditory-visual synesthetes. *Neuropsychologia.* 2012; **50**: 1471–7.

Cross References
Phosphene; Synaesthesia

Augmentation
The term augmentation may be used to describe different phenomena.

In Lambert-Eaton myasthenic syndrome (LEMS), augmentation refers to an increase in the strength of affected muscles detected in the first few seconds of maximal voluntary muscle contraction. This may also be known as Lambert's sign. Facilitation is another term used to describe the post-tetanic potentiation seen in LEMS.

Augmentation may also be used to refer to the paradoxical worsening of the symptoms of restless legs syndrome under dopaminergic treatment, manifesting as earlier symptom onset in the evenings or afternoons, shorter periods of rest required to provoke symptom onset, greater intensity of symptoms when they occur, spread of symptoms to other body parts such as the arms, and decreased duration of benefit from medication.

Reference
Trenkwalder C, Winkelmann J, Inoue Y, Paulus W. Restless legs syndrome – current therapies and management of augmentation. *Nat Rev Neurol.* 2015; **11**: 434–45.

Cross References
Facilitation; Lambert's sign

Aura
An aura is a brief feeling or sensation, lasting seconds to minutes, occurring immediately before the onset of a paroxysmal neurological event such as an epileptic seizure or a migraine attack (migraine with aura, "classical migraine"), "warning" of its imminent presentation. Migraine aura may also occur in isolation (migraine aura without headache, "migraine equivalent").

An aura indicates the focal onset of neurological dysfunction. Auras are exclusively subjective, and may be entirely sensory, such as the fortification spectra (teichopsia) of migraine, or more complex, labelled psychosensory or experiential, as in certain seizures. Epileptic auras may be classified into subgroups:

- *Somatosensory*:
    e.g. paraesthesia.
- *Visual*:
    Hallucinations, illusions; occipital or temporal origin; complex hallucinations and a "tunnel vision" phenomenon are exclusive to seizures of anteromedial temporal and occipitotemporal origin, whereas elementary hallucinations, illusions, and visual loss are common to both occipital and temporal lobe seizures.
- *Auditory*:
    May indicate an origin in the superior temporal gyrus.
- *Olfactory*:
    Parosmia may occur in seizures of medial temporal lobe origin (uncus; uncinate fits).
- *Gustatory*
- *Autonomic*
- *Abdominal*:
    Rising epigastic sensation ("visceral aura") of temporal lobe epilepsy.
- *Psychic*:
    Complex hallucinations or illusions that usually affect different senses, *e.g.* distortions of familiarity such as *déjà vu* or *jamais vu* auras of focal-onset epilepsy, indicative of temporal lobe and limbic onset respectively.

References
Bien CG, Benninger FO, Urbach H, Schramm J, Kurthen M, Elger CE. Localizing value of epileptic visual auras. *Brain*. 2000; **123**: 244–253.
Charles A, Hansen JM. Migraine aura: new ideas about cause, classification, and clinical significance. *Curr Opin Neurol*. 2015; **28**: 255–60.
Lüders H, Acharya J, Baumgartner C, et al. Semiological seizure classification. *Epilepsia*. 1998; **39**: 1006–13.

Cross References
"Alice in Wonderland" syndrome; *Déjà vu*; Fortification spectra; Hallucination; Illusion; *Jamais vu*; Parosmia; Seizure; "Tunnel vision"

Automatic Obedience
Automatic obedience may be seen in startle syndromes such as the jumping Frenchmen of Maine, latah, and myriachit, when a sudden shout of, for example, "jump" is followed by a jump. These are sometimes known as the startle-automatic obedience syndromes. Although initially classified (by Gilles de la Tourette) with tic syndromes, there are clear clinical and pathophysiological differences.

Reference
Lajonchere C, Nortz M, Finger S. Gilles de la Tourette and the discovery of Tourette syndrome. Includes a translation of his 1884 article. *Arch Neurol*. 1996; **53**: 567–74.

Cross Reference
Tic

Automatic Writing
Automatic writing is a behaviour characterised by increased writing activity. It has been suggested that it should refer specifically to behaviour which is permanently present or elicitable, characterised by compulsive, iterative and not necessarily complete, written reproduction of visually or orally perceived messages (*cf*. hypergraphia). This may be conceptualised as a particular, sometimes isolated, form of utilization behaviour in which the inhibitory functions of the frontal lobes are suppressed, perhaps due to a disconnection within frontal-subcortical circuits (for example following left inferior capsular genu infarction) leading to motor perseveration in writing.

References
Suzuki K, Miyamoto T, Miyamoto M, Hirata K. Transient automatic writing behavior following a left inferior capsular genu infarction. *Case Rep Neurol.* 2009; **1**: 8–14.
Van Vugt P, Paquier P, Kees L, Cras P. Increased writing activity in neurological conditions: a review and clinical study. *J Neurol Neurosurg Psychiatry.* 1996; **61**: 510–4.
Cross References
Hypergraphia; Utilization behaviour

Automatism
Automatisms are complex motor movements occurring in complex motor seizures, which resemble natural movements but occur in an inappropriate setting. These may occur during a state of impaired consciousness during or shortly after an epileptic seizure. There is usually amnesia for the event.

Automatisms occur in about one-third of patients with complex partial seizures, most commonly those of temporal or frontal lobe origin. Although there are qualitative differences between the automatisms seen in seizures arising from these sites, they are not of sufficient specificity to be of reliable diagnostic value; bizarre automatisms are more likely to be frontal.

Automatisms may take various forms:

- *Oro-facial movements*:
  e.g. lip smacking, chewing and swallowing movements, salivation (especially temporal lobe origin).
- *Gestural*:
  Hand fumbling, foot shuffling, tidying, or more complex actions such as undressing; upper limb movements are said to be more suggestive of temporal lobe origin, lower limb movements (kicking, cycling) of frontal lobe origin; pelvic thrusting (may also be seen in pseudoseizures).
- *Ambulatory*:
  Walking or running around (cursive seizures); prolonged wandering may be termed fugue or poriomania.
- *Emotional*:
  Laughing and, more rarely, crying (gelastic and dacrystic seizures, respectively, although crying may also be a feature of non-epileptic seizures), fear, anger.
- *Verbal*:
  Humming, whistling, grunting, speaking incoherently; vocalization is common in frontal lobe automatisms.

Automatic behaviour and fugue-like states may also occur in the context of narcolepsy, and must be differentiated from the automatisms of complex partial seizures, on the basis of history, examination and EEG findings.

References
Delgado-Escueto AV, Bascal FE, Treiman DM. Complex partial seizures on closed circuit television and EEGs: a study of 691 attacks in 79 patients. *Ann Neurol.* 1982; **11**: 292–300.
Lüders H, Acharya J, Baumgartner C, et al. Semiological seizure classification. *Epilepsia.* 1998; **39**: 1006–13.
Cross References
Absence; Aura; Pelvic thrusting; Poriomania; Seizure

Autophony
Autophony is the perception of the reverberation of ones own voice, which occurs with external or middle, but not inner, ear disease.

Autoscopy

Autoscopy or autoscopia (literally "seeing oneself") is a visual hallucination of ones own face, sometimes with upper body or entire body, likened to seeing oneself in a mirror (hence "mirror hallucination"). The hallucinated image is a mirror image, *i.e.* shows left-right reversal as in a mirror image. Unlike heautoscopy, there is a coincidence of egocentric and body-centred perspectives. Autoscopy may be associated with parieto-occipital space-occupying lesions, epilepsy, migraine, and depression.

References

Blanke O, Landis T, Spinelli L, Seeck M. Out-of-body experience and autoscopy of neurological origin. *Brain*. 2004; **127**: 243–58.

Brugger P. Reflective mirrors: perspective taking in autoscopic phenomena. *Cogn Neuropsychiatry*. 2002; **7**:179–94.

Garry G. A case of autoscopy in a patient with depressive illness. *Prog Neurol Psychiatry*. 2012; **16**(5): 17–8, 20–1.

Cross References

Hallucination; Heautoscopy

Autotopagnosia

Autotopagnosia, or somatotopagnosia, is a rare disorder of body schema characterized by inability to identify parts of the body, either to verbal command or by imitation; this is sometimes localized but may sometimes involve all parts of the body. This may be a form of category-specific anomia with maximum difficulty for naming body parts, or one feature of anosognosia. Finger agnosia and right-left disorientation are partial forms of autotopagnosia, all of which are most often seen following cerebrovascular events involving the left parietal area.

Reference

Ogden JA. Autotopagnosia: occurrence in a patient without nominal aphasia and with an intact ability to point to parts of animals and objects. *Brain*. 1985; **108**: 1009–22.

Cross References

Agnosia; Anosognosia; Finger agnosia; Gerstmann syndrome; Right-left disorientation; Somatoparaphrenia

B

Babinski's Sign (1)

Babinski's sign is a polysynaptic cutaneous reflex consisting of an extensor movement (dorsiflexion) of the big toe on eliciting the plantar response, due to contraction of extensor hallucis longus. There may be in addition fanning (abduction) of the other toes (fan sign; *signe de l'éventail*) but this is neither necessary nor sufficient for Babinski's sign to be judged present. There may be simultaneous contraction of other limb flexor muscles, consistent with the notion that Babinski's sign forms part of a flexion synergy (withdrawal) of the leg. The use of the term "negative Babinski sign" to indicate the normal finding of a downgoing (flexor; plantar flexion) big toe is incorrect, "flexor plantar response" being the appropriate description. The plantar response is most commonly performed by stroking the sole and/or lateral border of the foot, although many other variants are described (*e.g.* Chaddock's sign, Gordon's sign, Oppenheim's sign).

Babinski's sign is a normal finding in infants with immature (unmyelinated) corticospinal tracts; persistence beyond 3 years of age, or re-emergence in adult life, is pathological. In this context, Babinski's sign is considered a reliable ("hard") sign of corticospinal (pyramidal) tract dysfunction (upper motor neurone pathology), and may coexist with other signs of upper motor neurone dysfunction (*e.g.* weakness in a so-called pyramidal distribution, spasticity, hyperreflexia). However, if weakness of extensor hallucis longus is one of the features of upper motor neurone dysfunction, or from any other cause, Babinski's sign may be unexpectedly absent although anticipated on clinical grounds.

A diagnostic accuracy study found Babinski's sign had high specificity (0.99) but low sensitivity (0.51) for pyramidal tract dysfunction.

Other causes of Babinski's sign include hepatic coma, post epileptic seizure, deep sleep following prolonged induced wakefulness, and cataplectic attack. Hence it is not necessarily a consequence of a permanent and irreversible lesion of the pyramidal tracts.

In the presence of extrapyramidal signs, it is important to distinguish Babinski's sign, a "pyramidal sign", from pseudo-Babinski sign and striatal toe (spontaneous upgoing plantar).

References

Critchley M. The citadel of the senses and other essays. New York: Raven Press; 1986. p. 35, 65.
Isaza Jaramillo SP, Uribe Uribe CS, Garcia Jimenez FA, et al. Accuracy of the Babinski sign in the identification of pyramidal tract dysfunction. *J Neurol Sci.* 2014; **343**: 66–8.
Lance JW. The Babinski sign. *J Neurol Neurosurg Psychiatry.* 2002; **73**: 360–2.
Van Gijn J. The Babinski sign: a centenary. Utrecht: Universiteit Utrecht; 1996.

Cross References

Chaddock's sign; Gordon's sign; Hyperreflexia; Oppenheim's sign; Parkinsonism; Plantar response; Pseudo-Babinski sign; Spasticity; Striatal toe; Upper motor neurone (UMN) syndrome; Weakness

Babinski's Sign (2)

Babinski (1905) described the paradoxical elevation of the eyebrow in hemifacial spasm as orbicularis oris contracts and the eye closes, a synkinesis which is not reproducible by will. This observation indicated to Babinski the peripheral (facial nerve) origin of hemifacial spasm. It may assist in differentiating hemifacial spasm from other craniofacial movement disorders. It has a high prevalence (0.86) and specificity (1.00) in hemifacial spasm

© Springer International Publishing Switzerland 2016
A.J. Larner, *A Dictionary of Neurological Signs*,
DOI 10.1007/978-3-319-29821-4_2

Reference
Pawlowski M, Gess B, Evers S. The Babinski-2 sign in hemifacial spasm. *Mov Disord.* 2013;
28: 1298–300.
Cross Reference
Hemifacial spasm

Babinski's Trunk-Thigh Test
Babinski's trunk-thigh test, also known as the "rising sign", is suggested to be of use in distinguishing organic from functional paraplegia and hemiplegia (the abductor sign may also be of use in the former case, Hoover's sign in the latter).

The recumbent patient is asked to sit up with the arms folded on the front of the chest. In organic hemiplegia there is involuntary flexion of the paretic leg, which may automatically rise higher than the normal leg; in paraplegia both legs are involuntarily raised. In functional paraplegic weakness neither leg is raised, and in functional hemiplegia only the normal leg is raised.
Reference
Critchley M. The citadel of the senses and other essays. New York: Raven Press; 1986. p. 37.
Cross References
Abductor sign; Functional weakness and sensory disturbance; Hemiplegia; Hoover's sign;
Paraplegia

"Bag of Worms"
- see MYOKYMIA

Balaclava Helmet
A pattern of facial sensory loss resembling in distribution a balaclava helmet, involving the outer parts of the face but sparing the nose and mouth, may be seen with central brainstem lesions such as syringobulbia which progress upwards from the neck, such that the lowermost part of the spinal nucleus of the trigeminal nerve which serves the outer part of the face is involved whilst the upper part of the nucleus which serves the central part of the face is spared. This pattern of facial sensory impairment may also be known as onion peel or onion skin.
Cross Reference
Onion peel, Onion skin

Balint's Syndrome
Balint's syndrome, first described by a Hungarian neurologist in 1909, consists of:

- *Simultanagnosia* (*q.v.*; dorsal type):
  A constriction of visual attention, such that the patient is aware of only one object at a time; visual acuity is preserved, and patients can recognise single objects placed directly in front of them; they are unable to read or distinguish overlapping figures.
- *Spatial disorientation*:
  Loss of spatial reference and memory, leaving the patient "lost in space".
- *Disorders of oculomotor function*:
  Specifically visually guided eye movements (fixation, pursuit, saccades); Balint's "psychic paralysis of gaze", or "sticky fixation", refers to an inability to direct voluntary eye movements to visual targets, despite a full range of eye movements; this has also been characterised as a form of oculomotor apraxia. Accurate eye movements may be programmed by sound or touch. Loss of spontaneous blinking has also been reported.
- *Optic ataxia*:
  A failure to grasp or touch an object under visual guidance.

Not all elements may be present; there may also be co-existing visual field defects, hemispatial neglect, visual agnosia, or prosopagnosia.

Balint's syndrome results from bilateral lesions of the parieto-occipital junction causing a functional disconnection between higher order visual cortical regions and the frontal eye fields, with sparing of the primary visual cortex. Brain imaging, either structural (CT, MRI) or functional (SPECT, PET), may demonstrate this bilateral damage, which is usually of vascular origin, for example due to watershed or borderzone ischaemia, or top-of-the-basilar syndrome.

Balint syndrome has also been reported as a migrainous phenomenon, following traumatic brain injury and in association with Alzheimer's disease, brain tumour (butterfly glioma), radiation necrosis, progressive multifocal leukoencephalopathy, Marchiafava-Bignami disease with pathology affecting the corpus callosum, and X-linked adrenoleukodystrophy.

References
Husein M, Stein J. Rezso Balint and his most celebrated case. *Arch Neurol.* 1988; **45**: 89–93.
Rafal R. Bálint's syndrome: a disorder of visual cognition. In: D'Esposito M, editor. Neurological foundations of cognitive neuroscience. Cambridge: MIT Press; 2003. p. 27–40.
Cross References
Apraxia; Blinking; Ocular apraxia; Optic ataxia; Simultanagnosia

Ballism, Ballismus
Ballism or ballismus is a hyperkinetic involuntary movement disorder characterized by wild, flinging, throwing movements of a limb. These movements most usually involve one half of the body (hemiballismus), although they may sometimes involve a single extremity (monoballismus) or both halves of the body (paraballismus). The movements are often continuous during wakefulness but cease during sleep. Hemiballismus may be associated with limb hypotonia. Clinical and pathophysiological studies suggest that ballism is a severe form of chorea. It is most commonly associated with lesions of the contralateral subthalamic nucleus.
Reference
Milburn-McNulty P, Michael BD, Woodford HJ, Nicolson A. Hyperosmolar non-ketotic hyperglycaemia: an important and reversible cause of acute bilateral ballismus. *BMJ Case Rep.* 2012; **2012**: pii: bcr1120115084.
Cross References
Chorea, Choreoathetosis; Hemiballismus; Hypotonia, Hypotonus

Bathing Suit Sensory Loss
- see SUSPENDED SENSORY LOSS

Battle's Sign
Battle's sign is a haematoma (bruising) overlying the mastoid process, which indicates an underlying basilar skull fracture extending into the mastoid portion of the temporal bone. It appears 48–72 h after the trauma which causes the fracture. It is reported to have a very high positive predictive value for skull base fracture (100%) but less for intracranial lesions such as acute extradural or subdural haematoma, pneumocephalus, brain contusion, and brain swelling (66%).
Reference
Pretto Flores L, De Almeida CS, Casulari LA. Positive predictive values of selected clinical signs associated with skull base fractures. *J Neurosurg Sci.* 2000; **44**: 77–82.
Cross Reference
Raccoon eyes, Raccoon sign

Bed Cycling Test
In the bed cycling test, the patient lies supine, with hips flexed, and is asked to air cycle rapidly with eyes closed, 10 s forward, and 10 s backward. The test is visually rated. It is said to be able to detect a subtle unilateral cerebral lesion, and be analogous to forearm rolling.

Reference
Feil K, Boettcher N, Lezius F, et al. The bed cycling test: a bedside test for unilateral cerebral dysfunction. *Eur J Neurol.* 2015; **22**(Suppl 1): 179.
Cross References
Forearm and finger rolling; Thumb rolling test

Beevor's Sign
Beevor's sign is an upward movement of the umbilicus in a supine patient who is attempting either to flex the head onto the chest against resistance (*e.g.* the examiner's hand) or performing a sit-up. It indicates weakness of the rectus abdominis muscle below, but not above, the umbilicus. This may occur with a spinal lesion (*e.g.* tumour, syringomyelia) between T10 and T12 causing isolated weakness of the lower part of the muscle, or myopathies affecting abdominal muscles, particularly facioscapulohumeral muscular dystrophy. Lower cutaneous abdominal reflexes are also absent, having the same localising value.

Downward movement of the umbilicus ("inverted Beevor's sign") due to weakness of the upper part of rectus abdominis is less often seen.
References
Eger K, Jordan B, Habermann S, Zierz S. Beevor's sign in facioscapuloperoneal muscular dystrophy: an old sign with new implications. *J Neurol.* 2010; **257**: 436–8.
Tashiro K. Charles Edward Beevor (1854–1908) and Beevor's sign. In: Rose FC, editor. A short history of neurology: the British contribution 1660–1910. Oxford: Butterworth Heinemann; 1999. p. 222–5.
Cross Reference
Abdominal reflexes

Belle Indifférence
The term *la belle indifférence* has been used to refer to a patient's seeming lack of concern in the presence of serious symptoms. This was first defined in the context of "hysteria", as a typical conversion symptom, along with exaggerated emotional reactions, what might now be termed functional or somatoform illness. However, the sign is a poor discrimator against "organic" illness. Some patients' coping style is to make light of serious symptoms; they might be labelled stoical. Because of the lack of discrimination between conversion symptoms and organic disease, some authors have advocated the term be abandoned until a clearer definition emerges.

Patients with neuropathological lesions may also demonstrate a lack of concern for their disabilities, either due to a disorder of body schema (anosodiaphoria) or due to incongruence of mood (typically in frontal lobe syndromes, sometimes seen in multiple sclerosis).
Reference
Stone J, Smyth R, Carson A, Warlow C, Sharpe M. La belle indifference in conversion symptoms and hysteria: systematic review. *Br J Psychiatry.* 2006; **188**: 204–9.
Cross References
Anosodiaphoria; Frontal lobe syndromes; Functional weakness and sensory disturbance

Bell's Palsy
Bell's palsy is an idiopathic peripheral (lower motor neurone) facial weakness (prosopoplegia). It is thought to result from viral inflammation of the facial (VII) nerve. Other causes of lower motor neurone facial paresis may need to be excluded before a diagnosis of Bell's palsy can be made.

In the majority of patients with Bell's palsy (idiopathic facial paresis), spontaneous recovery occurs over 3 weeks to 2 months. Poorer prognosis is associated with older age (over 40 years) and if no recovery is seen within 4 weeks of onset. Meta-analyses suggest that steroids are associated with better outcome than no treatment, but that aciclovir alone has no benefit.

References
De Almeida JR, Al Khabori M, Guyatt GH, et al. Combined corticosteroid and antiviral treatment for Bell palsy: a systematic review and meta-analysis. *JAMA*. 2009; **302**: 985–93.
Quant EC, Jeste SS, Muni RH, Cape AV, Bhussar MK, Peleq AY. The benefits of steroids versus steroids plus antivirals for treatment of Bell's palsy: a meta-analysis. *BMJ*. 2009; **339**: b3354.
Cross References
Bell's phenomenon, Bell's sign; Facial paresis, Facial weakness; Lower motor neurone (LMN) syndrome

Bell's Phenomenon, Bell's Sign
Bell's phenomenon or sign is reflex upward rotation and slightly outward deviation of the eyeballs in response to closure or attempted closure of the eyelids. This is a synkinesis of central origin involving superior rectus and inferior oblique muscles. It may be very evident in a patient with Bell's palsy (idiopathic facial nerve paralysis) attempting to close the paretic eyelid.

The reflex indicates intact nuclear and infranuclear mechanisms of upward gaze, and hence that any defect of upgaze is supranuclear. However, in making this interpretation it should be remembered that perhaps 10–15% of the normal population do not show a Bell's phenomenon.

Bell's phenomenon is usually absent in progressive supranuclear palsy, and is only sometimes spared in Parinaud's syndrome
References
An JG, Guo CL. Bell's sign with lagophthalmos in leprosy. *QJM*. 2015; **108**: 167.
Bell C. On the motions of the eye, in illustration of the use of the muscles and nerves of the orbit. *Philos Trans R Soc Lond*. 1823; **113**: 166–86.
Cross References
Bell's palsy; Facial paresis, Facial weakness; Gaze palsy; Parinaud's syndrome; Supranuclear gaze palsy; Synkinesia, Synkinesis

Benediction Hand
Benediction hand (also sometimes known as Papal benediction sign, Benedictine hand, or orator's hand) describes a hand posture likened to that of a priest saying benediction, namely with index and middle finger extended and little and ring finger flexed.

Some confusion exists as to the aetiology of this clinical sign. It may result from median nerve lesions in the axilla or upper arm which cause weakness in all median nerve innervated muscles, including flexor digitorum profundus, such that on attempting to make a fist, there is impaired flexion of the index and middle fingers, complete and partial respectively, but with normal ring and little finger flexion (ulnar-nerve mediated). Alternatively, an ulnar-nerve lesion may result in clawing of the hand resembling this benediction posture. In light of the confusion, the term is perhaps best avoided, with clinical and neurophysiological efforts best directed toward defining the underlying peripheral nerve lesion.
Reference
Futterman B. Analysis of the Papal Benediction Sign: the ulnar neuropathy of St. Peter. *Clin Anat*. 2015; **28**: 696–701.
Cross References
Claw hand; Simian hand

Bent Spine Syndrome
- see CAMPTOCORMIA

Bielschowsky's Sign, Bielschowsky's Test
Bielschowsky's sign is head tilt towards the shoulder, typically toward the side contralateral to a trochlear (IV) nerve palsy. The intorsion of the unaffected eye brought about by the head tilt compensates for the double vision caused by the unopposed extorsion of the affected eye.

Very occasionally, head tilt is paradoxical, *i.e.* towards the involved side: presumably the greater separation of images thus produced allows one of them to be ignored or suppressed.

Bielschowsky's (head tilt) test consists of the examiner tipping the patient's head from shoulder to shoulder: with a unilateral trochlear (IV) nerve lesion this will improve or exacerbate double vision as the head is respectively tilted away from or towards the affected side. The test is usually negative in a skew deviation causing vertical divergence of the eyes.

This test may also be used as part of the assessment of vertical diplopia to see whether hypertropia changes with head tilt to left or right; increased hypertropia on left head tilt suggests a weak intortor of the left eye (superior rectus); increased hypertropia on right head tilt suggests a weak intortor of the right eye (superior oblique).

Reference
Hertzberg R. Bielschowsky's sign. Its genesis and other observations by Bielschowsky. *Aust J Ophthalmol.* 1982; **10**: 282–4.

Cross References
Diplopia; Hypertropia; Skew deviation

Binasal Hemianopia
Of the hemianopic visual field defects, binasal hemianopia, suggesting lateral compression of the optic chiasm, is less common than bitemporal hemianopia. Various causes are recorded including syphilis, glaucoma, drusen, chronically raised intracranial pressure, and it has also been observed in the absence of identifiable ocular or neurological defects.

Reference
Bryan BT, Pomeranz HD, Smith KH. Complete binasal hemianopia. *Proc (Bayl Univ Med Cent).* 2014; **27**: 356–8.

Cross References
Hemianopia; Visual field defects

Bitemporal Hemianopia
Bitemporal hemianopia due to optic chiasmal compression, for example by a pituitary lesion or craniopharyngioma, is probably the most common cause of a heteronymous hemianopia. Conditions mimicking bitemporal hemianopia include congenitally tilted discs ("pseudobitemporal hemianopia"), nasal sector retinitis pigmentosa, and papilloedema with greatly enlarged blind spots.

Cross References
Hemianopia; Visual field defects

Blepharohaematoma
- see RACCOON EYES, RACCOON SIGN

Blepharoptosis
- see PTOSIS

Blepharospasm
Blepharospasm is a focal dystonia of the orbicularis oculi resulting in repeated involuntary forced eyelid closure, with failure of voluntary eye opening. Usually bilateral in origin, it may be sufficiently severe to result in functional blindness. The condition typically begins in the sixth decade of life, and is more common in women than men. Blepharospasm may occur in isolation ("benign essential blepharospasm"), or in combination with other involuntary movements which may be dystonic (orobuccolingual dystonia or Meige syndrome; limb dystonia) or dyspraxic (eyelid apraxia), or in association with another neurological disorder such as Parkinson's disease. Other examples of "secondary blepharospasm" include drug therapy (neuroleptics, levodopa) and lesions of the brainstem, and more rarely cerebellum and striatum.

Like other forms of dystonia, blepharospasm may be relieved by sensory tricks (*geste antagoniste*) such as talking, yawning, singing, humming or touching the eyelid. This feature is helpful in diagnosis. Blepharospasm may be aggravated by reading, watching television, exposure to wind or bright light.

In one variant of blepharospasm, confined to the pretarsal parts of orbicularis oculi, contraction may be difficult to identify. There may be confusion with other causes of isolated bilateral ptosis such as myasthenia gravis or eyelid apraxia.

Blepharospasm is usually idiopathic but may be associated with lesions (usually infarction) of the rostral brainstem, diencephalon, and striatum; it has been occasionally reported with thalamic lesions. The pathophysiological mechanisms underlying blepharospasm are not understood, but may reflect dopaminergic pathway disruption causing disinhibition of brainstem reflexes.

Local injections of botulinum toxin into orbicularis oculi are the treatment of choice, the majority of patients deriving benefit and requesting further injection. Failure to respond to botulinum toxin may be due to concurrent eyelid apraxia or dopaminergic therapy with levodopa.

References
Hallett M, Daroff RB. Blepharospasm: report of a workshop. *Neurology*. 1996; **46**: 1213–8.
Hellman A, Torres-Russotto D. Botulinum toxin in the management of blepharospasm: current evidence and recent developments. *Ther Adv Neurol Disord*. 2015; **8**: 82–91.
Cross References
Blinking; Dystonia; Eyelid apraxia; Gaping; Sensory tricks; Yawning

Blindsight
Blindsight describes a rare phenomenon in which patients with bilateral occipital lobe damage affecting the primary visual cortex are nonetheless able to discriminate certain visual perceptual events within their "blind" fields, although entirely unaware of the presentation of visual stimuli. This "type-1 blindsight" (stimuli elicit no conscious experience) may be distinguished from "type-2 blindsight" in which experience may be sometimes elicited.

Reference
Weiskrantz L. Blindsight. A case study and implications. Oxford: Clarendon; 1986.
Cross References
Agnosopsia; Scotoma

Blind Spot
The blind spot is defined anatomically as the point on the retina at which axons from the retinal ganglion cells enter the optic nerve; since this area is devoid of photoreceptors there is a physiological blind spot. This area may be mapped clinically by confrontation with the examiner's blind spot, or mechanically. Minor enlargement of the blind spot is difficult to identify clinically; formal perimetry is often needed in this situation.

Enlargement of the blind spot (peripapillary scotoma) is observed with raised intracranial pressure causing papilloedema: this may be helpful in differentiating papilloedema from other causes of disc swelling such as optic neuritis, in which a central scotoma is the most common field defect. Enlargement of the blind spot may also be a feature of peripapillary retinal disorders including the acute idiopathic blind spot enlargement (big blind spot) syndrome.

Reference
Liu X, Chen B, Zhang M, Huang H. Clinical features and differential diagnosis of acute idiopathic blind spot enlargement syndrome. *Eye Sci*. 2014; **29**: 143–50.
Cross References
Disc swelling; Papilloedema; Scotoma; Visual field defects

Blinking

Involuntary blinking rate is decreased in idiopathic Parkinson's disease (and may be improved by dopaminergic therapy), and in progressive supranuclear palsy (Steele-Richardson-Olszewski syndrome) where the rate may be <5/min. In contrast, blink rate is normal in multiple system atrophy and dopa-responsive dystonia, and increased in schizophrenia and postencephalitic parkinsonism. These disparate observations are not easily reconciled with the suggestion that blinking might be a marker of central dopaminergic activity.

Loss of spontaneous blinking has been reported in Balint's syndrome. In patients with impaired consciousness, the presence of involuntary blinking implies an intact pontine reticular formation; absence suggests structural or metabolic dysfunction of the reticular formation. Blinking decreases in coma. Functional disorders may be accompanied by an increase in blinking.

Reference
Karson CN. Spontaneous eye-blink rates and dopaminergic systems. *Brain*. 1983; **106**: 643–53.

Cross References
Balint's syndrome; Blink reflex; Coma; Corneal reflex; Parkinsonism; Sighing; Yawning

Blink Reflex

The blink reflex consists of bilateral reflex contraction of the orbicularis oculi muscles. This may be induced by:

- *Mechanical stimulus*:
  Examples include: percussion over the supraorbital ridge (glabellar tap reflex, Myerson's sign, nasopalpebral reflex); touching the cornea (corneal reflex); stroking the eyelashes in unconscious patients with closed eyes ("eyelash reflex").
- *Visual stimulus*:
  Sudden visual stimulus approaching the eyes (menace reflex, threat reflex, visuopalpebral reflex).
- *Acoustic stimulus*:
  Sudden loud sounds (acousticopalpebral reflex, cochleopalpebral reflex).

The final common (efferent) pathway for these responses is the facial nerve nucleus and facial (VII) nerve, the afferent limbs being the trigeminal (V), optic (II), and auditory (VIII) nerves respectively. The corneal reflex is thought to be entirely subcortical, whilst the menace reflex has a cortical component.

Electrophysiological study of the blink reflex may demonstrate peripheral or central lesions of the trigeminal (V) nerve or facial (VII) nerve (afferent and efferent pathways, respectively). It has been reported that in the evaluation of sensory neuronopathy the finding of an abnormal blink reflex favours a non-paraneoplastic aetiology, since the blink reflex is normal in paraneoplastic sensory neuronopathies.

References
Auger RG, Windebank AJ, Lucchinetti CF, Chalk CH. Role of the blink reflex in the evaluation of sensory neuronopathy. *Neurology*. 1999; **53**: 407–8.
Liu GT, Ronthal M. Reflex blink to visual threat. *J Clin Neuro-ophthalmol*. 1992; **12**: 47–56.

Cross References
Balint's syndrome; Blinking; Corneal reflex; Glabellar tap reflex; Menace reflex

Body Part as Object

In this phenomenon, apraxic patients use a body part when asked to pantomime certain actions, such as using the palm when asked to demonstrate the use of a hair brush or comb, or fingers when asked to demonstrate use of scissors or a toothbrush.

References
Goodglass H, Kaplan E. Disturbance of gesture and pantomime in aphasia. *Brain*. 1963; **86**: 703–20.

Kato M, Meguro K, Sato M, et al. Ideomotor apraxia in patients with Alzheimer's disease: why do they use their body parts as objects? *Neuropsychiatry Neuropsychol Behav Neurol.* 2001; **14**: 45–52.
Cross References
Apraxia; Parapraxia, Parapraxis

"Bon-Bon Sign"
Involuntary pushing of the tongue against the inside of the cheek, the "bon-bon sign", is said to be typical of the stereotypic orolingual movements of tardive dyskinesia, along with chewing and smacking of the mouth and lips, and rolling of the tongue in the mouth. These signs may help to distinguish tardive dyskinesia from chorea, although periodic protrusion of the tongue (flycatcher, trombone tongue) is common to both.
Cross References
Buccolingual syndrome; Chorea, Choreoathetosis; Trombone tongue

Bouche De Tapir
Patients with facioscapulohumeral (FSH) muscular dystrophy have a peculiar and characteristic facies, with puckering of the lips when attempting to whistle. The pouting quality of the mouth, unlike that seen with other types of bilateral (neurogenic) facial weakness, has been likened to the face of the tapir (*Tapirus* sp.), a large herbivorous mammal with a prehensile snout.
Cross Reference
Facial paresis, Facial weakness

Bovine Cough
A bovine cough lacks the explosive character of a normal voluntary cough. It may result from injury to the distal part of the vagus nerve, particularly the recurrent laryngeal branches which innervate all the muscles of the larynx (with the exception of cricothyroid) with resultant vocal cord paresis. Because of its longer intrathoracic course, the left recurrent laryngeal nerve is more often involved. A bovine cough may be heard in patients with tumours of the upper lobes of the lung (Pancoast tumour) due to recurrent laryngeal nerve palsy. Bovine cough may also result from any cause of bulbar weakness, such as motor neurone disease, Guillain-Barré syndrome, and bulbar myopathies.
Reference
Arcasoy SM, Jett JR. Superior pulmonary sulcus tumors and Pancoast's syndrome. *N Engl J Med.* 1997; **337**: 1370–6.
Cross References
Bulbar palsy; Diplophonia; *Signe de rideau*

Bradykinesia
Bradykinesia is slowness of initiation of voluntary movement with progressive reduction in speed and amplitude of repetitive actions in the absence of weakness. It is one of the typical signs of parkinsonian syndromes, and a *sine qua non* for the diagnosis of idiopathic Parkinson's disease.

Bradykinesia in parkinsonian syndromes is often accompanied by other signs such as difficulty in the initiation of movement (akinesia, hypokinesia) and reduced amplitude of movement (hypometria) which may increase with rapid repetitive movements (fatigue). Bradykinesia may be susceptible to motivational modulation, and be overcome by reflexive movements or in moments of intense emotion (*kinesis paradoxica*).

Bradykinesia in parkinsonian syndromes reflects dopamine depletion in the basal ganglia. It may be improved by levodopa and dopaminergic agonists, less so by anticholinergic agents.

Slowness of voluntary movement may also be seen in other conditions, such as psychomotor retardation, frontal lobe lesions producing abulia, and in the condition of obsessive slowness.

References
Berardelli A, Rothwell JC, Thompson PD, Hallett M. Pathophysiology of bradykinesia in Parkinson's disease. *Brain*. 2001; **124**: 2131–46.
Gibb WRG, Lees AJ. The relevance of the Lewy body to the pathogenesis of idiopathic Parkinson's disease. *J Neurol Neurosurg Psychiatry*. 1988; **51**: 745–52.
Pal G, Goetz CG. Assessing bradykinesia in parkinsonian disorders. *Front Neurol*. 2013; **4**: 54.
Cross References
Abulia; Akinesia; Fatigue; Hypokinesia; Hypometria; *Kinesis paradoxica*; Parkinsonism; Psychomotor retardation

Bradylalia
Bradylalia may be used to describe slowness of speech, typically seen in the frontal-subcortical types of cognitive impairment, with or without extrapyramidal features, or in depression.
Cross References
Palilalia; Tachylalia

Bradyphrenia
The concept of bradyphrenia dates to Naville in 1922, characterizing a condition of slow cognition, apathy, and impaired concentration, originally in the context of encephalitis lethargica. Slowness of thought is typically seen in the frontal-subcortical types of cognitive impairment, *e.g.* progressive supranuclear palsy, vascular dementia, Huntington's disease. Such patients typically answer questions correctly but with long response times. Slowed cognition is a general mechanism of age-related cognitive performance, but in Parkinson's disease there may be additional cognitive decline and dementia.
Reference
Rogers D. Bradyphrenia in parkinsonism: a historical review. *Psychol Med*. 1986; **16**: 257–65.
Cross References
Abulia; Apathy; Dementia

Bragard's Test
- see LASÈGUE'S SIGN

Broca's Aphasia
Broca's aphasia is the classic "expressive aphasia", in distinction to the "receptive aphasia" of Wernicke; however, there are problems with this simple classification, since Broca's aphasics may show comprehension ("receptive") problems with complex material, particularly in relation to syntax; and certainly speech output ("expression") is not normal in Wernicke's aphasia.
    Considering each of the features suggested for the clinical classification of aphasias (see Aphasia), Broca's aphasia is typically characterized by:

- *Fluency*: slow, laboured, effortful speech (non-fluent) with phonemic paraphasias, agrammatism, and aprosody; the patient knows what s/he wants to say and usually recognises the paraphasic errors (*i.e.* patients can "self-monitor").
- *Comprehension*: comprehension for simple material is preserved, but there may be problems with more complex syntax.
- *Repetition*: impaired.
- *Naming*: impaired (anomia, dysnomia); may be aided by phonemic or contextual cueing (*cf.* Wernicke's aphasia).
- *Reading*: alexia with laboured oral reading, especially of function words and verb inflections. Silent reading may also be impaired (deep dyslexia) as reflected by poor text comprehension.
- *Writing*: similarly affected.

Aphemia was the name originally given by Broca to the language disorder he observed; subsequently this was named "Broca's aphasia". The term alalia was also once used. The terms "small Broca's aphasia", "mini-Broca's aphasia", and "Broca's area aphasia", have been reserved for a more circumscribed clinical and neuroanatomical deficit than Broca's aphasia, wherein the damage is restricted to Broca's area or its subjacent white matter. There is a mild and transient aphasia or anomia which may share some of the characteristics of aphemia/phonetic disintegration (*i.e.* a motor disorder of speech production with preserved comprehension of spoken and written language).

The syndrome of Broca's aphasia may emerge during recovery from a global aphasia. Broca's aphasia is sometimes associated with a right hemiparesis, especially affecting the arm and face; there may also be bucco-lingual-facial dyspraxia. Depression may be a concurrent feature.

Classically Broca's aphasia is associated with a vascular lesion of the third frontal gyrus in the inferior frontal lobe (Broca's area), but in practice such a circumscribed lesion is seldom seen. More commonly there is infarction in the perisylvian region affecting the insula and operculum (Brodmann areas 44 and 45), which may include underlying white matter and the basal ganglia (territory of the superior branch of the middle cerebral artery). Indeed this is more in keeping with the extent of the lesions seen in Broca's original patients when their brains were subjected to high resolution imaging.

Non-fluent aphasia is one of the classical phenotypes of frontotemporal lobar degeneration (the agrammatic variant of primary progressive aphasia); in addition to aphasia, there is marked speech apraxia.

References
Dronkers NF, Plaisant O, Iba-Zizen MT, Cabanis EA. Paul Broca's historic cases: high resolution MR imaging of the brains of Leborgne and Lelong. *Brain.* 2007; **130**: 1432–41.
Grodzinsky Y, Amunts K, editors. Broca's region. New York: Oxford University Press; 2006.
Cross References
Agrammatism; Agraphia; Alalia; Alexia; Aphasia; Aphemia; Aprosodia, Aprosody; Paraphasia; Recurrent utterances; Speech apraxia; Wernicke's aphasia

Brown-Séquard Syndrome
The Brown-Séquard syndrome is the consequence of anatomical or, more usually, functional hemisection of the spinal cord (spinal hemisection or hemicord syndrome), producing the following pattern of clinical findings:

- *Motor*:

    Ipsilateral spastic weakness, due to corticospinal tract involvement.
    Segmental lower motor neurone signs at the level of the lesion, due to root and/or anterior horn cell involvement.
- *Sensory*:

    A dissociated sensory loss, *i.e.*:
    Ipsilateral loss of proprioception, due to dorsal column involvement;
    Contralateral loss of pain and temperature sensation, due to crossed spinothalamic tract involvement.

Spinal cord lesions producing this syndrome may be either extramedullary (*e.g.* prolapsed cervical intervertebral disc, extrinsic spinal cord tumour) or intramedullary (*e.g.* multiple sclerosis, intrinsic spinal cord tumour, myelitis, radiation-induced myelopathy); the former group is said to be the more common cause.

References
Aminoff MJ. *Brown-Séquard. A visionary of science.* New York: Raven; 1993. p. 112–31.
Engelhardt P, Trostdorf E. Zur Differentialdiagnose des Brown-Séquard-Syndroms. *Nervenarzt.* 1997; **48**: 45–9.
Tattersall R, Turner B. Brown-Séquard and his syndrome. *Lancet.* 2000; **356**: 61–3.

Cross References
Dissociated sensory loss; Myelopathy; Proprioception; Spasticity; Weakness

Brudzinski's (Neck) Sign
Brudzinski described a number of signs, but the one most often used in clinical practice is the neck sign, which is sometimes evident in cases of meningeal irritation, for example due to meningitis. Passive flexion of the neck to bring the head onto the chest is accompanied by flexion of the thighs and legs. As with nuchal rigidity and Kernig's sign, Brudzinski's sign may be absent in elderly or immunosuppressed patients with meningeal irritation. Brudzinski's sign is reported to have low sensitivity (0.05) and does not accurately discriminate between adult patients with and without meningitis, although the sensitivity is better in children (0.66; specificity 0.74).

References
Curtis S, Stobart K, Vandermeer B, Simel DL, Klassen T. Clinical features suggestive of meningitis in children. A systematic review of prospective data. *Pediatrics* 2010; **126**: 952–60.
Thomas KE, Hasbun R, Jekel J, Quagliarello VJ. The diagnostic accuracy of Kernig's sign, Brudzinski's sign, and nuchal rigidity in adults with suspected meningitis. *Clin Infect Dis.* 2002; **35**: 46–52.
Ward MA, Greenwood TM, Kumar DR, Mazza JJ, Yale SH. Josef Brudzinski and Vladimir Mikhailovich Kernig: signs for diagnosing meningitis. *Clin Med Res.* 2010; **8**: 13–7.

Cross References
Kernig's sign; Meningism; Nuchal rigidity

Brueghel's Syndrome
Brueghel's syndrome [NB some texts give "Breughel's" syndrome] is the name given to a dystonia of the motor trigeminal nerve causing gaping or involuntary opening of the mouth, so named after the painting by Pieter Brueghel the Elder (*ca.* 1525–1569) entitled *De Gaper* (1558) which is thought to illustrate a typical case. Additional features may include paroxysmal hyperpnoea and upbeating nystagmus. Brueghel's syndrome should be distinguished from other syndromes of cranial dystonia featuring blepharospasm and oromandibular dystonia, better termed Meige's syndrome.

Reference
Gilbert GJ. Brueghel syndrome: its distinction from Meige syndrome. *Neurology.* 1996; **46**: 1767–9.

Cross References
Blepharospasm; Dystonia; Gaping

Bruit
Bruits arise from turbulent blood flow causing arterial wall vibrations which are audible at the body surface with the unassisted ear or with a stethoscope (diaphragm rather than bell, better for detecting higher frequency sounds). They are associated with stenotic vessels or with fistulae where there is arteriovenous (AV) shunting of blood. Dependent on the clinical indication, various sites may be auscultated: eye for orbital bruit in carotico-cavernous fistula; head for bruit of AV fistula; but probably the most frequently auscultated region is the carotid bifurcation, high up under the angle of the jaw, in individuals thought to have had a transient ischaemic attack or ischaemic stroke. Examination for carotid bruits in asymptomatic individuals is probably best avoided, other than in the clinical trial setting, since the optimal management of asymptomatic carotid artery stenosis remains controversial. Moreover, carotid bruit is of only moderate value for detecting a clinically relevant carotid stenosis (low sensitivity, high specificity), and the likelihood of detecting a bruit does not increase with increasing degrees of stenosis,

References
McColgan P, Bentley P, McCarron M, Sharma P. Evaluation of the clinical utility of a carotid bruit. *QJM.* 2012; **105**: 1171–7.
Sandercock PAG, Kavvadia E. The carotid bruit. *Pract Neurol.* 2002; **2**: 221–4.

Brushfield Spots
Brushfield spots are small grey-white specks of depigmentation that can be seen in the iri-des of some patients (90%) with Down's syndrome; they may also occur in normal individuals.

Bruxism
Bruxism is forcible grinding or gnashing of the teeth. This is common in children and is said to occur in 5-20% of the population during non-REM sleep (sleep bruxism, a parasomnia). Masseter hypertrophy may become apparent in persistent grinders. Bruxism may also occur in encephalopathic disorders (*e.g.* hepatic encephalopathy) and occasionally in disorders of the basal ganglia (multiple system atrophy, basal ganglia infarcts). Dysfunction of efferent and/or afferent thalamic and striatopallidal tracts has been suggested as the neural substrate.

If necessary, a rubber gum shield or bite may be worn in the mouth to protect the teeth. Botulinum toxin injections have also been tried.
Reference
Carra MC, Huynh N, Fleury B, Lavigne G. Overview on sleep bruxism for sleep medicine clinicians. *Sleep Med Clin.* 2015; **10**: 375–84.
Cross References
Encephalopathy; Masseter hypertrophy

Buccofacial Dyspraxia
- see OROFACIAL DYSPRAXIA

Buccolingual Syndrome
This is a form of tardive dyskinesia that involves involuntary movements of the facial muscles and protrusion of the tongue.
Cross References
"Bon-bon sign"; Dyskinesia

Bulbar Palsy
Bulbar palsy refers to weakness of the bulbar musculature of lower motor neurone origin. This may be differentiated clinically from bulbar weakness of upper motor neurone origin (pseudobulbar palsy). Clinical features of bulbar palsy include:

- Dysarthria of flaccid/nasal type.
- Dysphonia.
- Dysphagia, often with nasal regurgitation.
- Weak ("bovine") cough; risk of aspiration.
- +/− Wasted, fasciculating tongue.
- +/− Absent jaw jerk.
- +/− Absent gag reflex.

Bulbar palsy is usually neurogenic. Recognised causes include:
- Brainstem disorders affecting cranial nerve motor nuclei (intrinsic):
   Motor neurone disease (which may also cause a pseudobulbar palsy).
   Poliomyelitis.
   Glioma.
   Syringobulbia.
- Cranial nerve lesions outside the brainstem (there may be associated sensory signs):
   Infiltration by carcinoma, granuloma.
- Neuromuscular junction transmission defect:
   Myasthenia gravis.

A myogenic bulbar palsy may be seen in oculopharyngeal muscular dystrophy, inclusion body myositis, and polymyositis.

Cross References
Bovine cough; Dysarthria; Dysphagia; Dysphonia; Fasciculation; Gag reflex; Jaw jerk; Lower motor neurone (LMN) syndrome; Pseudobulbar palsy; Upper motor neurone (UMN) syndrome

Bulbocavernosus Reflex
The bulbocavernosus reflex is a test of the integrity of the S2, S3 and S4 spinal roots, elicited by squeezing the glans penis or clitoris (*i.e.* stimulating the dorsal nerve of the penis or clitoris) and looking for reflex contraction of the anal sphincter (this may be felt with a gloved finger in the rectum). The reflex may be abolished in cauda equina lesions.

Cross References
Cauda equina syndrome; Reflexes

Buphthalmos
Buphthalmos, literally ox-eye, consists of a large and bulging eye caused by raised intraocular pressure due to congenital or secondary glaucoma. This is one of the ophthalmological features of Sturge-Weber syndrome.

"Butt-First Manoeuvre"
- see GOWERS' SIGN

C

Cacogeusia
Cacogeusia is the sensation of a disagreeable taste, often associated with parosmia.
Cross References
Ageusia; Parosmia

Cacosmia
- see PAROSMIA

Caecocentral Scotoma
- see CENTRAL SCOTOMA, CENTROCAECAL SCOTOMA

Calf Head Sign
A consistent pattern of muscle enlargement or wasting, described as "calf heads on a trophy", has been observed in Miyoshi-type dysferlinopathy when the arms are raised with the shoulders abducted and the elbows flexed to 90°. Diamond on quadriceps sign may also be seen in dysferlinopathies.
Reference
Pradhan S. Calf-head sign in Miyoshi myopathy. *Arch Neurol.* 2006; **63**: 1414–7.
Cross Reference
Diamond on quadriceps sign

Calf Hypertrophy
Calf enlargement has many causes; it may reflect true hypertrophy (enlargement of muscle fibres) or, more commonly, pseudohypertrophy, due to infiltration with tissue elements other than muscle. Hypertrophy may be due to neuromuscular disorders producing:

- chronic partial denervation, *e.g.*:
    radiculopathy.
    peripheral neuropathy.
    spinal muscular atrophy.
    following paralytic poliomyelitis.
- continuous muscle activity *e.g.*:
    myotonia congenita.
    neuromyotonia (Isaac's syndrome).
    generalised myokymia.

Calf (and other muscle) hypertrophy is also a feature of limb girdle muscular dystrophy type 2I.
Calf pseudohypertrophy may be due to:

- Dystrophinopathies (Duchenne muscular dystrophy, Becker dystrophy), due to excess connective tissue.
- Infection/inflammation: myositis.
- Infiltration: amyloidosis, tumour, cysticercosis.

© Springer International Publishing Switzerland 2016
A.J. Larner, *A Dictionary of Neurological Signs*,
DOI 10.1007/978-3-319-29821-4_3

References
Coles A, Dick D. Unilateral calf hypertrophy. *J Neurol Neurosurg Psychiatry*. 2004; **75**: 1606.
Wilson H, Kidd D, Howard RS, Williams AJ, Spencer GT. Calf hypertrophy following paralytic poliomyelitis. *Postgrad Med J*. 2000; **76**: 179–81.
Cross References
Gowers' sign; Muscle hypertrophy; Myokymia; Myotonia; Neuromyotonia

Caloric Testing

Caloric tests examine the vestibulo-ocular reflexes (VOR). They are mainly used in two circumstances: to identify vestibular pathology in the assessment of dizziness/vertigo when clinical tests of VOR are unhelpful, and to assess brainstem integrity in coma.

Each labyrinth may be separately assessed by irrigating each outer ear. Head flexion to 30° above the horizontal allows maximum stimulation of the horizontal semicircular canals, whereas 60° below horizontal maximally stimulates the lateral semicircular canals. Water 7 °C above and below body temperature (*i.e.* 30 and 44 °C) is used, applied for 30–40 s. Induced nystagmus is then timed both with and without visual fixation (in the dark, Frenzel glasses). This method is cheap but has poor patient acceptability.

Normally, the eyes show conjugate deviation towards the ear irrigated with cold water, with corrective nystagmus in the opposite direction; with warm water the opposite pattern is seen. (The direction of nystagmus may thus be recalled by the mnemonic COWS: cold opposite, warm same.) Dysconjugate responses suggest brainstem damage or depression. A reduced duration of induced nystagmus is seen with canal paresis; enhancement of the nystagmus with removal of visual fixation suggests this is peripheral in origin (labyrinthine, vestibulocochlear nerve), whereas no enhancement suggests a central lesion.

In coma the deviation may be present but without corrective saccades, even at a time when the oculocephalic responses elicited by the doll's head manoeuvre are lost. As coma deepens even the caloric reflexes are lost as brainstem involvement progresses.

Reference
Rudge P, Bronstein AM. Investigations of disorders of balance. In: Hughes RAC, editor. Neurological Investigations. London: BMJ Publishing; 1997. p. 283–314.
Cross References
Coma; Nystagmus; Oculocephalic response; Vertigo; Vestibulo-ocular reflexes

Camptocormia

Camptocormia, or "bent spine syndrome", describes abnormal thoracolumbar spinal flexion, usually at least 45°. It is present on standing, walking or on exercise but is alleviated when sitting, lying, using a walking support, or standing against a wall.

Camptocormia was first conceptualised as a psychiatric phenomenon in men facing armed conflict (a "war neurosis"). It was subsequently realised that the axial postural deformity of reducible lumbar kyphosis could result from neurological disorders. The aetiology is heterogeneous, and includes muscle disease (paravertebral myopathy, nemaline myopathy), Parkinson's disease, dystonia, motor neurone disease, and, possibly, a paraneoplastic phenomenon. Cases with associated lenticular (putaminal) lesions have also been described. Camptocormia may be related in some instances to dropped head syndrome.

Treatment is dependent on cause, where this can be established. Therapeutic options to improve posture in Parkinson's disease may include apomorphine infusion, botulinum toxin injections, and deep brain stimulation.

References
Jankovic J. Camptocormia, head drop and other bent spine syndromes: heterogeneous etiology and pathogenesis of Parkinsonian deformities. *Mov Disord*. 2010; **25**: 527–8.

Lenoir T, Guedj N, Boulu P, Guigui P, Benoist M. Camptocormia: the bent spine syndrome, an update. *Eur Spine J.* 2010; **19**: 1229–37.
Srivanitchapoom P, Hallett M. Camptocormia in Parkinson's disease: definition, epidemiology, pathogenesis and treatment modalities. *J Neurol Neurosurg Psychiat.* 2016; **87**: 75–85.
Cross References
Dropped head syndrome; Dystonia

Camptodactyly
Camptodactyly, literally "bent finger", is a flexion deformity at the proximal interphalangeal joint, especially affecting the little fingers; this may be unilateral or bilateral. A distinction is sometimes drawn between camptodactyly and streblodactyly: in the latter, several fingers are affected by flexion contractures (streblo = twisted, crooked), but it is not clear whether the two conditions overlap or are separate. The term streblomicrodactyly has sometimes been used to designate isolated crooked little fingers.
Camptodactyly is not accompanied by any sensory or motor signs. The condition may be familial, and is more common in women. Camptodactyly may occur in isolation or as part of a developmental disorder with other dysmorphic features.
It is important to differentiate camptodactyly, a non-neurogenic cause of clawing, from neurological diagnoses such as:

- Ulnar neuropathy.
- C8/T1 radiculopathy.
- Cervical rib.
- Syringomyelia.

Awareness of the condition is important to avoid unnecessary neurological investigation.
Reference
Larner AJ. Camptodactyly: a 10-year series. *Eur J Dermatol.* 2011; **21**: 771–5.
Cross Reference
Claw hand

Capgras Syndrome
This is one of the classical delusional syndromes of psychiatry, first described by Capgras and Reboul-Lachaux in 1923, in which patients recognise a close family relative, or other loved object, but believe them to be have been replaced by an exact alien or "double" (illusion of doubles).
Initially described in patients with psychiatric disorders, it may also occur in traumatic, metabolic and neurodegenerative disorders (*e.g.* Alzheimer's disease, dementia with Lewy bodies). Neurologists have sometimes encompassed this phenomenon under the term reduplicative paramnesia.
Some believe this syndrome to be the "mirror image" of prosopagnosia, in which faces are not recognised but emotional significance is. Capgras' syndrome may be envisaged as a Geschwindian disconnection syndrome, in which the visual recognition system is disconnected from the limbic system, hence faces can be recognised but no emotional significance ascribed to them.
References
Devinsky O. Behavioral neurology. The neurology of Capgras syndrome. *Rev Neurol Dis.* 2008; **5**: 97–100.
Josephs KA. Capgras syndrome and its relationship to neurodegenerative disease. *Arch Neurol.* 2007; **64**: 1762–6.
Cross References
Cotard's syndrome; Disconnection syndromes; Prosopagnosia; Reduplicative paramnesia

Carpal Compression Test
- see DURKAN'S COMPRESSION TEST

Carphologia, Carphology
Carphologia or carphology is an aimless plucking at clothing or bedclothes, as if picking off pieces of thread; the related phenomenon of floccillation is an aimless plucking at the air. This may sometimes be seen in psychiatric illness, delirium, Alzheimer's disease, or vascular dementia particularly affecting the frontal lobe. Some have characterised carphologia as a form of akathisia.

One study has suggested a very high specificity (0.98) for these signs in delirium, indicating that their presence is highly suggestive for this diagnosis.

References
Holt R, Teale EA, Mulley GP, Young J. A prospective observational study to investigate the association between abnormal hand movements and delirium in hospitalized older people. *Age Ageing*. 2015; **44**: 42–5.
Larner AJ. Carphologia, or floccillation. *Adv Clin Neurosci Rehabilit*. 2007; **7**(4): 25.

Cross References
Akathisia; Delirium; Dementia

Carpopedal Spasm
- see *MAIN D'ACCOUCHEUR*

Catalepsy
This term has been used to describe increased muscle tone, leading to the assumption of fixed postures which may be held for long periods of time without apparent fatigue; it may be possible for the examiner to position an extremity into any posture, in which it then remains for some time. Clearly this term is either cognate or overlaps with "waxy flexibility" which is a feature of catatonic syndromes.

Catalepsy may be induced by neuroleptic medications with antidopaminergic action, suggesting that it originates in extrapyramidal pathways. Catalepsy may be feigned (see, for example, Dr Arthur Conan Doyle's story of The Resident Patient in *The Memoirs of Sherlock Holmes*, first published in 1894).

Catalepsy should not be confused with the term cataplexy, a syndrome in which muscle tone is transiently lost.

Reference
Perkin GD. Catalepsy. *J Neurol Neurosurg Psychiatry*. 1995; **59**: 86.

Cross References
Cataplexy; Catatonia

Cataplexy
Cataplexy is a sudden loss of limb tone which may lead to falls (drop attacks) without loss of consciousness, usually lasting less than 1 min. Attacks may be precipitated by strong emotion (laughter, anger, embarrassment, surprise). Sagging of the jaw and face may occur, as may twitching around the face or eyelids. During an attack there is electrical silence in anti-gravity muscles, which are consequently hypotonic, and transient areflexia. Rarely status cataplecticus may develop, particularly after withdrawal of tricyclic antidepressant medication.

Cataplexy may occur as part of the narcoleptic syndrome of excessive and inappropriate daytime somnolence, hypnagogic hallucinations and sleep paralysis (Gélineau's original description of narcolepsy in 1877 included an account of "astasia" which corresponds to cataplexy). Symptomatic cataplexy occurs in certain neurological diseases including brainstem lesions, von Economo's disease (postencephalitic parkinsonism), Niemann-Pick disease type C, and Norrie's disease. The pathophysiology of cataplexy may involve the activation during wakefulness of brainstem pathways which in REM sleep suppress muscle tone.

Cataplexy is included in the differential diagnosis of syncope since, although there is no loss of consciousness, retrograde amnesia may occur in syncope leading to presentation as "unexplained falls".

Therapeutic options for cataplexy are limited, but include: tricyclic antidepressants such as protriptyline, imipramine and clomipramine; serotonin reuptake inhibitors such as fluoxetine; noradrenaline and serotonin reuptake inhibitors such as venlafaxine; and gamma-hydroxybutyrate.

Reference

Dauvilliers Y, Siegel JM, Lopez R, Torontali ZA, Peever JH. Cataplexy – clinical aspects, pathophysiology and management strategy. *Nat Rev Neurol*. 2014; **10**: 386–95.

Cross References

Areflexia; Hypersomnolence; Hypotonia, Hypotonus

Catathrenia

Catathrenia is expiratory groaning during sleep, especially its later stages. Although sufferers are unaware of the condition, it does alarm relatives and bed partners. There are no associated neurological abnormalities, and no identified neurological or otorhinolaryngological cause.

Catathrenia was categorised with the parasomnias in the International Classification of Sleep Disorders (ICSD2, 2005), but in ICSD-3 it was categorised as a respiratory disorder. Some studies have shown concurrent sleep breathing disorder with inspiratory flow limitation and a small anatomical upper airway, sometimes responding to continuous positive airway pressure (CPAP) or surgery despite the absence of obstructive sleep apnoea. Different subtypes of catathrenia may therefore exist.

References

Iriarte J, Campo A, Alegre M, Fernandez S, Urrestarazu E. Catathrenia: respiratory disorder or parasomnia? *Sleep Med*. 2015; **16**: 827–30.
Vetrugno R, Provini F, Plazzi G, Vignatelli L, Lugaresi E, Montagna P. Catathrenia (nocturnal groaning): a new type of parasomnia. *Neurology*. 2001; **56**: 681–3.

Catatonia

Catatonia is a clinical syndrome, first described by Kahlbaum in 1874, characterized by a state of unresponsiveness but with maintained, immobile, body posture (sitting, standing; *cf.* stupor), mutism, and refusal to eat or drink, with or without staring, grimacing, limb rigidity, maintained abnormal postures (waxy flexibility or *flexibilitas cerea*), negativism, echophenomena (imitation behaviour), stereotypy, and urinary incontinence or retention.

Catatonia is categorized in DSM-5, and scales to measure the severity of catatonia have been described (*e.g.* Northoff Catatonia Scale, Bush-Francis Catatonia Rating Scale). After recovery patients are often able to recall events which occurred during the catatonic state (*cf.* stupor). "Lethal catatonia", in which accompanying fever and collapse lead to death, was described in the 1930s, and seems to resemble neuroleptic malignant syndrome; the name "malignant catatonia" has been proposed for this syndrome. Catatonia may be confused clinically with abulia.

Kraeplin classified catatonia as a subtype of schizophrenia but most catatonic patients in fact suffer a mood or affective disorder. Furthermore, although initially thought to be exclusively a feature of psychiatric disease, catatonia is now recognised as a feature of structural or metabolic brain disease (the original account contains descriptions suggestive of extrapyramidal disease):

- Psychiatric disorders:
    Manic-depressive illness.
    Schizophrenia.

- Neurological disorders:

  Cerebrovascular disease (posterior circulation).
  Tumours (especially around the third ventricle, corpus callosum).
  Head trauma.
  Encephalitis (*e.g.* NMDA-receptor antibody linked).
  Neurosyphilis.
  Extrapyramidal disorders.
  Epilepsy.
- Systemic illnesses:

  Endocrine: hyperthyroidism, Addison's disease, Cushing's disease, diabetic ketoacidosis.
  Metabolic: uraemia, hypercalcaemia, hepatic encephalopathy.
  Others: systemic lupus erythematosus.

Various subtypes of catatonia are enumerated by some authorities, including:

- Retarded catatonia (Kahlbaum's syndrome).
- Excited catatonia (manic delirium, Bell's mania).
- Malignant catatonia, lethal catatonia: also encompasses the neuroleptic malignant syndrome and the serotonin syndrome.
- Periodic catatonia.

Catatonia of psychiatric origin often responds to lorazepam; zolpidem is also an option. Electroconvulsive therapy (ECT) may be tried if pharmacological treatment fails.

References

Daniels J. Catatonia: clinical aspects and neurobiological correlates. *J Neuropsychiatry Clin Neurosci.* 2009; **21**: 371–80.

Fink M, Taylor MA. Catatonia: a clinician's guide to diagnosis and treatment. Cambridge: Cambridge University Press; 2003.

Francis A. Catatonia: diagnosis, classification, and treatment. *Curr Psychiatry Rep.* 2010; **12**: 180–5.

Kahlbaum K. Catatonia. Levij Y, Pridan T (trans.). Baltimore: Johns Hopkins University Press; 1973.

Muqit MMK, Rakshi JS, Shakir RA, Larner AJ. Catatonia or abulia? A difficult differential diagnosis. *Mov Disord.* 2001; **16**: 360–2.

Cross References

Abulia; Akinetic mutism; Imitation behaviour; Mutism; Negativism; Rigidity; Stereotypy; Stupor

Cauda Equina Syndrome

A cauda equina syndrome results from pathological processes affecting the spinal roots below the termination of the spinal cord around L1/L2, hence it is a syndrome of multiple radiculopathies. Depending on precisely which roots are affected, this may produce symmetrical or asymmetrical sensory impairment in the buttocks (saddle anaesthesia; sacral anaesthesia) and the backs of the thighs, radicular pain, and lower motor neurone type weakness of the foot and/or toes (even a flail foot). Weakness of hip flexion (L1) does not occur, and this may be useful in differentiating a cauda equina syndrome from a conus lesion which may otherwise produce similar features. Sphincters may also be involved, resulting in incontinence, or, in the case of large central disc herniation at L4/L5 or L5/S1, acute urinary retention. Causes of a cauda equina syndrome include:

- Central disc herniation.
- Tumour: primary (ependymoma, meningioma. Schwannoma), metastasis.
- Haematoma.
- Abscess.

- Lumbosacral fracture.
- Inflammatory disease, *e.g.* sarcoidosis (rare).
- Ankylosing spondylitis (rare).

The syndrome needs to be considered in any patient with acute (or acute-on-chronic) low back pain, radiation of pain to the legs, altered perineal sensation, and altered bladder function. Missed diagnosis of acute lumbar disc herniation may be costly, from the point of view of both clinical outcome and resultant litigation.

References
Lavy C, James A, Wilson-MacDonald J, Fairbank J. Cauda equina syndrome. *BMJ*. 2009; **338**: 881–4.
Markham DE. Cauda equina syndrome: diagnosis, delay and litigation risk. *J Med Defence Union*. 2004; **20**(1): 12–5.
Todd NV. Neurological deterioration in cauda equina syndrome is probably progressive and continuous. Implications for clinical management. *Br J Neurosurg*. 2015; **29**: 630–4.

Central Scotoma, Centrocaecal Scotoma
These visual field defects are typical of retinal or optic nerve pathology. They may be mapped by confrontation testing or automatically.

- *Central scotoma*:
  Field defect occupying the macula, due to involvement of the macula or the papillomacular bundle; this is the typical (but not exclusive) finding in optic neuritis, but may also be seen with disease of the macula, optic nerve compression, Leber's hereditary optic neuropathy. Examination for a concurrent contralateral superior temporal defect should be undertaken: such junctional scotomas may be seen with lesions at the anterior angle of the chiasm.
- *Centrocaecal or caecocentral scotoma*:
  Field defect involving both the macula and the blind spot; seen in optic nerve disease, such as Leber's hereditary optic neuropathy, toxic or nutritional optic neuropathies (said to be typical of vitamin B_{12} deficiency optic neuropathy), sometimes in optic neuritis.

Cross References
Junctional scotoma, Junctional scotoma of Traquair; Scotoma; Visual field defects

Cerebellar Syndromes
Differing clinical pictures may be seen with pathology in different parts of the cerebellum. Broadly speaking, a midline cerebellar syndrome (involving the vermis) may be distinguished from a hemispheric cerebellar syndrome (involving the hemispheres). Their clinical characteristics are:

- *Midline cerebellar syndrome*:
  Gait ataxia but with little or no limb ataxia, hypotonia, or nystagmus (because the vestibulocerebellum is spared), or dysarthria; causes include alcoholic cerebellar degeneration, tumour of the midline (*e.g.* medulloblastoma), paraneoplastic cerebellar degeneration.
- *Hemispheric cerebellar syndrome*:
  Limb ataxia (*e.g.* ataxia on finger-nose and/or heel-shin testing), dysdiadochokinesia, dysmetria, dysarthria, nystagmus; usual causes are infarcts, haemorrhages, demyelination, and tumours.
- *Pancerebellar syndrome*:
  Affecting all parts of the cerebellum, and showing a combination of the above signs (*e.g.* cerebellar degenerations).

References
Grimaldi G, Manto M. Topography of cerebellar deficits in humans. *Cerebellum*. 2012; **11**: 336–51.
Holmes G. The Croonian lectures on the clinical symptoms of cerebellar disease and their interpretation. *Lancet*. 1922; **i**: 1177–82; 1231–7; **ii**: 59–65; 111–5.
Manto MU, Pandolfo M, editors. The cerebellum and its disorders. Cambridge: Cambridge University Press; 2011.
Cross References
Asynergia; Ataxia; Dysarthria; Dysdiadochokinesia; Dysmetria; Hemiataxia; Hypotonia, Hypotonus; Nystagmus

Cervical Dystonia
- see TORTICOLLIS

Chaddock's Sign
Chaddock's sign, or the external malleolar sign, is a variant method for eliciting the plantar response, by application of a stimulus in a circular direction around the external malleolus, or the lateral aspect of the foot, moving from heel to little toe. The same reflex may have been described by Kisaku Yoshimura, some 5 years before Chaddock's report. A "reversed Chaddock method" has also been described, in which the dorsum of the foot is stroked from medial to lateral direction. Extension of the hallux (upgoing plantar response, Babinski's sign) is pathological, indicating corticospinal tract (upper motor neurone) pathology. The development of Babinski's sign always predates that of Chaddock's sign.

References
Chaddock CG. A preliminary communication concerning a new diagnostic nervous sign. *Interst Med J*. 1911; **18**: 742–6.
Koehler PJ. Foot eponyms leave their mark. *World Neurol*. 2010; **25**(5): 4.
Van Gijn J. The Babinski sign: a centenary. Utrecht: Universiteit Utrecht; 1996.
Cross References
Babinski's sign (1); Gordon's sign; Oppenheim's sign; Plantar response; Upper motor neurone (UMN) syndrome

Charcot Joint
Charcot joint (neuropathic joint, Charcot neuroarthropathy) describes a destructive arthropathy seen following repeated injury to an anaesthetic joint in patients with impaired or absent pain sensation. There is trophic change, with progressive destruction of articular surfaces with disintegration and reorganisation of joint structure. Although the destruction is painless, the Charcot joint itself may be painful. There may be concurrent skin ulceration.

Charcot joints were originally described in the context of tabes dorsalis (knees, shoulders, elbows, hips, ankles) but they may also be seen in:

- Syringomyelia (elbow).
- Hereditary sensory (and autonomic) neuropathies (HSAN, "congenital insensitivity to pain"; ankles).
- Leprosy.
- Diabetes mellitus.

Reference
Chisholm KA, Gilchrist JM. The Charcot joint: a modern neurologic perspective. *J Clin Neuromuscul Dis*. 2011; **13**: 1–13.
Cross References
Analgesia; *Main succulente*

Charles Bonnet Syndrome
Described by the Swiss naturalist and philosopher Charles Bonnet in 1760, this syndrome consists of well-formed (complex), elaboarate and often stereotyped visual hallucinations, of variable frequency and duration, in a partially sighted (usually elderly) individual who has insight into their unreality (hence "pseudohallucinations"). They may disappear on eye closure. Predisposing visual disorders include cataract, macular degeneration and glaucoma. There are no other features of psychosis or neurological disease such as dementia.

The pathogenesis of the visual hallucinations is uncertain. Reduced stimulation of the visual system leading to increased cortical hyperexcitability is one possible explanation (the deafferentation hypothesis), although the syndrome may occasionally occur in people with normal vision. Functional magnetic resonance imaging suggests ongoing cerebral activity in ventral extrastriate visual cortex.

Treatment consists primarily of reassurance. Pharmacological treatment with atypical anti-psychotics or anticonvulsants may be tried but there is no secure evidence base.

An auditory equivalent may exist in hearing-impaired individuals.

References
Ffytche DH, Howard RJ, Brammer MJ, David A, Woodruff P, Williams S. The anatomy of conscious vision: an fMRI study of visual hallucinations. *Nat Neurosci*. 1998; **1**: 738–42.
Flournoy T. Le cas de Charles Bonnet. Hallucinations visuelles chez un vieillard opéré de la cataracte. *Archives de Psychologie*. 1902; **1**: 1–23.
Jacob A, Prasad S, Boggild M, Chandratre S. Charles Bonnet syndrome – elderly people and visual hallucinations. *BMJ*. 2004; **328**: 1552–4.
Menon GJ, Rahman I, Menon SJ, Dutton GN. Complex visual hallucinations in the visually impaired: the Charles Bonnet syndrome. *Surv Ophthalmol*. 2003; **48**: 58–72.
Teunisse RJ, Cruysberg JRM, Verbeek A, Zitman FG. The Charles Bonnet syndrome: a large prospective study in the Netherlands. A study of the prevalence of the Charles Bonnet syndrome and associated factors in 500 patients attending the University Department of Ophthalmology at Nijmegen. *Br J Psychiat*. 1995; **166**: 254–7.
Cross References
Hallucination; Pseudohallucination

Chasm
- see YAWNING

Cheiro-Oral Syndrome
- see PSEUDORADICULAR SYNDROME

Cherry Red Spot at the Macula
The appearance of a "cherry red spot at the macula", caused by the contrast of a red macula against retinal pallor, occurs in a number of metabolic storage disorders, including:

• sialidosis (type I = cherry red spot-myoclonus syndrome).
• gangliosidoses (*e.g.* Tay-Sachs disease: Tay's sign).
• metachromatic leukodystrophy.
• Niemann-Pick disease (especially type A).

Storage of sphingolipids or other substances in ganglion cells in the perimacular region gives rise to the appearance.

Reference
Kivlin JD, Sanborn GE, Myers GG. The cherry-red spot in Tay-Sachs and other storage diseases. *Ann Neurol*. 1985; **17**: 356–60.
Cross Reference
Maculopathy

Cheyne-Stokes Breathing
- see PERIODIC RESPIRATION

"Chicken Wings"
In facioscapulohumeral (FSH) muscular dystrophy, the bulk of the deltoid and forearm muscles is normally well preserved, whilst biceps and triceps are wasted (and may be weak), thus giving rise to an appearance of the upper limbs sometimes labelled as "chicken wings" or "Popeye arms".
Cross Reference
Winging of the scapula

Chorea, Choreoathetosis
Chorea describes an involuntary movement disorder characterized by jerky, restless, purposeless movements (literally dance-like) which tend to flit from one part of the body to another in a rather unpredictable way, giving rise to a fidgety appearance. There may also be athetoid movements (slow, sinuous, writhing), jointly referred to as choreoathetosis. Severe proximal choreiform movements of large amplitude ("flinging") are referred to as ballism or ballismus. When, as is often the case, such movements are confined to one side of the body they are referred to as hemichorea-hemiballismus. There may be concurrent abnormal muscle tone, either hypotonia or rigidity. Hyperpronation of the upper extremity may be seen when attempting to maintain an extended posture.

The pathophysiology of chorea (as for ballismus) is unknown; movements may be associated with lesions of the contralateral subthalamic nucleus, caudate nucleus, putamen, and thalamus. One model of basal ganglia function suggests that reduced basal ganglia output to the thalamus disinhibits thalamic relay nuclei leading to increased excitability in thalamocortical pathways which passes to descending motor pathways resulting in involuntary movements.

Recognised causes of chorea and choreoathetosis are many, including:

- Inherited disorders:
    Autosomal dominant:

        Huntington's disease.
        Spinocerebellar ataxias.
        Dentatorubral-pallidoluysian atrophy (DRPLA).
        Benign hereditary chorea (BHC).

    Autosomal recessive:

        Aminoacidopathies.
        Ataxia telangiectasia (AT).
        Basal ganglia calcification.
        Lesch-Nyhan syndrome.
        Lysosomal disorders.
        Neuroacanthocytosis.
        Neurodegeneration with brain iron accumulation (Hallervorden-Spatz disease).
        Porphyria.
        Tuberous sclerosis.
        Urea cycle disorders.
        Wilson's disease.

    Others:

        Paroxysmal dyskinesias: paroxysmal kinesigenic choreoathetosis (PKC) and paroxysmal dystonic choreoathetosis (PDC).
        Leigh's syndrome.
        Mitochondrial disease.

- Drug-induced:

    Neuroleptics.
    Anti-parkinsonian medication: levodopa therapy in later stages of idiopathic Parkinson's disease.
    Propofol.
    Anti-epileptic drugs.
    Oral contraceptives.
    Amphetamines and tricyclic antidepressants (rare).

- Toxic/metabolic:

    Alcohol.
    Anoxia.
    Carbon monoxide poisoning.
    Cocaine.
    Heavy metal poisoning.
    Hyperthyroidism.
    Hypoparathyroidism.
    Pregnancy: chorea gravidarum.
    Hyper- or hypo- natraemia, magnesaemia, calcaemia; hyperosmolality.
    Hyper- or hypoglycaemia.
    Non-Wilsonian acquired hepatocerebral degeneration.
    Nutritional.

- Infection:

    Sydenham's chorea (post-infectious, rheumatic chorea, St Vitus dance, PANDAS).
    Brainstem encephalitis, Encephalitis lethargica.
    Prion disease: Creutzfeldt-Jakob disease, variant CJD.

- Immunological:

    Systemic lupus erythematosus.
    Henoch-Schonlein purpura.
    Neurosarcoidosis.
    Multiple sclerosis.
    Behçet's disease (rare).
    Vasculitis.
    Hashimoto's encephalopathy.

- Vascular:

    Infarction (including Binswanger's encephalopathy).
    Haemorrhage.
    Arteriovenous malformation.
    Polycythaemia rubra vera (hyperviscosity).
    Migraine.
    Cerebral palsy.

- Tumours:

    Primary and secondary (rare).

- Others:

    Trauma.
    Physiological chorea of infancy.
    "Senile chorea".
    Post pump (cardiac bypass) chorea.
    Psychogenic.

Where treatment is necessary, treatment of cause is optimal. Symptomatic treatment with antidopaminergic agents such as dopamine receptor antagonists (*e.g.* neuroleptics, sulpiride, risperidone) and dopamine depleting agents (*e.g.* tetrabenazine, reserpine) may help, although they may cause parkinsonism, akathisia, neuroleptic malignant syndrome, and sedation. Chronic neuroleptic use may also cause chorea, but these movements are repetitive and predictable, unlike "classic" chorea.

References

Barker R. Chorea: diagnosis and management. *Adv Clin Neurosci Rehabilit*. 2003; **3**(4): 19–20.
Cardoso F, Seppi K, Mair KJ, et al. Seminar on chorea. *Lancet Neurol*. 2006; **5**: 589–602.
Wild EJ, Tabrizi SJ. The differential diagnosis of chorea. *Pract Neurol*. 2007; **7**: 360–73.
Piccolo I, Defanti CA, Soliveri P, Volonte MA, Cislaghi G, Girotti F. Cause and course in a series of patients with sporadic chorea. *J Neurol*. 2003; **250**: 429–35.
Walker RH, editor. The differential diagnosis of chorea. Oxford: Oxford University Press; 2011.

Cross References

Athetosis; Ballism, Ballismus; Dyskinesia; Hypotonia, Hypotonus; Milkmaid's grip; Pseudochoreoathetosis; Rigidity; Trombone tongue

Chromaesthesia

- see SYNAESTHESIA

Chronognosia

This name has been sometimes given to a primary disturbance of the sense of time. Luria claimed it was associated with deep-seated temporal and temporo-diencephalic lesions, possibly right-sided lesions in particular. It occurs in some patients with Alzheimer's disease who get up and dress, make tea, or phone relatives in the small hours, oblivious to the actual time, much to the exasperation of their loved ones. Whether this is a true agnosia remains open to investigation.

Reference

Luria AR. Higher cortical function in man, 2nd edn. New York: Basic Books; 1980, p. 402.

Cross Reference

Agnosia

Chvostek's Sign

Chvostek's sign is contraction of facial muscles provoked by lightly tapping over the facial nerve as it crosses the zygomatic arch. Chvostek's sign is observed in hypocalcaemic states, such as hypoparathyroidism and the respiratory alkalosis associated with hyperventilation. There may be concurrent posturing of the hand, known as *main d'accoucheur* because of its resemblance to the posture adopted for manual delivery of a baby.

The pathophysiology of this mechanosensitivity of nerve fibres is uncertain, but is probably related to increased discharges in central pathways. Although hypocalcaemia might be expected to impair neuromuscular junction transmission and excitation-contraction coupling (since Ca^{2+} ions are required for these processes) this does not in fact occur.

Reference

Athappan G, Ariyamuthu VK. Images in clinical medicine. Chvostek's sign and carpopedal spasm. *New Engl J Med*. 2009; **360**: e24.

Cross References

Main d'accoucheur; Spasm

Ciliospinal Response

The ciliospinal response consists of rapid bilateral pupillary dilatation and palpebral elevation in response to a painful stimulus in the mantle area, for example pinching the skin of the neck.

Reference

Reeves AG, Posner JB. The ciliospinal response in man. *Neurology*. 1969; **19**: 1145–52.

Cross Reference

Pupillary reflexes

Cinematic Vision
Cinematic vision is a form of metamorphopsia, characterized by distortion of movement, with action appearing as a series of still frames as if from a movie. Causes include migraine aura, partial seizures, and schizophrenic psychosis.
Cross Reference
Metamorphopsia

Circumlocution
Circumlocution may be used to refer to:

- A discourse that wanders from the point, only eventually to return to the original subject matter, as seen in fluent aphasias.
- A response to word-finding difficulties, as in early Alzheimer's disease or non-fluent aphasias: in response to familiar pictures, patients may comment that the name is on the tip-of-the-tongue but they cannot access it, and therefore give alternatives, *e.g.* "gardener's friend" or "beetle" for ladybird. This phenomenon has also been called periphrasis.

References
Allison RS. The senile brain. A clinical study. London: Edward Arnold; 1962, p. 79, 138.
Astell AJ, Harley TA. Tip of the tongue states in lexical access in dementia. *Brain Lang*. 1996; **54**: 196–215.
Cross References
Anomia; Aphasia; Dementia

Clapham's Sign
Clapham's sign describes contraction of the facial muscles observed following mechanical stretch of the cheek in patients with facial (VII) nerve palsy or transection, indicating preserved activity in the excitation-contraction apparatus of facial muscles.
Reference
Clapham L, Thomas S, Allen D, Arunachalam R, Cole J. Facial muscle contraction in response to mechanical stretch after severe facial nerve injury: Clapham's sign. *J Laryngol Otol*. 2011; **125**: 732–7.
Cross Reference
Facial paresis, Facial weakness

Clapping Test
- see APPLAUSE SIGN

Clasp-Knife Phenomenon
Clasp-knife phenomenon is the name sometimes applied to the sudden "give" encountered when passively moving a markedly spastic limb. Since the clasp-knife phenomenon is a feature of spasticity, the term "clasp-knife rigidity" is probably best eschewed to avoid possible confusion.
Cross References
Rigidity; Spasticity

Claudication
Claudication (literally limping, Latin *claudicatio*) refers to intermittent symptoms of pain secondary to ischaemia. Claudication of the legs on walking is a symptom of peripheral vascular disease. Claudiaction of the jaw, tongue, and limbs (especially upper) may be a feature of giant cell (temporal) arteritis. Jaw claudication is said to occur in 40% of patients with giant cell arteritis and is the presenting complaint in 4%; tongue claudication occurs in 4% and is rarely the presenting feature. Presence of jaw claudication is one of the clinical features which increase the likelihood of a positive temporal artery biopsy. Jaw claudication may also occur in other causes of external carotid artery occlusive disease.

Reference
Caselli RJ, Hunder GG, Whisnant JP. Neurologic disease in biopsy-proven giant cell (temporal) arteritis. *Neurology*. 1988; **38**: 352–9.
Cross Reference
Jaw claudication

Claw Foot
Claw foot, or *pied en griffe*, is an abnormal posture of the foot, occurring when weakness and atrophy of the intrinsic foot muscles allows the long flexors and extensors to act unopposed, producing shortening of the foot, heightening of the arch, flexion of the distal phalanges and dorsiflexion of the proximal phalanges (*cf*. pes cavus). This may occur in chronic neuropathies of early onset which involve motor fibres, such as hereditary motor and sensory neuropathies.
Cross Reference
Pes cavus

Claw Hand
Claw hand, or *main en griffe*, is an abnormal posture of the hand with hyperextension at the metacarpophalangeal joints (5th, 4th, and, to a lesser extent, 3rd finger) and flexion at the interphalangeal joints. This results from ulnar nerve lesions above the elbow, or injury to the lower part of the brachial plexus (Dejerine-Klumpke type), producing wasting and weakness of hypothenar muscles, interossei, and ulnar (medial) lumbricals, allowing the long finger extensors and flexors to act unopposed.
Reference
Yildirim FB, Sarikcioglu L. Augusta Dejerine-Klumpke (1859-1927) and her eponym. *J Neurol Neurosurg Psychiatry*. 2008; **79**: 102.
Cross References
Benediction hand; Camptodactyly

Clonus
Clonus is rhythmic, involuntary, repetitive, muscular contraction and relaxation. It may be induced by sudden passive stretching of a muscle or tendon, most usually the Achilles tendon (ankle clonus) or patella (patellar clonus). Ankle clonus is best elicited by holding the relaxed leg underneath the moderately flexed knee, then quickly dorsiflexing the ankle and holding it dorsiflexed. A few beats of clonus is within normal limits but sustained clonus is pathological.

Clonus reflects hyperactivity of muscle stretch reflexes and may result from self reexcitation. It is a feature of upper motor neurone disorders affecting the corticospinal (pyramidal) system. Patients with disease of the corticospinal tracts may describe clonus as a rhythmic jerking of the foot, for example when using the foot pedals of a car.

Clonus may also be observed as part of a generalized (primary or secondary) epileptic seizure, either in isolation (clonic seizure) or much more commonly following a tonic phase (tonic-clonic seizure). The clonic movements usually involve all four limbs and decrease in frequency and increase in amplitude over about 30–60 s as the attack progresses. Rather different "clonic" movements may occur in non-epileptic seizures. A few clonic jerks may also be observed in syncopal attacks, leading the uninitiated to diagnose "seizure" or "convulsion".
Reference
Boyraz I, Uysal H, Koc B, Sarman H. Clonus: definition, mechanism, treatment. *Medicinski Glasnik (Zenica)*. 2015; **12**: 19–26.
Cross References
Myoclonus; Seizure; Upper motor neurone (UMN) syndrome

Closed Fist Sign
This is one of the provocative tests for carpal tunnel syndrome: it is positive if paraesthesia develops in the distribution of the median nerve after maintaining fist closure for 60 s.
References
D'Arcy CA, McGee S. Does this patient have carpal tunnel syndrome? *JAMA*. 2000; **283**: 3110–7.
Hi ACF, Wong S, Griffith J. Carpal tunnel syndrome. *Pract Neurol*. 2005; **5**: 210–7.
Cross References
"Flick sign"; Phalen's sign; Tinel's sign

"Closing-In" Sign
Copying of drawings which are close to or superimposed on the original has been referred to as the "closing-in" sign. It may be seen in patients with Alzheimer's disease with deficits in visuospatial function. This has sometimes been characterised as one aspect of the "constructional apraxia" of Alzheimer's disease which may be useful in differentiating it from subcortical vascular dementia. It is also seen in non-demented Parkinson's disease patients in whom it is said to be related to frontal monitoring defects.
References
De Lucia N, Trojano L, Vitale C, Grossi D, Barone P, Santangelo G. The closing-in phenomenon in Parkinson's disease. *Parkinson Relat Disord*. 2015; **21**: 793–6.
Kwak YT. "Closing-in" phenomenon in Alzheimer's disease and subcortical vascular dementia. *BMC Neurol*. 2004; **4**: 3.

Cluster Breathing
Damage at the pontomedullary junction may result in a breathing pattern characterised by a cluster of breaths following one another in an irregular sequence. This sign may be of localizing value in comatose patients.
Cross Reference
Coma

Co-activation Sign
This sign is said to be characteristic of psychogenic tremors, namely increased tremor amplitude with loading (*cf.* reduced amplitude of organic tremor with loading), perhaps due to muscle coactivation to maintain oscillation.
Reference
Deuschl G, Koster B, Lucking CH, Scheidt C. Diagnostic and pathophysiological aspects of psychogenic tremors. *Mov Disord*. 1998; **13**: 294–302.
Cross Reference
Entrainment test; Tremor

Cochleopalpebral Reflex
- see BLINK REFLEX

Cock Walking
- see TOE WALKING

Cogan's (Lid Twitch) Sign
Cogan's sign is a twitching of the upper eyelid seen a moment after the eyes are moved from downgaze to the primary position. Twitches may also be seen with eye closure after sustained upgaze. These phenomena are said to be characteristic signs of ocular myasthenia gravis, and in one study were found in 60% of myasthenics. They may also occur occassionally in other oculomotor brainstem disorders such as Miller Fisher syndrome, but are not seen in healthy individuals. Hence the sign is neither sensitive nor specific.

Cogan's lid twitch sign should not be confused with either Cogan's syndrome, an autoimmune disorder of episodic vertigo, tinnitus, hearing loss and interstitial keratitis; or the oculomotor apraxia of Cogan, a congenital lack of lateral gaze.

References
Cogan DG. Myasthenia gravis: a review of the disease and a description of lid twitch as a characteristic sign. *Arch Ophthalmol*. 1965; **74**: 217–21.
Van Stavern GP, Bhatt A, Haviland J, Black EH. A prospective study assessing the utility of Cogan's lid twitch sign in patients with isolated unilateral or bilateral ptosis. *J Neurol Sci*. 2007; **256**: 84–5.

Cross References
Fatigue; Ice pack test; Ocular apraxia

Cogwheeling, Cogwheel Phenomenon, Cogwheel Rigidity
- see RIGIDITY; SACCADIC INTRUSION, SACCADIC PURSUIT

"Cold Hands Sign"
In multiple system atrophy (MSA), the hands may be cold, dusky and violaceous with poor circulatory return after blanching by pressure, suggesting defective neurovascular control of the distal extremities as one feature of the autonomic dysfunction in MSA. The findings are not present in idiopathic Parkinson's disease.

Reference
Klein C, Brown R, Wenning G, Quinn N. The "cold hands sign" in multiple system atrophy. *Mov Disord*. 1997; **12**: 514–8.

Collapsing Weakness
Collapsing weakness, or "give-way" weakness, suggesting intermittent voluntary effort, is often taken as a sign that weakness is of functional origin. Although sometimes labelled as "volitional weakness", it is not clear that such weakness is in any conscious sense willed, and it is therefore probably better to use a non-committal term such as "apparent weakness". Such collapsing weakness has also been recorded following acute brain lesions such as stroke.

References
Gould R, Miller BL, Goldberg MA, Benson DF. The validity of hysterical signs and symptoms. *J Nerv Mental Dis*. 1986; **174**: 593–7.
Stone J, Zeman A, Sharpe M. Functional weakness and sensory disturbance. *J Neurol Neurosurg Psychiatry*. 2002; **73**: 241–5.

Cross References
Functional weakness and sensory disturbance; Spasticity; Weakness; "Wrestler's sign"

Collier's Sign
Collier's sign ("posterior fossa stare", "tucked lid" sign), first described in 1927, is elevation and retraction of the upper eyelids, baring the sclera above the cornea, with the eyes in the primary position or looking upward. This may be seen with upper dorsal midbrain supranuclear lesions, *e.g.* "top of the basilar syndrome", Parinaud's syndrome. There may be accompanying paralysis of vertical gaze (especially upgaze) and light-near dissociation of pupillary reflexes. The sign is thought to reflect damage to the posterior commissure levator inhibitory fibres.

References
Collier J. Nuclear ophthalmoplegia with special reference to retraction of the lids and ptosis and to lesions of the posterior commissure. *Brain*. 1927; **50**: 488–98.
Galetta SL, Gray LG, Raps EC, Schatz NJ. Pretectal eyelid retraction and lag. *Ann Neurol*. 1993; **33**: 554–7.

Cross References
Lid retraction; Light-near pupillary dissociation; Parinaud's syndrome

Colour Anomia
- see ACHROMATOPSIA; ANOMIA

Coma

Coma is characterized by absent wakefulness and awareness. It is a state of unrousable unresponsiveness lasting >6 h in which a person:

- cannot be awakened;
- fails to respond normally to painful stimuli, light, or sound;
- lacks a normal sleep-wake cycle;
- does not initiate voluntary actions.

These are all important points of differentiation from vegetative state and minimally conscious state. These terms are now preferred to older (obsolete) terminology such as stupor or obtundation, which lack precise definition.

Description of the individual aspects of neurological function in unconscious patients, such as eye movements, limb movements, vocalization, and response to stimuli, conveys more information than the use of terms such as coma, stupor or obtundation, or the use of a lumped "score", such as the Glasgow Coma Scale. These signs should be documented serially to assess any progression of coma. Assessment of the depth of coma may be made by observing changes in eye movements and response to central noxious stimuli: roving eye movements are lost before oculocephalic responses; caloric responses are last to go. The switch from flexor to extensor posturing (decorticate *vs.* decerebrate rigidity) also indicates increasing depth of coma.

There are many causes of coma, which may be broadly categorised as structural or toxic-metabolic; the latter are generally more slowly progressive and produce symmetrical signs, whereas structural lesions more often have an abrupt onset and some focal asymmetric findings on examination, but these distinctions are not absolute. Recognised causes of coma include:

- Structural:
     Vascular insults (subarachnoid haemorrhage, cerebral infarction or haemorrhage, CADASIL).
     Trauma.
     Tumour.
     Hydrocephalus.
     Vasculitides, leukodystrophies, leukoencephalopathies.
- Toxic-metabolic:
     Drugs/toxins.
     Metabolic causes: *e.g.* hypoxia, hypercapnia, hypoglycaemia.
     Infections: *e.g.* meningitis, encephalitis, sepsis.
     Epilepsy.

Unrousability which results from psychiatric disease, or which is being feigned ("pseudo-coma"), also needs to be differentiated.

A number of neurobehavioural states may be mistaken for coma, including abulia, akinetic mutism, catatonia, and the locked-in syndrome. EEG features may assist in differential diagnosis: prominent rhythmic beta activity raises the possibility of drug intoxication.

References

Posner JB, Saper CB, Schiff ND, Plum F. Plum and Posner's diagnosis of stupor and coma, 4th edn. Oxford: Oxford University Press; 2007.
Royal College of Physicians. Prolonged disorders of consciousness: national clinical guidelines. London: Royal College of Physicians; 2013, p. 3.

Teasdale G, Jennett B. Assessment of coma and impaired consciousness: a practical scale. *Lancet*. 1974; **2**: 81–4.
Wijdicks EFM. Coma. *Pract Neurol*. 2010; **10**: 51–60.
Cross References
Abulia; Akinetic mutism; Caloric testing; Catatonia; Decerebrate rigidity; Decorticate rigidity; Locked-in syndrome; Minimally conscious state; Obtundation; Oculocephalic response; Roving eye movements; Stupor; Vegetative states; Vestibulo-ocular reflexes

"Compulsive Grasping Hand"
This name has been given to involuntary left hand grasping related to all right hand movements in a patient with a callosal haemorrhage. This has been interpreted as a motor grasp response to contralateral hand movements, and a variant of anarchic or alien hand. The description seems to differ from that of behaviours labelled as forced groping and the alien grasp reflex.
Reference
Kumral E. Compulsive grasping hand syndrome: a variant of anarchic hand. *Neurology*. 2001; **57**: 2143–4.
Cross References
Alien grasp reflex; Alien hand, Alien limb; Forced groping; Intermanual conflict

Conduction Aphasia
Conduction aphasia (Wernicke's *Leitungsaphasia*) is defined as a fluent aphasia with paraphasic errors (especially phonemic/literal) during speech, repetition and naming. In its "pure" form, there is dissociation between relatively preserved auditory and reading comprehension of language and impaired repetition (in which the phenomenon of *conduit d'approche* may occur) and naming. Reading comprehension is good or normal, and is better than reading aloud which is impaired by paraphasic errors.

Conduction aphasia was traditionally explained as due to a disconnection between sensory (Wernicke) and motor (Broca) areas for language, involving the arcuate fasciculus in the supramarginal gyrus. Certainly the brain damage (usually infarction) associated with conduction aphasia most commonly involves the left parietal lobe (lower postcentral and supramarginal gyri) and the insula, but it is variable, and it is possible that the cortical injury may be responsible for the clinical picture.

Conduction aphasia is most often seen during recovery from Wernicke's aphasia, and clinically there is often evidence of some impairment of comprehension. If isolated, the prognosis for conduction aphasia is good.
References
Ardila A. A review of conduction aphasia. *Curr Neurol Neurosci Rep*. 2010; **10**: 499–503.
Benson DF, Sheremata WA, Bouchard R, Segarra JM, Price D, Geschwind N. Conduction aphasia. A clinicopathological study. *Arch Neurol*. 1973; **28**: 339–46.
Bernal B, Ardila A. The role of the arcuate fasciculus in conduction aphasia. *Brain*. 2009; **132**: 2309–16.
Damasio H, Damasio AR. The anatomical basis of conduction aphasia. *Brain*. 1980; **103**: 337–50.
Cross References
Anomia; Aphasia; Broca's aphasia; *Conduit d'approche*; Paraphasia; Transcortical aphasias; Wernicke's aphasia

Conduit D'approche
Conduit d'approche, or "homing-in" behaviour, is a verbal output phenomenon applied to patients with conduction aphasia attempting to repeat a target word, in which multiple phonemic approximations of the word are presented, with gradual improvement until the target

word is achieved. This phenomenon suggests that an acoustic image of the target word is preserved in this condition.

A similar phenomenon may be observed in patients with optic aphasia attempting to name a visual stimulus. A similar behaviour is seen in so-called speech apraxia, in which patients repeatedly approximate to the desired output before reaching it.

The term may also be used to refer to a parapraxis in which patients attempt to perform a movement several times before achieving the correct movement.

Cross References
Aphasia; Conduction aphasia; Optic aphasia; Parapraxia, Parapraxis; Speech apraxia

Confabulation
The old definition of confabulation as the falsification of episodic memory occurring in clear consciousness, often in association with amnesia (in other words, paramnesias related as true events) has proven increasingly deficient, not least because most amnesic patients, suffering from medial temporal lobe/hippocampal lesions, do not confabulate, and poor memory alone cannot explain confabulation.

Schnider has developed a fourfold schema of intrusions, momentary confabulations, fantastic confabulations, and behaviourally spontaneous confabulations, of which the latter are clinically the most challenging. Anterior limbic structures are thought culpable, and the pathogenesis includes a wide variety of diseases, and there may be associated phenomena such as amnesia, disorientation, false recognition syndromes including the Capgras delusion, and anosognosia.

Psychophysical and neuroimaging studies suggest that confabulators have reality confusion and a failure to integrate contradictory information due to the failure of a filtering process, 200–300 ms after stimulus presentation and before recognition and re-encoding, which normally permits suppression of currently irrelevant memories.

References
Hirstein W, editor. Confabulation. Views from neuroscience, psychiatry, psychology, and philosophy. Oxford: Oxford University Press; 2009.
Schnider A. The confabulating mind. How the brain creates reality. Oxford: Oxford University Press; 2008.
Cross References
Amnesia; Asomatognosia; Capgras syndrome; Cortical blindness; Delusion; Paramnesia

Conflict of Intentions
- see NEGATIVISM

Confusion
Confusion, understood as the inability to think with one's customary clarity and coherence, is a feature of delirium (acute confusional syndrome), but also of other situations (encephalopathies, attentional disorders).

There is a lack of correlation of meaning when this term is used by different health professionals, for which reason it may be regarded as an unhelpful term.

References
Simpson CJ. Doctors' and nurses' use of the word confusion. *Br J Psychiatry*. 1984; **145**: 441–3.
Mesulam MM. Attentional and confusional states. *Continuum (Minneap Minn)*. 2010; **16**: 128–39.
Wei LA, Fearing MA, Sternberg EJ, Inouye SK. The Confusion Assessment Method: a systematic review of current usage. *J Am Geriatr Soc*. 2008; **56**: 823–30.
Cross Reference
Attention; Delirium

Congenital Nystagmus
Congenital nystagmus is a pendular nystagmus with the following characteristics:

- Usually noted at birth or in early infancy; sometimes may only become apparent in adult life.
- Irregular waveforms.
- Conjugate.
- Almost always horizontal.
- Accentuated by fixation, attention, anxiety.
- Decreased by convergence, active eyelid closure.
- Often a null point or region.
- No complaint of oscillopsia.
- It may appear with blindness of childhood onset.

   Acquired pendular nystagmus may be a result of neurological disease which may present in childhood, such as Pelizaeus-Merzbacher disease, or in adulthood, such as mitochondrial disease, multiple sclerosis, and Whipple's disease.
Cross References
Nystagmus; Oscillopsia

Consensual Light Reflex
- see PUPILLARY REFLEXES

Constructional Apraxia
- see APRAXIA

Contracture
The term contracture may be used in various contexts:

- Clinically, to describe an acquired restriction of joint mobility (prenatally acquired restriction of joint mobility is called arthrogryposis). This may be due to a variety of factors, including prolonged muscle spasticity with or without muscle fibrosis (*i.e.* without pathological muscle shortening), and ligamentous restrictions. This often occurs in the context of limb immobilisation or inactivity, for example in a flexed posture. Injections of botulinum toxin to abolish muscle spasticity may be required to assess whether there is concurrent ligamentous restriction, and thus to plan optimum treatment, which may involve surgery. Contractures of muscular origin may be seen in conditions such as Emery-Dreifuss disease (especially elbow, Achilles tendon, posterior part of neck), Bethlem myopathy and Ullrich congenital muscular dystrophy associated with mutations in genes encoding the peptide chains of collagen VI, limb girdle muscular dystrophy type 2A associated with mutations in the calpain 3 gene, and Duchenne muscular dystrophy.
- Clinically, to describe a hard, contracted muscle which is painful to straighten, and lasting for several hours following exercise in a metabolic myopathy such as McArdle's disease (myophosphorylase deficiency, glycogen storage disease type V); this may be associated with EMG silence.
- Physiologically, to describe a prolonged painful muscle spasm with EMG silence, as observed in myotonia and paramyotonia.

   Contractures may be distinguished from cramps by their longer duration, the fact that they cannot be resolved by passively stretching the affected muscle, and by the accompanying EMG electrical silence.

References
Bonne G, Lampe AK. Muscle diseases with prominent muscle contractures. In: Karpati G, Hilton-Jones D, Bushby K, Griggs RC, editors. Disorders of voluntary muscle, 8th edn. Cambridge: Cambridge Univesrity Press; 2010. p. 299–313.
Meinck HM. Cramps, spasms, startles and related symptoms. In: Schmitz B, Tettenborn B, Schomer DL, editors. The paroxysmal disorders. Cambridge: Cambridge University Press; 2010. p. 130–44.
Cross References
Cramp; Myotonia; Paramyotonia; Paraplegia; Spasm; Spasticity

Convergence-Retraction Nystagmus
- see NYSTAMGUS; PARINAUD'S SYNDROME

Converse Ocular Bobbing
- see OCULAR BOBBING

Coprolalia
Coprolalia is the use of expletives or other obscene language. This may be

- Vocal: involuntary utterance of obscenities.
- Mental: compulsion to think obscenities.

The former is a complex vocal tic most characteristically seen in Tourette syndrome although it actually occurs in less than half of affected individuals. Other recognized disease associations are:

- Lesch-Nyhan syndrome.
- Postencephalitic parkinsonism.
- Neuroacanthocytosis.
- Cingulate cortical seizures.

The pathophysiology of coprolalia is unknown but may be related to frontal (cingulate and orbitofrontal) dysfunction, for which there is some evidence in Tourette syndrome.
Reference
Eddy CM, Cavanna AE. "It's a curse!": coprolalia in Tourette syndrome. *Eur J Neurol*. 2013; **20**: 1467–70.
Cross Reference
Tic

Copropraxia
Copropraxia is a complex motor tic comprising obscene gesturing, sometimes seen in Tourette syndrome.
Cross References
Coprolalia; Tic

Corectopia
Corectopia is pupillary displacement, which may be seen with midbrain lesions, including transtentorial herniation and top-of-the-basilar syndrome, peripheral oculomotor nerve palsies, and focal pathology in the iris.
Reference
Lindbauer N, Strenger V, Urban C. Teaching NeuroImages: dorsal midbrain (Parinaud) syndrome with corectopia. *Neurology*. 2012; **79**: e154

Corneal Reflex

The corneal reflex consists of a bilateral blink response elicited by touching the cornea lightly, for example with a piece of cotton wool. As well as observing whether the patient blinks, the examiner should also ask whether the stimulus was felt: a difference in corneal sensitivity may be the earliest abnormality in this reflex. Synkinetic jaw movement may also be observed: the corneomandibular reflex.

The afferent limb of the corneal reflex is via the trigeminal (V) nerve, the efferent limb via the facial (VII) nerve to orbicularis oculi. The fibres subserving the corneal reflex seem to be the most sensitive to trigeminal nerve compression or distortion: an intact corneal reflex with a complaint of facial numbness leads to suspicion of a non-organic cause. Reflex impairment may be an early sign of a cerebellopontine angle lesion, such as vestibular schwannoma, which may also cause ipsilateral lower motor neurone type facial (VII) weakness and ipsilateral sensorineural hearing impairment (VIII). Trigeminal nerve lesions cause both ipsilateral and contralateral corneal reflex loss.

Cerebral hemisphere (but not thalamic) lesions causing hemiparesis and hemisensory loss may also be associated with a decreased corneal reflex.

The corneal reflex has a high threshold in comatose patients, and is usually preserved until late (unless coma is due to drug overdose), in which case its loss is a poor prognostic sign.

Reference

Parker HL. Tumours of the nervus acusticus. Signs of involvement of the fifth cranial nerve. *Arch Neurol Psychiatry*. 1928; **20**: 309–18.

Cross References

Blink reflex; Coma; Cerebellopontine angle syndrome; Corneomandibular reflex; Facial paresis, Facial weakness; Holmes-Adie pupil, Holmes-Adie syndrome; Menace reflex

Corneomandibular Reflex

The corneomandibular reflex, also known as the corneopterygoid reflex or Wartenberg's reflex or sign, consists of anterolateral jaw movement following corneal stimulation. In one study, the corneomandibular reflex was observed in about three-quarters of patients with motor neurone disease (MND) who displayed no other pathological reflexes, a frequency much higher than that seen in patients with stroke causing hemiparesis or pseudobulbar palsy. It was therefore suggested to be a sensitive indicator of upper motor neurone involvement in MND.

References

Heliopoulos I, Vadikolias K, Tsivgoulis G, Mikroulis D, Tsakaldimi S, Piperidou C. Corneomandibular reflex (Wartenberg reflex) in coma: a rarely elicited sign. *JAMA Neurol*. 2013; **70**: 794–5.

Okuda B, Kodama N, Kawabata K, Tachibana H, Sugita M. Corneomandibular reflex in ALS. *Neurology*. 1999; **52**: 1699–701.

Cross References

Corneal reflex; Pseudobulbar palsy

Corneopterygoid Reflex

- see CORNEOMANDIBULAR REFLEX

Corrective Gesture

- see SENSORY TRICKS

Cortical Blindness

Cortical blindness (*Rindblindheit*) is loss of vision due to bilateral visual cortical damage, usually hypoxic-ischaemic in origin, or due to bilateral subcortical lesions affecting the optic radiations. A small central field around the fixation point may be spared (macula sparing). Pupillary reflexes are presereved but optokinetic nystagmus cannot be elicited.

Cortical blindness may result from:

- Bilateral (sequential or simultaneous) posterior cerebral artery occlusion.
- "Top of the basilar syndrome".
- Migraine.
- Cerebral anoxia.
- Bacterial endocarditis.
- Wegener's granulomatosis.
- Following coronary or cerebral angiography (may be transient).
- Epilepsy (transient).
- Ciclosporin therapy, *e.g.* following organ transplantation.

If acute in onset (*i.e.* vascular), cortical blindness may ultimately evolve to prosopagnosia via visual object agnosia.

Patients with cortical blindness may deny their visual defect (Anton's syndrome, visual anosognosia) and may confabulate about what they "see".

Cross References
Anosognosia; Confabulation; Macula sparing, Macula splitting; Optokinetic nystagmus, Optokinetic response; Prosopagnosia; Pupillary reflexes; Visual agnosia

Cotard's Syndrome
Cotard's syndrome is a delusional syndrome, first described in the 1890s, and characterised by the patient's denial of their own existence, or of part of their body. The patient may assert that they are dead, and able to smell rotten flesh or feel worms crawling over their skin. Cotard described this as *délire des negations*, delusion of negation.

Although this may occur in the context of psychiatric disease, especially depression and schizophrenia, it may also occur in association with organic brain abnormalities, specifically lesions of the nondominant temporoparietal cortex, or migraine. I have also encountered this in a patient with behavioural variant frontotemporal dementia presenting in his 70s.

Some envisage Cotard's syndrome as a more pervasive form of the Capgras syndrome, originating similarly as a consequence of Geschwindian disconnection between the limbic system and all sensory areas, leading to a loss of emotional contact with the world.

Antidepressant treatment and/or ECT may sometimes be helpful in Cotard syndrome of psychiatric origin.

References
Cotard J. Etudes sur les maladies cerebrales et mentales. Paris: Bailliere; 1891.
Pearn J, Gardner-Thorpe C. Jules Cotard (1840-1889): his life and the unique syndrome which bears his name. *Neurology*. 2002; **58**: 1400–3.
Ramirez-Bermudez J, Aguilar-Venegas LC, Crail-Melendez D, Espinola-Nadurille M, Nente F, Mendez MF. Cotard syndrome in neurological and psychiatric patients. *J Neuropsychiat Clin Neurosci*. 2010; **22**: 409–16.

Cross References
Capgras syndrome; Delusion; Disconnection syndromes

Coup De Poignard
Coup de poignard, or dagger thrust, refers to a sudden precordial pain, as may occur in myocardial infarction or aortic dissection, also described with spinal subarachnoid haemorrhage.

Reference
Barton CW. Subarachnoid haemorrhage presenting as acute chest pain: a variant of le coup de poignard. *Ann Emerg Med*. 1988; **17**: 977–8.

Coup De Sabre

Coup de sabre is a localized form of scleroderma manifest as a linear, atrophic lesion on the forehead which may be mistaken for a scar. This lesion may be associated with hemifacial atrophy and epilepsy, and neuroimaging may show cerebral hemiatrophy and intracranial calcification. Whether these changes reflect inflammation or a neurocutaneous syndrome is not known.

Reference

Duyff RF, Vos J. A "scar" and epilepsy: coup de sabre. *J Neurol Neurosurg Psychiatry*. 1998; **65**: 568.

Cross Reference

Hemifacial atrophy

Cover Tests

The simple cover and cover-uncover tests may be used to demonstrate manifest and latent strabismus (heterotropia and heterophoria) respectively.

The cover test demonstrates tropias: the uncovered eye is forced to adopt fixation; any movement therefore represents a manifest strabismus (heterotropia).

The cover-uncover test demonstrates phorias: any movement of the covered eye to re-establish fixation as it is uncovered represents a latent strabismus (heterophoria).

The alternate cover or cross cover test, in which the hand or occluder moves back and forth between the eyes, repeatedly breaking and re-establishing fixation, is more dissociating, preventing binocular viewing, and therefore helpful in demonstrating whether or not there is strabismus. It should be performed in the nine cardinal positions of gaze to determine the direction that elicits maximal deviation. However, it does not distinguish between tropias and phorias, for which the cover and cover-uncover tests are required.

Cross References

Heterophoria; Heterotropia

Cramp

Cramps are defined as involuntary contractions of a number of muscle units which results in a hardening of the muscle with pain due to a local lactic acidosis. Cramps are not uncommon in normal individuals but in a minority of cases they are associated with an underlying neurological or metabolic disorder. Cramps need to be distinguished from spasticity, neuromyotonia and myokymia. Recognised associations of cramp include:

- Normal individuals:

    Especially during periods of dehydration with salt loss; pregnancy.
    Benign cramp syndrome, there is a family history of cramps.

- Metabolic causes:

    Hypothyroidism.
    Uraemia, haemodialysis.
    Hypocalcaemia; hyperventilation (with secondary hypocalcaemia).

- Neurological causes:

    Chronic peripheral neuropathy.
    Metabolic myopathies (*e.g.* myophosphorylase deficiency, lactate dehydrogenase (LDH) deficiency, with exercise intolerance and myoglobinuria).
    Muscular dystrophies (especially Becker, Duchenne).
    Motor neurone disease.
    Post-polio syndrome.
    Stiff man syndrome.

Treatment involves addressing any underlying metabolic abnormality. Symptomatic treatment of cramps may include use of quinine sulphate, vitamin B, naftidrofuryl, and calcium channel antagonists such as diltiazem; carbamazepine, phenytoin, and procainamide have also been tried.

References
De Carvalho M, Swash M. Cramps, muscle pain, and fasciculations: not always benign? *Neurology*. 2004; **63**: 721–3.
Katzberg HD, Khan AH, So YT. Assessment: symptomatic treatment for muscle cramps (an evidence-based review): report of the therapeutics and technology subcommittee of the American Academy of Neurology. *Neurology*. 2010; **74**: 691–6.
Meinck HM. Cramps, spasms, startles and related symptoms. In: Schmitz B, Tettenborn B, Schomer DL, editors. The paroxysmal disorders. Cambridge: Cambridge University Press; 2010. p. 130–44.
Cross References
Contracture; Fasciculation; Myokymia; Myotonia; Neuromyotonia; Spasm; Stiffness

Cremasteric Reflex
The cremasteric reflex is a superficial or cutaneous reflex: stimulation of the skin of the upper inner aspect of the thigh from above downwards (*i.e.* the L1, L2 dermatomes, via the ilioinguinal and genitofemoral nerves) resulting in contraction of the cremaster muscle causing elevation of the testicle.

The cremasteric reflex is lost when the corticospinal pathways are damaged above T12, or following lesions of the genitofemoral nerve. It may also be absent in elderly men, or with local pathology such as hydrocele, varicocele, orchitis or epididymitis.
Cross References
Abdominal reflexes; Reflexes

Crocodile Tears
Crocodile tears (also known as gustatory epiphora, or Bogorad's syndrome) reflect inappropriate unilateral lacrimation during eating, such that tears may spill down the face (epiphora). This autonomic synkinesis is a striking but rare consequence of aberrant reinnervation of the facial (VII) nerve, usually after a Bell's palsy, when fibres originally supplying the salivary glands are re-routed to the lacrimal gland via the greater superficial petrosal nerve.
Cross References
Bell's palsy; Epiphora; Synkinesia, Synkinesis

Crossed Adductor Reflex
Contralateral adductor muscle contraction in response to a tap on the adductor tendon may be found with a corticospinal tract lesion, hence a sign of upper motor neurone pathology, although it is a normal finding in infants.
Cross References
Reflexes; Upper motor neurone (UMN) syndrome

Crossed Aphasia
Aphasia from a right-sided cerebral lesion in a right-handed patient, crossed aphasia, is rare, presumably a reflection of crossed or mixed cerebral dominance. It may occur transiently during a focal epileptic seizure or migraine aura.
References
Bogousslavsky J. "The adventure": Charles-Ferdinand Ramuz's extraordinary stroke diary. *Eur Neurol*. 2009; **61**: 138–42.
Mariën P, Paghera B, De Deyn PP, Vignolo LA. Adult crossed aphasia in dextrals revisited. *Cortex*. 2004; **40**: 41–74.
Cross Reference
Aphasia

Crossed Apraxia
This name is given to apraxia in right-handed patients with right-sided lesions; apraxia is more commonly associated with left-sided brain injury.

Reference
Raymer AM, Merians AS, Adair JC, et al. Crossed apraxia: implications for handedness. *Cortex*. 1999; **35**: 183–99.
Cross Reference
Apraxia

Crossed Gerstmann Syndrome
- see GERSTMANN SYNDROME

Crossed Straight Leg Raising
- see LASÈGUE'S SIGN

Cross-Over
In the line bisection task for the detection of unilateral spatial neglect, in which the subjective midline is placed more towards the ipsilesional extreme of the line compared to the objective midline, especially with longer lines (length effect), with shorter lines there is a paradoxical deviation towards the contralesional side, a sign called cross-over.
Reference
Chatterjee A. Cross-over, completion and confabulation in unilateral spatial neglect. *Brain*. 1995; **118**: 455–65.
Cross Reference
Neglect

Crying
- see AUTOMATISM; PATHOLOGICAL CRYING, PATHOLOGICAL LAUGHTER; SEIZURES

Cuirasse
- see SUSPENDED SENSORY LOSS

Curtaining
Curtaining occurs when a ptotic eyelid is elevated resulting in ptosis (falling like a curtain) of the contralateral normal eyelid. As with enhanced ptosis, curtaining is explained by the action of Hering's law of equal innervation to paired yoked muscles (*i.e.* the eyelids). Recognised causes of curtaining include myasthenia gravis, Miller Fisher syndrome, and botulism.
Cross References
Enhanced ptosis; Ptosis

Cushing Reflex, Cushing Response
This is the triad of increasing systolic and pulse pressure with bradycardia and slow irregular respiration associated with increased intracranial pressure which may lead to cerebral herniation and fatal brainstem compression, for example with posterior fossa masses or subarachnoid haemorrhage.
Reference
Fodstad H, Kelly PJ, Buchfelder M. History of the Cushing reflex. *Neurosurgery*. 2006; **59**: 1132–7.

Czarnecki's Sign
Aberrant regeneration of the oculomotor (III) nerve to the iris sphincter may lead to gaze-evoked segmental constriction of the pupil, Czarnecki's sign, which may be visible only with slit-lamp examination.
Reference
Cox TA, Goldberg RA, Rootman J. Tonic pupil and Czarnecki's sign following third nerve palsy. *J Clin Neuroophthalmol*. 1991; **11**: 55–6.

D

Dalrymple's Sign
Dalrymple's sign is increased width of the palpebral fissure, often seen in hyperthyroidism.
Cross Reference
Lid retraction

Dazzle
Dazzle describes a painless intolerance of the eyes to bright light (*cf*. photophobia). It may be peripheral in origin (retinal disease; opacities within cornea, lens, vitreous); or central (lesions anywhere from optic nerve to occipitotemporal region).
Cross Reference
Photophobia

Decerebrate Rigidity
Decerebrate rigidity is a posture observed in comatose patients in which there is extension and pronation of the upper extremities, extension of the legs, and plantar flexion of the feet (= extensor posturing), which is taken to be an exaggeration of the normal standing position. Painful stimuli may induce opisthotonos, hyperextension and hyperpronation of the upper limbs.

Decerebrate rigidity occurs in severe metabolic disorders of the upper brainstem (anoxia/ischaemia, trauma, structural lesions, drug-intoxication). A similar picture was first observed by Sherrington (1898) following section of the brainstem of cats at the collicular level, below the red nuclei, such that the vestibular nuclei were intact. The action of the vestibular nuclei, unchecked by higher centres, may be responsible for the profound extensor tone.

Decerebrate rigidity indicates a deeper level of coma than decorticate rigidity; the transition from the latter to the former is associated with a worsening of prognosis.
Reference
Posner JB, Saper CB, Schiff ND, Plum F. Plum and Posner's diagnosis of stupor and coma. 4th ed. Oxford: Oxford University Press; 2007.
Cross References
Coma; Decorticate rigidity; Opisthotonos

De Clérambault Syndrome
- see DELUSION

Decomposition of Movement
- see ASYNERGIA

Decorticate Rigidity
Decorticate rigidity is a posture observed in comatose patients in which there is adduction of the shoulders and arms, and flexion of the elbows and wrists (= flexor posturing). The lesion responsible for decorticate rigidity is higher in the neuraxis than that causing decerebrate rigidity, often being diffuse cerebral hemisphere or diencephalic disease, although, despite the name, it may occur with upper brainstem lesions. Common causes are anoxia/ischaemia, trauma, and drugs.
Cross References
Coma; Decerebrate rigidity

© Springer International Publishing Switzerland 2016
A.J. Larner, *A Dictionary of Neurological Signs*,
DOI 10.1007/978-3-319-29821-4_4

Déjà Entendu
A sensation of familiarity akin to *déjà vu* but referring to auditory (literally "already heard") rather than visual experiences.

Déjà Vécu
- see *DÉJÀ VU*

Déjà Vu
Déjà vu (literally "already seen") is a subjective, inappropriate impression of familiarity for a present experience in relation to an undefined past. However, since the term has passed into the vernacular, not every patient complaining of "*déjà vu*" has a pathological problem. The term may be used colloquially to indicate familiar events or experiences (Yoga Berra: "It's déjà vu all over again!"). Recurrent hallucinations or vivid dream-like imagery may also enter the differential diagnosis. A phenomenon of slight confusion in which all is not clear although it is familiar has sometimes been labelled "*prèsque vu*".

Epileptic *déjà vu* is a complex aura of focal onset epilepsy; specifically, it is indicative of temporal lobe onset of seizures, and is said by some authors to be the only epileptic aura of reliable lateralising significance (right). Epileptic *déjà vu* may last longer and be more frequent than other causes, and may be associated with other features such as depersonalization and derealization, strong emotion such as fear, epigastric aura, or olfactory hallucinations. *Déjà vécu* ("already lived") has been used to denote a broader experience than *déjà vu* but the clinical implications are similar.

Déjà vu has also been reported to occur in several psychiatric disorders, such as anxiety, depression, and schizophrenia.

References
Warren-Gash C, Zeman A. Déjà vu. *Pract Neurol*. 2003; **3**: 106–9.
Wild E. Déjà vu in neurology. *J Neurol*. 2005; **252**: 1–7.
Cross References
Aura; Hallucination; *Jamais vu*

Délire Des Négations
- see COTARD'S SYNDROME

Delirium
Delirium, also sometimes known as acute confusional state, acute organic reaction, acute brain syndrome, or toxic-metabolic encephalopathy, is a neurobehavioural syndrome of which the cardinal feature is a deficit of attention, the ability to focus on specific stimuli. Diagnostic criteria also require a concurrent alteration in level of awareness, which may range from lethargy to hypervigilance, although delirium is not primarily a disorder of arousal or alertness (*cf.* coma, stupor, obtundation). Other features commonly observed in delirium include:

- impaired cognitive function: disorientation in time and place.
- perceptual disorders: illusions, hallucinations.
- behavioural disturbances: agitation, restlessness, aggression, wandering, which may occur as a consequence of perceptual problems (hyperalert type); or unresponsiveness, withdrawal (hypoalert or quiet type).
- language: rambling incoherent speech, logorrhoea.
- altered sleep-wake cycle: "sundowning" (restlessness and confusion at night)
- tendency to marked fluctuations in alertness/activity, with occasional lucid intervals.
- delusions: often persecutory.

Hence this abnormal mental state shows considerable clinical heterogeneity. Subtypes or variants are described, one characterised by hyperactivity ("agitated"), the other by withdrawal and apathy ("quiet").

The course of delirium is usually brief (seldom more than a few days, often only hours). On recovery the patient may have no recollection of events, although islands of recall may be preserved, corresponding with lucid intervals (a useful, if retrospective, diagnostic feature).

Delirium is often contrasted with dementia, a "chronic brain syndrome", in which attention is relatively preserved, the onset is insidious rather than acute, the course is stable over the day rather than fluctuating, and which generally lasts months to years. However, it should be noted that delirium is often superimposed on dementia, especially in the elderly. Dementia is a predisposing factor for the development of delirium, perhaps reflecting impaired cerebral reserve.

The pathophysiology of delirium is not well understood. Risk factors for the development of delirium may be categorised as either predisposing or precipitating.

- *Predisposing factors* include:

    Age: frailty, physiological age rather than chronological.
    Sex: men > women.
    Neurological illness: dementia.
    Burden of co-morbidity; dehydration.
    Drugs: especially anticholinergic medication.
    Primary sensory impairment (hearing, vision).

- *Precipitating factors* include:

    Drugs/toxins: benzodiazepines, opiates.
    Alcohol, especially withdrawal from, as in delirium tremens.
    Intercurrent illness:

    > Infection: primary CNS (encephalitis, meningitis), or systemic (urinary tract, chest, septicaemia).
    > Metabolic: hypoxia, hypo-/hyperglycaemia, hepatic failure, uraemia, porphyria.
    > CNS disorders: head injury, cerebrovascular disease, epilepsy (*e.g.* some forms of status), inflammatory disorders (*e.g.* collagen vascular disease).
    > Iatrogenic events: surgery (especially cardiac, orthopaedic).

These precipitating factors merit treatment in their own right, and investigations should be tailored to identify these aetiological factors. The EEG may show non-specific slowing in delirium, the degree of which is said to correlate with the degree of impairment, and reverses with resolution of delirium.

It is suggested that optimal nursing of delirious patients should aim at environmental modulation to avoid both under- and over-stimulation; a side room is probably best (if possible). Drug treatment is not mandatory, the evidence base for pharmacotherapy is slim. However, if the patient poses a risk to him/herself, other patients, or staff which cannot be addressed by other means, regular low dose oral haloperidol may be used, probably in preference to atypical neuroleptics, benzodiazepines (lorazepam), or cholinesterase inhibitors. Prevention of delirium by screening patients for risk factors is advocated.

References

Fong TG, Davis D, Growdon ME, Albuquerque A, Inouye SK. The interface between delirium and dementia in elderly adults. *Lancet Neurol.* 2015; **14**: 823–32.
Inouye SK. Current concepts: delirium in older persons. *N Engl J Med.* 2006; **354**: 1157–65.
Siddiqi N, House AO, Holmes JD. Occurrence and outcome of delirium in medical in-patients: a systematic literature review. *Age Ageing.* 2006; **35**: 350–64.

Cross References

Agraphia; Attention; Coma; Delusion; Dementia; Hallucination; Illusion; Logorrhoea; Obtundation; Stupor; "Sundowning"

Delusion

A delusion is a fixed false belief, not amenable to reason (*i.e.* held despite evidence to the contrary), and not culturally sanctioned. There are a number of common forms of delusion, including:

- persecutory (paranoia).
- reference: important events or people being influenced by a patient's thoughts, ideas.
- grandiose/expansive: occurs particularly in mania.
- guilt/worthlessness: occurs particularly in depression.
- hypochondria.
- thought broadcast and thought insertion.
- control by an external agency.

Specific, named, delusional syndromes are those of:

- *Capgras*: the "delusion of doubles", a familiar person or place is thought to be an impostor, or double; this resembles the reduplicative paramnesia described in neurological disorders such as Alzheimer's disease.
- *Fregoli*: a familiar person is identified in other people, even though they bear no resemblance; this may occur in schizophrenia.
- *De Clérambault* (erotomania): the belief (usually of a single woman) that a famous person is secretly in love with her ("hope"), followed by the belief that that person is persecuting her ("resentment"); may occur in schizophrenia.

Delusions are a feature of primary psychiatric disease (psychoses such as schizophrenia; neuroses such as depression), but may also be encountered in neurological disease with secondary psychiatric features ("organic psychiatry"), *e.g.* delirium, and dementing syndromes such as Alzheimer's disease, dementia with Lewy bodies.

References
Moore DP, Puri BK. Textbook of clinical neuropsychiatry and behavioral neuroscience. 3rd ed. London: Hodder Arnold; 2012.
Tekin S, Cummings JL. Hallucinations and related conditions. In: Heilman KM, Valenstein E, editors. Clinical neuropsychology. 4th ed. Oxford: Oxford University Press; 2003. p. 479–94.

Cross References
Delirium; Dementia; Ekbom's syndrome; Hallucination; Illusion; Intermetamorphosis; Misidentification syndromes; Reduplicative paramnesia

Delusional Parasitosis
- see EKBOM'S SYNDROME

Dementia

Dementia is a syndrome characterised by loss of intellectual (cognitive) functions sufficient to interfere with social and occupational functioning. Cognition encompasses multiple functions including language, memory, perception, praxis, attentional mechanisms and executive function (planning, reasoning). These elements may be affected selectively or globally: older definitions of dementia requiring global cognitive decline have now been superseded. Amnesia may or may not, depending on the classification system used, be a *sine qua non* for the diagnosis of dementia. Attentional mechanisms are largely preserved, certainly in comparison with delirium, a condition which precludes meaningful neuropsychological assessment because of profound attentional deficits. Multiple neuropsychological tests are available to test different areas of cognition.

Although more common in the elderly, dementia can also occur in the presenium, and in children who may lose cognitive skills as a result of hereditary metabolic disorders. Failure to develop cognitive skills is termed learning disability. The heterogeneity of dementia is further exemplified by the fact that it may be acute or insidious in onset, and its course may be progressive, stable, or, in some instances, reversible ("dysmentia").

A distinction is drawn by some authors between cortical and subcortical dementia: in the former the pathology is predominantly cortical and neuropsychological findings are characterized by amnesia, agnosia, apraxia, and aphasia (*e.g.* Alzheimer's disease); in the latter pathology is predominantly frontal-subcortical and neuropsychological deficits include psychomotor retardation, attentional deficits, with relative preservation of memory and language; movement disorders may also be apparent (*e.g.* progressive supranuclear palsy, Huntington's disease). However, not all authors subscribe to this distinction, and considerable overlap may be observed clinically.

Cognitive deficits also occur in affective disorders such as depression, usually as a consequence of impaired attentional mechanisms. This syndrome is often labelled as "pseudodementia" since it is potentially reversible with treatment of the underlying affective disorder. It may be difficult to differentiate dementia originating from depressive or neurodegenerative disease, since depression may also be a feature of the latter. Impaired attentional mechanisms may account for the common complaint of not recalling conversations or instructions immediately after they happen (aprosexia). Behavioural abnormalities are common in dementias due to degenerative brain disease, and may require treatment in their own right.

Recognised causes of a dementia syndrome include:

- Neurodegenerative diseases:

    Alzheimer's disease, frontotemporal lobar degenerations (encompassing behavioural variant frontotemporal dementia and the agrammatic and semantic variants of primary progressive aphasia, the latter two previously known as primary nonfluent aphasia and semantic dementia), Parkinson's disease dementia; dementia with Lewy bodies, Huntington's disease, progressive supranuclear palsy, corticobasal degeneration, prion disease, Down's syndrome, dementia pugilistica.

- Cerebrovascular disease:

    focal strategic infarcts (*e.g.* paramedian thalamic infarction), multiple infarcts, subcortical vascular disease, Binswanger's disease.

- Inflammatory disorders: multiple sclerosis, systemic lupus erythematosus.
- Structural disease: normal pressure hydrocephalus, subdural haematoma, tumours, dural arteriovenous fistula.
- Infection: HIV dementia, neurosyphilis, Whipple's disease.
- Metabolic causes: Wernicke-Korsakoff syndrome, vitamin B_{12} deficiency, hypothyroidism, hyperparathyroidism/hypercalcaemia, leucodystrophies, Wilson's disease.

Cognitive dysfunction may be identified in many other neurological illnesses.

Investigation of patients with dementia aims to identify its particular cause. Because of the possibility of progression, reversible causes are regularly sought though very rarely found. A focus on early identification at the pre-dementia stage, variously defined as mild cognitive impairment, cognitive impairment no dementia, or mild cognitive disorder, is now promoted, although disease-modifying treatments are lacking. Specific treatments for established dementia are few: cholinesterase inhibitors have been licensed for the treatment of mild to moderate Alzheimer's disease and may find a role in other conditions, such as Parkinson's disease dementia, dementia with Lewy bodies and vascular dementia, for behavioural as well as mnestic features. Memantine is licensed in some jurisdictions for moderate to severe dementia.

References
Ames D, Burns A, O'Brien J, editors. Dementia. 4th ed. London: Hodder Arnold; 2010.
Clarfield AM. The decreasing prevalence of reversible dementia: an updated meta-analysis. *Arch Intern Med.* 2003; **163**: 2219–29.

Dickerson B, Atri A, editors. Dementia. Comprehensive principles and practice. Oxford: Oxford University Press; 2014.
Larner AJ. Neuropsychological neurology. The neurocognitive impairments of neurological disorders. 2nd ed. Cambridge: Cambridge University Press; 2013.
Cross References
Agnosia; Amnesia; Aphasia; Apraxia; Aprosexia; Attention; Delirium; Dysmentia; Pseudodementia; Psychomotor retardation

De Musset's Sign
- see HEAD TREMOR

Depersonalisation
Depersonalisation, a form of dissociation, is the experience of feeling detached or alienated from oneself, such that the body feels strange, lacking control, or being viewed from the outside. There may be concurrent derealisation. Depersonalisation is a very common symptom in the general population, and may contribute to neurological presentations described as dizziness, numbness, and forgetfulness, with the broad differential diagnoses that such symptoms encompass. Such symptoms may also occur in the context of meditation and self-suggestion.
Reference
Stone J. Dissociation: what is it and why is it important? *Pract Neurol.* 2006; **6**: 308–13.
Cross References
Derealization; Dissociation

Derealisation
Derealisation, a form of dissociation, is the experience of feeling that the world around is unreal. There may be concurrent depersonalization.
Reference
Stone J. Dissociation: what is it and why is it important? *Pract Neurol.* 2006; **6**: 308–13.
Cross References
Depersonalsation; Dissociation

Dermatomal Sensory Loss
Dermatome refers to the area of skin innervated by a particualr neural element, such as a nerve root or spinal segment. Mapping out an area of sensory loss or impairment may correspond to a particular dermatome and hence assist in localisation. Few neurology textbooks neglect to include a dermatomal map of the body, but it should be realised that these maps are only approximate and adjacent dermatomes may show significant overlap.
Reference
Apok V, Gurusinghe NT, Mitchell JD, Emsley HCA. Dermatomes and dogma. *Pract Neurol.* 2011; **11**: 100–5.
Cross Reference
Radiculopathy

Dermo-Optical Perception
Dermo-optical perception, or fingertip sight, describes the rare ability to read print, describe pictures, and recognise colours purely by way of touch. This may be a form of paroptic vision; other forms have been decribed, for example though the nose. Experiments have suggested that in some cases fingertip sight for colours may be due to minute differences in surface texture or reflected heat, but correct identification of colours through a glass plate by some subjects would seem to rule out these mechanisms.

Colour-touch synaesthesia might also account for some of these phenomena, whose exact physiology remains uncertain.
Reference
Brugger P, Weiss PH. Dermo-optical perception: the non-synesthetic "palpability of colors" a comment on Larner (2006). *J Hist Neurosci.* 2008; **17**: 253–5.

Cross Reference
Synaesthesia

Developmental Signs
- see FRONTAL RELEASE SIGNS; PRIMITIVE REFLEXES

Diagonistic Dyspraxia
This term referes to a dissociative phenomenon observed after callosotomy, probably identical to intermanual conflict.
Reference
Akelaitis AJ. Studies on the corpus callosum, IV: diagonistic dyspraxia in epileptics following partial and complete section of the corpus callosum. *Am J Psychiatry*. 1944–1945; **101**: 594–9.
Cross References
Alien hand, Alien limb; Intermanual conflict

Diamond on Quadriceps Sign
Diamond on quadriceps sign may be seen in patients with dysferlinopathies (limb girdle muscular dystrophy type 2B, Miyoshi myopathy): with the knees slightly bent so that the quadriceps are in moderate action, an asymmetric diamond shaped bulge may be seen, with wasting above and below, indicative of the selectivity of the dystrophic process in these conditions.
Reference
Pradhan S. Diamond on quadriceps: a frequent sign in dysferlinopathy. *Neurology*. 2008; **70**: 322.
Cross Reference
Calf head sign

Diaphoresis
Diaphoresis describes sweating, either physiological as in sympathetic activation (*e.g.* during hypotension, hypoglycaemia), or pathological (hyperhidrosis, *q.v.*). Diaphoresis may be seen in syncope, delirium tremens, or may be induced by certain drugs (*e.g.* cholinesterase inhibitors) or drug withdrawal (*e.g.* opiates in dependent individuals). Anticholinergics decrease diaphoresis but increase core temperature, resulting in a warm dry patient.
Cross Reference
Hyperhidrosis

Diaphragm Weakness
Diaphragm weakness is a feature of certain myopathies such as acid maltase deficiency, and of cervical cord lesions (C3–C5) affecting phrenic nerve function. Forced vital capacity measured in the supine and sitting positions is often used to assess diaphragmatic function, a drop of 25% being taken as indicating diaphragmatic weakness.
Reference
Allen SM, Hunt B, Green M. Fall in vital capacity with posture. *Br J Diseases Chest*. 1985; **79**: 267–71.
Cross Reference
Paradoxical breathing

Digital Reflex
- see HOFFMANN'S SIGN; TRÖMNER'S SIGN

Diplophonia
Diplophonia, the simultaneous production of two pitch levels when phonating, occurs in unilateral vocal cord paralysis because each vocal fold has a different vibration frequency.
Cross References
Bovine cough; Dysphonia

Diplopia

Diplopia is double vision, *viz.*, seeing two images of a single object. The spatial and temporal characteristics of the diplopia may help to ascertain its cause.

Diplopia may be monocular, in which case ocular causes are most likely (although monocular diplopia may be cortical or functional in origin), or binocular, implying a divergence of the visual axes of the two eyes. With binocular diplopia, it is of great importance to ask the patient whether the images are separated horizontally, vertically, or obliquely (tilted), since this may indicate the extraocular muscle(s) most likely to be affected. Whether the two images are separate or overlapping is important when trying to ascertain the direction of maximum diplopia.

The experience of diplopia may be confined to, or particularly noticeable during, the performance of particular activities, reflecting the effect of gaze direction; for example, diplopia experienced on coming downstairs may reflect a trochlear (IV) nerve palsy; or only on looking to the left may reflect a left abducens (VI) nerve palsy. Double vision experienced on looking at a distant object after looking down (*e.g.* reading) may occur with bilateral abducens (VI) nerve palsies. The effect of gaze direction on diplopia should always be sought, since images are most separated when looking in the direction of a paretic muscle. Conversely, diplopia resulting from the breakdown of a latent tendency for the visual axes to deviate (latent strabismus, squint) results in diplopia in all directions of gaze.

Examination of the eye movements should include asking the patient to look at a target, such as a pen, in the various directions of gaze (versions) to ascertain where diplopia is maximal. Ductions are tested monocularly with the opposite eye covered. Then, each eye may be alternately covered to try to demonstrate which of the two images is the false one, namely that from the non-fixing eye. The false image is also the most peripheral image. Thus in a left abducens (VI) nerve palsy, diplopia is maximum on left lateral gaze; when the normal right eye is covered the inner image disappears; the non-fixing left eye is responsible for the remaining false image, which is the more peripheral and which disappears when the left eye is covered.

Other clues to the cause of diplopia include the presence of any other neurological signs, for example ptosis (unilateral: oculomotor (III) nerve palsy; bilateral: myasthenia gravis), or head tilt or turn (to the right suggests a weak right lateral rectus muscle suggesting a right abducens (VI) nerve palsy; tilt to the left shoulder suggests a right trochlear (IV) nerve palsy, = Bielschowsky's sign).

Manifest squints (heterotropia) are obvious but seldom a cause of diplopia if longstanding. Latent squints may be detected using the cover-uncover test, when the shift in fixation of the eyes indicates an imbalance in the visual axes; this may account for diplopia if the normal compensation breaks down. This produces diplopia in all directions of gaze (comitant). Patients may with an effort be able to fuse the two images.

Transient diplopia (minutes to hours) suggests the possibility of myasthenia gravis. There are many causes of persistent diplopia, including the breakdown of a latent strabismus, development of oculomotor (III), trochlear (IV) or abducens (VI) nerve palsy (singly or in combination), orbital myopathy (thyroid), and mass lesions of the orbit (tumour, pseudotumour).

Divergence of the visual axes or ophthalmoplegia without diplopia suggests a longstanding problem, such as amblyopia or chronic progressive external ophthalmoplegia. Some eye movement disorders are striking for the lack of associated diplopia, *e.g.* internuclear ophthalmoplegia.

References

Danchaivijitr C, Kennard C. Diplopia and eye movement disorders. *J Neurol Neurosurg Psychiatry*. 2004; **75**(Suppl IV): iv24–31.

Low L, Shah W, MacEwen CJ. Double vision. *BMJ*. 2015; **351**: h5385.

Rucker JC, Tomsak RL. Binocular diplopia. A practical approach. *Neurologist*. 2005; **11**: 98–110.

Yee RD. Approach to the patient with diplopia. In: Biller J, editor. Practical neurology. 2nd ed. Philadelphia: Lippincott Williams & Wilkins; 2002. p. 147–61.

Cross References
Abducens (VI) nerve palsy; Amblyopia; Bielschowsky's sign, Bielschowsky's test; Cover tests; Heterophoria; Heterotropia; Internuclear ophthalmoplegia (INO); Oculomotor (III) nerve palsy

Directional Hypokinesia
Directional hypokinesia describes a reluctance to move towards contralesional space seen in the neglect syndrome.
Cross Reference
Motor neglect; Neglect

Disc Swelling
Swelling or oedema of the optic nerve head may be visualized by ophthalmoscopy. It produces haziness of the nerve fibre layer obscuring the underlying vessels; there may also be disc haemorrhages and loss of spontaneous retinal venous pulsation at the disc margin. Whether vision is affected is dependent upon the precise cause of disc swelling.

The clinical history, visual acuity and visual fields may help determine the cause of disc swelling.

Disc swelling due to raised intracranial pressure (papilloedema, *q.v.*) may occur without specific visual complaint but with an enlarged blind spot on visual field testing. Local inflammation of the optic nerve (papillitis) may be associated with marked impairment of vision, as for example in optic neuritis.

Disc swelling due to oedema must be distinguished from pseudopapilloedema, elevation of the optic disc not due to oedema, in which the nerve fibre layer is clearly seen.

Recognised causes of disc swelling include:

- *Unilateral*:
  Optic neuritis.
  Acute ischaemic optic neuropathy (arteritic, non-arteritic).
  Orbital compressive lesions, *e.g.* optic nerve sheath meningioma (Foster Kennedy syndrome).
  Graves' ophthalmopathy (through compression of retinal veins by myositis).
  Central retinal vein occlusion.
  Infiltration: carcinoma, lymphoma, granuloma.
  Raised intracranial pressure (papilloedema; more usually bilateral).

- *Bilateral*:
  Raised intracranial pressure (papilloedema).
  Malignant hypertension.
  Hypercapnia.
  High CSF protein, as in Guillain-Barré syndrome.
  Any of the unilateral causes.

Cross References
Foster Kennedy syndrome; Papilloedema; Pseudopapilloedema; Retinal venous pulsation; Visual field defects

Disinhibition
Disinhibited behaviour is impulsive, showing poor judgment and insight, and may transgress normal cultural or social bounds. There is a loss of normal emotional and/or behavioural control. The disinhibited patient may be inappropriately jocular (*witzelsucht*), short-tempered (verbally abusive, physically aggressive), distractible (impaired attentional mechanisms), and show emotional lability. A Disinhibition Scale encompassing various domains (motor, intellectual, instinctive, affective, sensitive) has been described.

Disinhibition is a feature of frontal lobe, particularly orbitofrontal, dysfunction. This may be due to neurodegenerative disorders (behavioural variant frontotemporal dementia, Alzheimer's disease), mass lesions, or be a feature of epileptic seizures.

Cross References
Attention; Emotionalism, Emotional lability; Frontal lobe syndromes; Osculation; *Witzelsucht*

Dissociated Sensory Loss

Dissociated sensory loss refers to impairment of selected sensory modalities with preservation, or sparing, of others. It is usually an indication of an intramedullary spinal cord lesion. For example, a focal central cord pathology such as syringomyelia will, in the early stages, selectively involve decussating fibres of the spinothalamic pathway within the ventral commissure, thus impairing pain and temperature sensation (often in a suspended, "cape-like", "bathing suit", "vest-like", or cuirasse distribution), whilst the dorsal columns are spared, leaving proprioception intact. The anterior spinal artery syndrome also leaves the dorsal columns intact. Conversely, pathologies confined, largely or exclusively, to the dorsal columns (classically tabes dorsalis and subacute combined degeneration of the cord from vitamin B_{12} deficiency, but probably most commonly seen with compressive cervical myelopathy) impair proprioception, sometimes sufficient to produce pseudoathetosis or sensory ataxia, whilst pain and temperature sensation is preserved. A double dissociation of sensory modalities on opposite sides of the trunk is seen in the Brown-Séquard syndrome.

Small fibre peripheral neuropathies may selective affect the fibres which transmit pain and temperature sensation, leading to a glove-and-stocking impairment to these modalities. Neuropathic (Charcot) joints and skin ulceration may occur in this situation; tendon reflexes may be preserved.

Cross References
Analgesia; Ataxia; Brown-Séquard syndrome; Charcot joint; *Main succulente*; Myelopathy; Proprioception; Pseudoathetosis; Sacral sparing

Dissociation

Dissociation is an umbrella term for a wide range of symptoms involving feelings of disconnection from the body (depersonalsation) or the surroundings (derealization). Common in psychiatric disorders (depression, anxiety, schizophrenia), these symptoms are also encountered in neurological conditions (epilepsy, migraine, presyncope), conditions such as functional weakness and non-epilepetic attacks, and in isolation by a significant proportion of the general population. Symptoms of dizziness and blankness may well be the result of dissociative states rather than neurological disease.

Reference
Stone J. Dissociation: what is it and why is it important? *Pract Neurol.* 2006; **6**: 308–13.
Cross References
Depersonalsation; Derealization

Divisional Palsy

The oculomotor (III) nerve divides into superior and inferior divisions, usually at the superior orbital fissure. The superior division or ramus supplies the superior rectus and levator palpebrae superioris muscles; the inferior division or ramus supplies medial rectus, inferior rectus and inferior oblique muscles. Isolated dysfunction of these muscle groups allows diagnosis of divisional palsy and suggests pathology at the superior orbital fissure or anterior cavernous sinus. However, occasionally the division may occur more proximally, at the fascicular level (*i.e.* within the midbrain) or within the subarachnoid space, giving a false-localising divisional palsy. This may reflect the topographic arrangement of axons within the oculomotor nerve.

Reference
Larner AJ. Proximal superior division oculomotor nerve palsy from metastatic subarachnoid infiltration. *J Neurol.* 2002; **249**: 343–4.
Cross References
"False-localising signs"; Oculomotor (III) nerve palsy

Dix-Hallpike Positioning Test
- see HALLPIKE MANOEUVRE, HALLPIKE TEST

Doll's Eye Manoeuvre, Doll's Head Manoeuvre
This test of the vestibulo-ocular reflex (VOR) is demonstrated by rotating the patient's head and looking for a conjugate eye movement in the opposite direction. Although this can be done in a conscious patient focusing on a visual target, smooth pursuit eye movements may compensate for head turning; hence the head impulse test (*q.v.*) may be required. The manoeuvre is easier to do in the unconscious patient, when testing for the integrity of brainstem reflexes.

A slow (0.5–1.0 Hz) doll's head manoeuvre may be used in conscious patients to assess vestibulo-ocular reflexes. Whilst directly observing the eyes, "catch up" saccades may be seen in the absence of VOR. Measuring visual acuity with head movement compared to visual acuity with the head still (dynamic visual acuity, or illegible E test), two to three lines may be dropped if VOR is impaired. On ophthalmoscopy, the disc moves with the head if VOR is lost.
Reference
Roberts TA, Jenkyn LR, Reeves AG. On the notion of doll's eyes. *Arch Neurol.* 1984; **41**: 1242–3.
Cross References
Bell's phenomenon, Bell's sign; Caloric testing; Coma; Head impulse test; Oculocephalic response; Supranuclear gaze palsy; Vestibulo-ocular reflexes

"Dorsal Guttering"
Dorsal guttering refers to the marked prominence of the extensor tendons on the dorsal surface of the hand when intrinsic hand muscles (especially interossei) are wasted, as may occur in an ulnar nerve lesion, a lower brachial plexus lesion, or a T1 root lesion. Benign extramedullary tumours at the foramen magnum may also produce this picture (remote atrophy, a "false-localising sign"). In many elderly people the extensor tendons are prominent in the absence of significant muscle wasting.
Cross References
"False-localising signs"; Wasting

"Double Elevator Palsy"
This name has been given to monocular elevation paresis (apparent hypotropia). This may be congenital or acquired, the latter may occur in association with pretectal supranuclear lesions (*e.g.* pineal mass lesion) either contralateral or ipsilateral to the paretic eye interrupting efferents from the rostral interstitial nucleus of the medial longitudinal fasciculus to the superior rectus and inferior oblique subnuclei. Bell's phenomenon may be preserved.
Reference
Thömke F, Hopf HC. Acquired monocular elevation paresis. An asymmetric up-gaze palsy. *Brain.* 1992; **115**: 1901–10.
Cross References
Bell's phenomenon, Bell's sign; Hypotropia

Downbeat Nystagmus
- see NYSTAGMUS

Dressing Apraxia
- see APRAXIA

Drooling
- see SIALORRHOEA

Dropped Head Syndrome
Dropped head syndrome (head droop or head drop) refers to forward flexion of the head on the neck, such that the chin falls on to the chest (*cf.* antecollis) and the head cannot be voluntarily extended. This syndrome has a broad differential diagnosis, encompassing disorders which may cause axial truncal muscle weakness, especially of upper thoracic and paraspinous muscles.

- Neuropathy/Neuronopathy:
  Motor neurone disease (the author has also seen this syndrome in a patient with frontotemporal lobar degeneration with motor neurone disease, FTLD/MND). Guillain-Barré syndrome, chronic inflammatory demyelinating polyneuropathy. Paraneoplastic motor neuronopathy.
- Neuromuscular junction disorder:
  Myasthenia gravis.
- Myopathy:
  Polymyositis.
  Myotonic dystrophy.
  Myopathy with rimmed vacuoles.
  "Dropped head syndrome", or "isolated neck extensor myopathy", a condition of uncertain aetiology but which may on occasion be steroid-responsive ("bent spine syndrome" or camptocormia may be related forms of axial myopathy).
- Extrapyramidal disorders:
  Parkinson's disease.
  Multiple system atrophy.
  Progressive supranuclear palsy.

Of these, probably MND and myasthenia gravis are the most common causes.
Treatment of the underlying condition may be possible, hence investigation is mandatory. If not treatable (*e.g.* MND), a head brace may keep the head upright.
References
Katz JS, Wolfe GI, Burns DK, Bryan WW, Fleckenstein JL, Barohn RJ. Isolated neck extensor myopathy. A common cause of dropped head syndrome. *Neurology*. 1996; **46**: 917–21.
Nicholas RS, Lecky BRF. Dropped head syndrome: the differential diagnosis. *J Neurol Neurosurg Psychiatry*. 2002; **73**: 218 (abstract 26).
Rose MR, Levin KH, Griggs RC. The dropped head plus syndrome: quantitation of response to corticosteroids. *Muscle Nerve*. 1999; **22**: 115–8.
Swash M. Dropped-head and bent-spine syndromes: axial myopathies? *Lancet*. 1998; **352**: 758.
Cross References
Antecollis; Camptocormia; Myopathy

Drusen
Drusen are hyaline bodies that are typically seen on and around the optic nerve head, and may be mistaken for papilloedema ("pseudopapilloedema"). Drusen are thought to result from altered axonal flow with axonal degeneration. They occur sporadically or may be inherited in an autosomal dominant fashion, and are common, occurring in 2% of the population. In children the drusen are buried whilst in adults they are on the surface of the disc.

Drusen are usually asymptomatic but can cause visual field defects (typically an inferior nasal visual field loss) or occasionally transient visual obscurations, but not changes in visual acuity which require investigation for an alternative cause. When there is doubt whether papilloedema or drusen is the cause of a swollen optic nerve head, retinal fluorescein angiography is required.

Reference
Arbabi EM, Fearnley TE, Carrim ZI. Drusen and the misleading optic disc. *Pract Neurol.* 2010; **10**: 27–30.
Cross References
Disc swelling; Papilloedema; Pseudopapilloedena; Visual field defects

Durkan's Compression Test
Durkan's compression test, sometimes called the carpal compression test, is a provocative test for carpal tunnel syndrome. With the wrist in a supine position on a table, the examiner places three fingers over the carpal tunnel and compresses the area for 30 s. If the patient reports tingling, numbness, or altered sensation in the thumb or index finger, middle finger, or radial half of the ring finger, then the test is positive and suggestive of a diagnosis of carpal tunnel syndrome.
Cross References
Phalen's sign; Tinel's sign

Dynamic Aphasia
Dynamic aphasia refers to an aphasia characterized by difficulty initiating speech output, ascribed to executive dysfunction. There is a reduction in spontaneous speech, but on formal testing there are no paraphasias, minimal anomia, preserved repetition, reading, and automatic speech. "Incorporational echolalia", when the patient uses the examiner's question to help form an answer, may be observed.

Dynamic aphasia has been conceptualised as a variant of transcortical motor aphasia, and may be seen with lesions of dorsolateral prefrontal cortex ("frontal aphasia"). It has also been reported in progressive supranuclear palsy, and postulated to be a variant of primary progressive aphasia. A division into pure and mixed forms has been suggested, with additional phonological, lexical, syntactical and articulatory impairments in the latter.
Reference
Robinson GA. Primary progressive dynamic aphasia and Parkinsonism: generation, selection and sequencing deficits. *Neuropsychologia.* 2013; **51**: 2534–47.
Cross References
Aphasia; Echolalia; Transcortical aphasias

Dysaesthesia
Dysaesthesia (or dysesthesia) refers to an unpleasant, abnormal or unfamiliar, sensation, often with a burning and/or "electrical" quality. Some authorities reserve the term for provoked positive sensory phenomena, as opposed to spontaneous sensations (paraesthesia). Dysaesthesia differs from paraesthesia in its unpleasant quality, but may overlap in some respects with allodynia, hyperalgesia and hyperpathia (the latter phenomena are provoked by stimuli, either non-noxious or noxious).

There are many causes of dysaesthesia, both peripheral (including small fibre neuropathies, neuroma, nerve trauma) and central (*e.g.* spinal multiple sclerosis).

Dysaesthetic sensations may be helped by agents such as carbamazepine, amitriptyline, gabapentin and pregabalin.
Cross References
Allodynia; Hyperalgesia; Hyperpathia; Paraesthesia

Dysarthria
Dysarthria is a disorder of speech, as opposed to language (*cf.* aphasia), because of impairments in the actions of the speech production apparatus *per se*, due to paralysis, ataxia, tremor or spasticity, in the presence of intact mental function, comprehension and memory for words. In its most extreme form, anarthria, there is no speech output.

Dysarthria is a symptom which may be caused by a number of different conditions, all of which ultimately affect the function of pharynx, palate, tongue, lips and larynx, be that at the level of the cortex, lower cranial nerve nuclei or their motor neurones, neuromuscular junction or bulbar muscles themselves. Dysarthrias affect articulation in a highly reliable and consistent manner, the errors reflecting the muscle group involved in the production of specific sounds. There are various syndromes of dysarthria, which have been classified as follows:

- *Flaccid or nasal dysarthria*:
    hypernasal, breathy, whining output, as in bulbar palsy, *e.g.* myasthenia gravis.
- *Spastic dysarthria*:
    slow, strained ("strangled") output, monotonous, as in pseudobulbar palsy; may coexist with Broca's aphasia.
- *Ataxic or cerebellar dysarthria*:
    altered rhythm of speech, uneven irregular output, slurred speech (as if inebriated), improper stresses; seen in acute cerebellar damage due to asynergia of speech muscle contractions (*cf.* scanning speech).
- *Hypokinetic dysarthria*:
    monotonic pitch, hypophonic volume, as in parkinsonism.
- *Hyperkinetic dysarthria*:
    several varieties are described, including choreiform (as in Huntington's disease), dystonic (as in tardive dyskinesia, and other dystonic syndromes), tremulous (tremor syndromes), and the dysarthria with vocal tics (including coprolalia) in Tourette syndrome.
- *Mixed dysarthria*:
    combination of any of above.

    Recognised causes of dysarthria include:
- Muscle disease:
    e.g. oculopharyngeal muscular dystrophy: nasal speech; weak pharynx/drooling.
- Neuromuscular disorder:
    e.g. myasthenia gravis: nasal speech; fatiguability (development of hypophonia with prolonged conversation, or counting).
- Lower motor neurone disease = bulbar palsy:
    e.g. motor neurone disease (rasping monotones, wasted and fasciculating tongue), poliomyelitis, Guillain-Barré syndrome, diphtheria.
- Upper motor neurone disease = pseudobulbar palsy:
    e.g. motor neurone disease (spastic tongue), cerebrovascular disease.
- Cortical dysarthria:
    damage to left frontal cortex, usually with associated right hemiparesis; may be additional aphasia.
- Extrapyramidal disease:
    e.g. hypokinetic disorders: Parkinson's disease: slow, hypophonic, monotonic; multiple system atrophy (may have vocal cord palsy).
    e.g. hyperkinetic disorders: Huntington's disease: loud, harsh, variably stressed, and poorly co-ordinated with breathing; myoclonus of any cause (hiccup speech); dystonia of any cause.
- Ataxic dysarthria:
    disease of or damage to the cerebellum: slow, slurred, monotonous, with inco-ordination of speech with respiration; may therefore be quiet and then explosive; unnatural separation of syllables; slow tongue movements.

- Acquired stuttering:

   involuntary repetition of letters or syllables, may be acquired with aphasia; developmental stutter, the more common cause, usually affects the beginnings of words and with plosive sounds, whereas the acquired form may be evident throughout sentences and affect all speech sounds.

   Treatment of the underlying cause may improve dysarthria (*e.g.* nasal dysarthria of myasthenia gravis). Baclofen has been suggested for dysarthria of upper motor neurone type. Speech and language therapy may provide symptomatic benefit.

References

Darley FL, Aronson AE, Brown JR. Motor speech disorders. Philadelphia: Saunders; 1975.
LaMonte MP, Erskine MC, Thomas BE. Approach to the patient with dysarthria. In: Biller J, editor. Practical neurology. 2nd ed. Philadelphia: Lippincott Williams & Wilkins; 2002. p. 236–43.
Murdoch BE, editor. Dysarthria. A physiological approach to assessment and treatment. Cheltenham: Stanley Thornes; 1998.

Cross References

Anarthria; Aphasia; Asynergia; Broca's aphasia; Bulbar palsy; Coprolalia; Dysphonia; Fatigue; Lower motor neurone (LMN) syndrome; Parkinsonism; Pseudobulbar palsy; Scanning speech; Stutter; Upper motor neurone (UMN) syndrome

Dysautonomia

Dysautonomia describes autonomic nervous system dysfunction which may result from either pre- or post-ganglionic lesions of either the sympathetic or parasympathetic pathways, or both (pandysautonomia).

   Clinical features of dysautonomia include:

- Visual blurring; pupillary areflexia.
- Orthostatic hypotension.
- Cardiac arrhythmia.
- Abdominal pain, diarrhoea, vomiting, constipation, ileus, pseudo-obstruction.
- Sweating dysfunction (*e.g.* anhidrosis).

   Autonomic dysfunction may be:

- Congenital.
- Acquired:

   acute (*e.g.* after a viral infection such as infectious mononucleosis).
   subacute (*e.g.* the "autonomic-only" form of Guillain-Barré syndrome).
   chronic (*e.g.* pure autonomic failure, multiple system atrophy, certain hereditary neuropathies).

   As regards aetiology, in addition to hereditary (genetic) and neurodegenerative disorders, autoimmune forms of autonomic neuropathy are described, for example a pandysautonomia associated with antibodies to ganglionic neuronal nicotinic acetylcholine receptors (*cf.* antibodies to muscarinic acetylcholine receptors in myasthenia gravis) which may respond well to immunomodulatory therapies.

References

Goldstein DS, Holmes C, Dendi R, Li ST, Brentzel S, Vernino S. Pandysautonomia associated with impaired ganglionic neurotransmission and circulating antibody to the neuronal nicotinic receptor. *Clin Auton Res*. 2002; **12**: 281–5.
Mathias CJ, Bannister R, editors. Autonomic failure. A textbook of clinical disorders of the autonomic nervous system. 5th ed. Oxford: Oxford University Press; 2013.

Dyscalculia
- see ACALCULIA

Dyschromatopsia
- see ACHROMATOPSIA

Dysdiadochokinesia
Dysdiadochokinesia, or adiadochokinesia, is a difficulty in performing rapid alternating movements, for example pronation/supination of the arms, tapping alternately with the palm and dorsum of the hand, tapping the foot on the floor.

Dysdiadochokinesia is a sign of cerebellar dysfunction, especially hemisphere disease, and may be seen in association with asynergia, ataxia, dysmetria, and excessive rebound phenomenon. It may reflect the impaired checking response seen in cerebellar disease. Dysdiadochokinesia may also be seen with disease of the frontal lobes ("frontal apraxia") or basal ganglia.
Cross References
Asynergia; Apraxia; Ataxia; Cerebellar syndromes; Dysmetria; Rebound phenomenon

Dysexecutive Syndrome
The term executive function encompasses a range of cognitive processes including sustained attention, fluency and flexibility of thought, problem solving skills, planning and regulation of adaptive and goal-directed behaviour. Some authors prefer to use these individual terms, rather than "lump" them together as executive function. Deficits in these various functions, the dysexecutive syndrome, are typically seen with lateral prefrontal cortex lesions.
Reference
Knight RT, D'Esposito M. Lateral prefrontal syndrome: a disorder of executive control. In: D'Esposito M, editor. Neurological foundations of cognitive neuroscience. Cambridge: MIT Press; 2003. p. 259–79.
Cross References
Attention; Frontal lobe syndromes

Dysgeusia
Dysgeusia is a complaint of distorted taste perception. It may occur along with anosmia as a feature of upper respiratory tract infections, and has also been described with various drug therapies, in psychiatric diseases, and as a feature of zinc deficiency.
Reference
Henkin RI, Patten BM, Pe RK, Bronzert DA. A syndrome of acute zinc loss. Cerebellar dysfunction, mental changes, anorexia and taste and smell dysfunction. *Arch Neurol.* 1975; **32**: 745–51.
Cross References
Ageusia; Anosmia

Dysgraphaesthesia
- see AGRAPHOGNOSIA; GRAPHAESTHESIA

Dysgraphia
- see AGRAPHIA

Dyskinesia
Dyskinesia may be used as a general term for excessive involuntary movements, encompassing tremor, myoclonus, chorea, athetosis, tics, stereotypies, and hyperekplexia. The term may be qualified to describe a number of other syndromes of excessive movement, *e.g.*:

- *Drug-induced dyskinesia*:
  Fluid, restless, fidgety movements seen in patients with Parkinson's disease after several years of levodopa therapy, and often described according to their relationship to timing of tablets (*e.g.* peak dose, diphasic), although others are unpredictable (freezing, yo-yo-ing). In MPTP-induced parkinsonism, dyskinesias tend to occur early, hence it may be the depth of dopamine deficiency rather than chronicity of treatment which is the key determinant; reduction in overall levodopa use (increased frequency of smaller doses, controlled-release preparations, addition of dopamine agonists) may reduce these effects; amantadine is sometimes helpful.

- *Tardive dyskinesia*:
  A form of drug-induced dyskinesia developing after long-term use of neuroleptic (dopamine antagonist) medication, typically involving orolingual musculature (buccolingual syndrome, rabbit syndrome, "bon-bon sign") and occasionally trunk and arms; usually persists after withdrawal of causative therapy; clonazepam, baclofen, and tetrabenazine may sometimes help.

- *Paroxysmal dyskinesias*:
  Paroxysmal kinesigenic choreoathetosis/dystonia (PKC; usually responds to carbamazepine), and paroxysmal non-kinesigenic dystonia/choreoathetosis (PDC; does not respond to carbamazepine).

- *Focal dyskinesias*:
  Orofacial dyskinesia, belly-dancer's dyskinesia, moving ear syndrome.

References
Fahn S. The paroxysmal dyskinesias. In: Marsden CD, Fahn S, editors. Movement disorders. 3rd ed. Oxford: Butterworth-Heinemann; 1994. p. 310–45.
Schelosky LD. Paroxysmal dyskinesias. In: Schmitz B, Tettenborn B, Schomer DL, editors. The paroxysmal disorders. Cambridge: Cambridge University Press; 2010. p. 113–29.
Wojcieszek J. Drug-induced movement disorders. In: Biller J, editor. Iatrogenic neurology. Boston: Butterworth-Heinemann; 1998. 215–31.

Cross References
Athetosis; "Bon-bon sign"; Chorea, Choreoathetosis; Dystonia; Hyperekplexia; Moving ear; Myoclonus; Parkinsonism; Stereotypy; Tic; Yo-yo-ing

Dyslexia
Dyslexia is difficulty or impairment in reading, usually applied to developmental abnormalities of reading ability. A loss of previously acquired reading ability is probably better termed alexia.

Cross Reference
Alexia

Dysmentia
The term dysmentia has been suggested as an alternative to dementia, to emphasize the possibility that cognitive impairment and decline may be amenable to treatment and prevention, thereby reversing the therapeutic nihilism sometimes associated with the diagnostic label of dementia.

Reference
Chiu E. What's in a name: dementia or dysmentia? *Int J Geriatr Psychiatry*. 1994; **9**: 1–4.

Cross Reference
Dementia

Dysmetria
Dysmetria, or past-pointing, is a disturbance in the control of range of movement in voluntary muscular action, and is one feature of the impaired checking response seen in cerebellar lesions (especially cerebellar hemisphere lesions).

Dysmetria may also be evident in saccadic eye movements: hypometria (undershoot) is common in parkinsonism; hypermetria (overshoot) is more typical of cerebellar disease (lesions of dorsal vermis and fastigial nuclei).

In cerebellar disorders, dysmetria reflects the asynergia of co-ordinated muscular contraction.

References
Bötzel K, Rottach K, Büttner U. Normal and pathological saccadic dysmetria. *Brain.* 1993; **116**: 337–53.
Büttner U, Straube A, Spuler A. Saccadic dysmetria and "intact" smooth pursuit eye movements after bilateral deep cerebellar nuclei lesions. *J Neurol Neurosurg Psychiatry.* 1994; **57**: 832–4.

Cross References
Asynergia; Cerebellar syndromes; Dysdiadochokinesia; Parkinsonism; Rebound phenomenon; Saccades

Dysmorphopsia
The term dysmorphopsia has been proposed for impaired vision for shapes, a visual recognition defect in which visual acuity, colour vision, tactile recognition and visually-guided reaching movements are intact. These phenomena have been associated with bilateral lateral occipital cortical damage (*e.g.* after carbon monoxide poisoning) and are thought to reflect a selective loss of the magnocellular visual pathway. Whether this condition is an agnosia for shape or visual form, or a perceptual problem ("pseudoagnosia"), remains a subject of debate and the term dysmorphopsia has been suggested as a compromise between the different strands of thought.

Reference
Milner AD, Perrett DI, Johnston RS, et al. Perception and action in "visual form agnosia". *Brain.* 1991; **114**: 405–28.

Cross References
Agnosia; Visual agnosia; Visual form agnosia

Dysnomia
- see ANOMIA

Dysphagia
Dysphagia is difficulty swallowing. This may have local mechanical causes which are usually gastroenterological in origin (tumour; peptic ulceration/stricture, in which case there may be additional pain on swallowing – odynophagia) but sometimes vascular (aberrant right subclavian artery – dysphagia lusoria) or due to connective tissue disease (systemic sclerosis).

Dysphagia of neurological origin may be due to pathology occurring anywhere from cerebral cortex to muscle. Neurological control of swallowing is bilaterally represented and so unilateral upper motor neurone lesions may cause only transient problems. Poststroke dysphagia is common, but there is evidence of cortical reorganization (neuroplasticity) underpinning recovery. Bilateral upper motor neurone lesions cause persistent difficulties. Dysphagia of neurological origin may be accompanied by dysphonia, palatal droop, and depressed or exaggerated gag reflex.

Dysphagia may be:

- *Neurogenic*:
  CNS:
  Cerebrovascular disease: hemisphere, brainstem stroke.
  Extrapyramidal disease: Parkinson's disease, progressive supranuclear palsy, Huntington's disease, Wilson's disease, tardive dyskinesia, dystonia.

Inflammatory disease: multiple sclerosis.
Neoplasia: primary, secondary; cerebral, brainstem (skull base).
Other structural disorders of the brainstem: syringobulbia, cerebellar disease.
Developmental disorders: cerebral palsy syndromes, Chiari malformations.
Neuronopathy:
  Motor neurone disease.
Neuropathy:
  Guillain-Barré syndrome.
  Autonomic neuropathy (diabetes mellitus, amyloidosis, Chagas' disease, auto-
  nomic failure, Riley Day syndrome).
  Lower motor neurone pathology: bulbar palsy, isolated vagus (X) nerve palsy,
  jugular foramen syndrome.
Neuromuscular:
  Myasthenia gravis.

- *Myogenic*:
  Inflammatory muscle disease: polymyositis, inclusion body myositis.
  Myotonia: myotonic dystrophy.
  Muscular dystrophy: oculopharyngeal muscular dystrophy.
  Symptomatic oesophageal peristalsis ("nutcracker oesophagus").

- *Functional*:
  "Hysterical", globus hystericus (diagnosis of exclusion).

Gastrointestinal causes of dysphagia include:

- *Intrinsic*:
  Oesophageal carcinoma.
  Metastatic or extrinsic tumour spread.
  Peptic (post-inflammatory) stricture.
  Hiatus hernia.

- *Extrinsic*:
  Thoracic aortic aneurysm.
  Abnormal origin of right subclavian artery (dysphagia lusoria).
  Posterior mediastinal mass.
  Large goitre.
  Retropharyngeal mass.

If swallowing is compromised with a risk of aspiration, feeding may need to be undertaken via nasogastric tube, percutaneous gastrostomy or jejunostomy placed endoscopically
(PEG or PEJ), or even parenterally.

Reference
Abdel Jalil AA, Katzka DA, Castell DO. Approach to the patient with dysphagia. *Am J Med*.
2015; **128**: 1138.e17–23.

Cross References
Bulbar palsy; Dysphonia; Gag reflex; Jugular foramen syndrome; Pseudobulbar palsy

Dysphasia
"The inaccuracy of applying an absolute negation [i.e. aphasia] to a partial effect [of lan-
guage] has led to the suggestion of 'dysphasia' as a substitute. The term does not, however,
seem likely to come into use, a matter of little regret, since the word has not the merit of
unimpeachable exactness, and it has an unfortunate resemblance in sound to 'dysphagia'."
Reference
Gowers WR. Manual of diseases of the nervous system. Vol. 2; 2nd ed. London: J&A
Churchill; 1893. p. 110n1

Cross Reference
Aphasia

Dysphonia
Dysphonia is a disorder of the volume, pitch or quality of the voice resulting from dysfunction of the larynx, *i.e.* a disorder of phonation or sound generation. Hence this is a motor
speech disorder and could be considered as a type of dysarthria if of neurological origin.
    Dysphonia manifests as hoarseness, or a whispering breathy quality to the voice.
Diplophonia may occur. At the extreme, there may be complete loss of the voice (aphonia).
    Recognised causes of dysphonia include:

- infection (laryngitis).
- structural abnormalities, *e.g.* polyp, nodule, papilloma of vocal cord.
- neurological causes:
    Focal dystonic syndrome: spasmodic dysphonia or laryngeal dystonia (either
    abductor or adductor); the voice may have a strained and harsh quality, with low
    volume and pitch, vocal tremor, and irregularly distributed stoppages; with con-
    tinuing speech, or if holding a single note, the voice may fade away entirely. These
    syndromes may be amenable to treatment with botulinum toxin.
    Flaccid dysphonia, due to superior laryngeal nerve or vagus nerve (recurrent laryn-
    geal nerve) palsy, bulbar palsy.

Reference
Blitzer A, Brin MF, Stewart CF. Botulinum toxin management of spasmodic dysphonia
(laryngeal dystonia): a 12-year experience in more than 900 patients. *Laryngoscope*. 2015; **125**:
1751–7.
Cross References
Aphonia; Bulbar palsy; Diplophonia; Dysarthria; Dystonia; Hypophonia; Vocal tremor,
Voice tremor

Dyspraxia
Dyspraxia is difficulty or impairment in the performance of a skilled voluntary motor act
despite an intact motor system and level of consciousness. This may be developmental in
origin ("clumsy child"), but in adult practice reflects a loss of function, hence apraxia is a
better term.
Cross Reference
Apraxia

Dysprosodia, Dysprosody
- see APROSODIA, APROSODY

Dyssynergia
- see ASYNERGIA

Dystaxia
- see ATAXIA

Dystextia
Dystextia is a neologism coined to describe difficulty writing mobile phone texts. Acute dystextia has been described in the context of dominant hemisphere stroke with concurrent
aphasia and in migraine. It may reflect not only linguistic difficulties but also visual and
motor problems (as for agraphia). The tendency of predictive text functions to garble meaning, and the peculiar argot used by frequent users of mobile texts, should not be forgotten
when considering the possibility of dystextia.

References
Burns B, Randall M. "Dystextia": onset of difficulty writing mobile phone texts determines the time of acute ischaemic stroke allowing thrombolysis. *Pract Neurol*. 2014; **14**: 256–7.
Cawood TJ, King T, Sreenan S. Dystextia – a sign of the times? *Irish Med J*. 2006; **99**: 157.
Cross References
Agraphia; Aphasia; Dystypia

Dystonia
Dystonia, a term first used by Oppenheim in 1911, is a motor syndrome of sustained involuntary muscle contractions causing twisting and repetitive movements, sometimes tremor, and/or abnormal postures. Dystonic movements may initially appear with voluntary movement of the affected part ("action dystonia") but may eventually occur with voluntary movement elsewhere in the body ("overflow"). The severity of dystonia may be reduced by sensory tricks (*geste antagoniste*), using tactile or proprioceptive stimuli to lessen or eliminate posturing; this feature is unique to dystonia. Dystonia may develop after muscle fatiguing activity, and patients with focal dystonias show more rapid fatigue than normals. Dystonic disorders may be classified according to:

- *Age of onset*: the most significant predictor of prognosis: worse with earlier onset.
- *Distribution*: focal, segmental, multifocal, generalised; hemidystonia.
- *Aetiology*: primary/idiopathic *vs*. secondary/symptomatic.

Primary/idiopathic dystonias include:

- Primary torsion dystonia (idiopathic torsion dystonia).
- Severe generalized dystonia (dystonia musculorum deformans).
- Segmental, multifocal and focal dystonias (*e.g.* torticollis, blepharospasm, writer's cramp).
- Dopa-responsive dystonia (DRD; Segawa's syndrome).
- Myoclonic dystonia.

Secondary/symptomatic dystonia: the differential diagnosis is broad, with more than 40 known causes, including:

- Heredodegenerative disorders: Wilson's disease, Huntington's disease, neurodegeneration with brain iron accumulation, mitochondrial disorders, X-linked dystonia-parkinsonism (lubag).
- Paroxysmal dystonias/dyskinesias: paroxysmal kinesigenic choreoathetosis/dystonia (PKC; usually responds to carbamazepine), and paroxysmal non-kinesigenic dystonia/choreoathetosis (PDC; does not respond to carbamazepine).
- Metachromatic leukodystrophy.
- Gangliosidoses (GM1, GM2).
- Perinatal cerebral injury.
- Encephalitis.
- Head trauma.
- Multiple sclerosis.
- Drugs/toxins, *e.g.* antipsychotic, antiemetic, and antidepressant drugs.
- Psychogenic.

Appropriate investigations to exclude these symptomatic causes (especially Wilson's disease) are appropriate.
The pathogenesis of dystonia is incompletely understood. Different mechanisms may apply in different conditions. Peripheral focal dystonias such as torticollis and writer's cramp have been suggested to result from abnormal afferent information relayed from "stiff" muscle spindles. The genetic characterisation of various dystonic syndromes may facilitate understanding of pathogenesis.

From the therapeutic point of view, one of the key questions relates to response to levodopa: dopa-responsive dystonia (DRD) responds very well to levodopa (and response fluctuations do not develop over time; *cf.* Parkinson's disease). Other treatments which are sometimes helpful include anticholinergics, dopamine antagonists, dopamine agonists, and baclofen. Drug-induced dystonia following antipsychotic, antiemetic, or antidepressant drugs is often relieved within 20 min by intramuscular biperiden (5 mg) or procyclidine (5 mg). Botulinum toxin may be very helpful in some focal dystonias (*e.g.* blepharospasm). Surgery for dystonia using deep brain stimulation is still at the experimental stage.

References

Fahn S, Marsden CD, Calne DB. Classification and investigation of dystonia. In: Marsden CD, Fahn S, editors. Movement disorders 2. London: Butterworth; 1987. p. 332–58.

Moore P, Naumann M, editors. Handbook of botulinum toxin treatment. 2nd ed. Oxford: Blackwell Scientific; 2003.

Phukan J, Albanese A, Gasser T, Warner T. Primary dystonia and dystonia-plus syndromes: clinical characteristics, diagnosis, and pathogenesis. *Lancet Neurol.* 2011; **10**: 1074–85.

Van Harten PN, Hoek HW, Kahn RS. Acute dystonia induced by drug treatment. *BMJ.* 1999; **319**: 623–6.

Warner TT, Bressman SB, editors. Clinical diagnosis and management of dystonia. Abingdon: Informa Healthcare; 2007.

Cross References

Anismus; Blepharospasm; Dysphonia; Eyelid apraxia; Fatigue; Gaping; Hemidystonia; Sensory tricks; Torticollis; Writer's cramp

Dystypia

Dystypia describes a specific impairment in typewriting, particular using a personal computer, in the absence of aphasia, agraphia, apraxia or other neuropsychological deficit. Two types have been suggested according to whether typing errors are predominantly linguistic (frontal type) or spatial (parietal type)

References

Cook FA, Makin SD, Wardlaw J, Dennis MS. Dystypia in acute stroke not attributable to aphasia or neglect. *BMJ Case Rep.* 2013; **2013**. pii: bcr2013200257.

Otsuki M, Nakagawa Y, Imamura H, Ogata A. Dystypia: frontal type and parietal type. *J Neurol.* 2011; **258**(Suppl 1): S189 (abstract P696).

Cross References

Agraphia; Aphasia; Dystextia

E

Ear Click
- see PALATAL MYOCLONUS; TINNITUS

Eastchester Clapping Sign
The Eastchester clapping sign is advocated as an early and sensitive sign of hemispatial ego-centric neglect. Patients are asked to clap: those with neglect perform one handed motions which stop at the midline. Hemiplegic patients without neglect reach across the midline and clap against their plegic hand.

Reference
Ostrow LW, Llinas RH. Eastchester clapping sign: a novel test of parietal neglect. *Ann Neurol.* 2009; **66**: 114–7.

Cross Reference
Neglect

Echolalia
Echolalia is the involuntary repetition of an interviewer's speech utterances (as opposed to the voluntary mickey-taking which characterises an irritating game typical of childhood, but sometimes indulged in by adults). This may be observed in a variety of clinical situations:

- Transcortical sensory aphasia:

  In the context of a fluent aphasia with repetition often well or normally preserved, usually as a result of a vascular lesion of the left hemisphere although an analogous situation may be encountered in Alzheimer's disease; "incorporational echolalia", when the patient uses the examiner's question to help form an answer, may be observed as a feature of "dynamic aphasia" which bears resemblance to transcortical motor aphasia, but may result from a frontal lesion; this has also been reported in progressive supranuclear palsy.

- Transcortical motor aphasia:

  "Effortful echolalia" has been reported in the context of infarction of the left medial frontal lobe, including the supplementary motor area, showing that neither the ability to repeat nor fluent speech is required for echolalia.

- Tourette syndrome:

  As a complex vocal tic, along with coprolalia.

- Alzheimer's disease, frontotemporal lobar degeneration, Creutzfeldt-Jakob disease:

  As a symptom of cognitive impairment/dementia.

- Epilepsy:

  From a left frontal lobe (supplementary motor area) focus.

- Schizophrenia:

  As a catatonic symptom.

- Early infantile autism, mental retardation:

  As a reflection of pathological mental development.

© Springer International Publishing Switzerland 2016
A.J. Larner, *A Dictionary of Neurological Signs*,
DOI 10.1007/978-3-319-29821-4_5

- Frontal lobe lesions:
    As a feature of imitation behaviour.
- Normal children:
    At a particular stage of language acquisition.

References
Hadano K, Nakamura H, Hamanaka T. Effortful echolalia. *Cortex*. 1998; **34**: 67–82.
Mendez MF. Prominent echolalia from isolation of the speech area. *J Neuropsychiatry Clin Neurosci*. 2002; **14**: 356–7.
Cross References
Aphasia; Coprolalia; Dynamic aphasia; Imitation behaviour; Jargon aphasia; Logorrhoea; Palilalia; Transcortical aphasias

Echolocation
More usually associated with bats and dolphins, humans can also echolocate, either passively (*e.g.* by listening for echoes bouncing off furniture) or actively by making tongue clicks and listening for echoes, a skill which allows some blind individuals to undertake activities such as mountain biking. Compensatory enhancement (cross-modal plasticity) underlies this faculty.
Reference
Thaler L, Arnott SR, Goodale MA. Neural correlates of natural human echolocation in early and late blind echolocation experts. *PLoS One*. 2011; **6**: e20162.

Echophenomena
A number of echophenomena are described in the neurological literature: echolalia, echopraxia, echolocation. The term echophenomena has sometimes been used interchangeably with imitation behaviour.
Reference
Larner AJ. Neurological signs: echo phenomena. *Adv Clin Neurosci Rehabil*. 2015; **15**(3): 16.
Cross Reference
Imitation behaviour

Echopraxia
Echopraxia is the involuntary, automatic, imitation of an interviewer's movements. This may be observed as a feature of apraxic syndromes such as corticobasal degeneration, as a complex motor tic in Tourette syndrome, and in frontal lobe disorders (imitation behaviour), and rarely as an ictal phenomenon.
Reference
Pridmore S, Brüne M, Ahmadi J, Dale J. Echopraxia in schizophrenia: possible mechanisms. *Aust N Z J Psychiatry*. 2008; **42**: 565–71.
Cross References
Copropraxia; Imitation behaviour; Tic

Écriture En Double Miroir
- see MIRROR WRITING

Ectropion
- see LID RETRACTION

Eidetic Memory
Eidetic, or "photographic", memory is an enhancement of memory function to prodigious capacity, beyond hypermnesia. Synaesthesia may be linked to eidetic memory, synaesthesia being used as a mnemonic aid.

Reference
Luria AR. The mind of a mnemonist. New York: Basic Books; 1968.
Cross Reference
Synaesthesia

Eight-And-A-Half Syndrome
The combination of a facial (VII) nerve palsy with a one-and-a-half syndrome due to a pontine lesion has been labelled the eight-and-a-half syndrome. Recognised causes include infarction and inflammation (*e.g.* multiple sclerosis). Patients may develop oculopalatal myoclonus months to years after the onset of the ocular motility problem.
References
Eggenberger EJ. Eight-and-a-half syndrome: One-and-a-half syndrome plus cranial nerve VII palsy. *J Neuroophthalmol*. 1998; **18**: 114–6.
Nandhagopal R, Krishnamoorthy SG. Eight-and-a-half syndrome. *J Neurol Neurosurg Psychiatry*. 2006; **77**: 463.
Wolin MJ, Trent RG, Lavin PJM, Cornblath WT. Oculopalatal myoclonus after the one-and-a-half syndrome with facial nerve palsy. *Ophthalmol*. 1996; **103**: 177–80.
Cross References
Facial paresis, Facial weakness; Myoclonus; One-and-a-half syndrome; Palatal myoclonus

Ekbom's Syndrome
Ekbom's syndrome or delusional parasitosis (not to be confused with Willis-Ekbom syndrome or disease, better known as restless legs syndrome) is a condition in which patients believe with absolute certainty that insects, maggots, lice or other vermin infest their skin or other parts of the body. Sometimes other psychiatric features may be present, particularly if the delusions are part of a psychotic illness such as schizophrenia or depressive psychosis. Females are said to be more commonly affected. Clinical examination may sometimes show evidence of skin picking, scratching, or dermatitis caused by repeated use of antiseptics. The patient may produce skin fragments or other debris as "evidence" of infestation. Treatment should be aimed at the underlying condition if appropriate; if the delusion is isolated, antipsychotics such as pimozide may be tried.
References
Enoch MD, Ball HN. Uncommon psychiatric syndromes. 4th ed. London: Arnold; 2001. p. 209–23.
Karroum E, Konofal E, Arnulf I. Karl-Axel Ekbom (1907-1977). *J Neurol*. 2009; **256**: 683–4.
Lombardi C, Belli D, Passalacqua G. When allergology meets psychiatry: delusional parasitosis (Ekbom's syndrome). *Eur Ann Allergy Clin Immunol*. 2011; **43**: 89–91.
Cross Reference
Delusion

Emotionalism, Emotional Lability
Emotionalism, or emotional lability, or emotional incontinence, implies both frequent and unpredictable changes in emotional expression, for example tearfulness followed shortly by elation, and an inappropriate expression of emotion, for example uncontrollable ("uninhibited" or disinhibited) laughter or crying. A distinction may be drawn between the occurrence of these phenomena spontaneously or without motivation, or in situations which although funny or sad are not particularly so. Also, a distinction may be made between such phenomena when there is congruence of mood and affect, sometimes labelled with terms such as moria or *witzelsucht* (*e.g.* laughing when feeling happy or elated), and when there is no such congruence (e.g. laughing when not feeling happy or elated), sometimes labelled as pathological, forced, or inappropriate laughter and crying.
    The neurobehavioural state of emotional lability reflects frontal lobe (especially orbitofrontal) lesions, often vascular in origin, and may coexist with disinhibited behaviour. It is more common in vascular dementia than Alzheimer's disease. It may also be seen in delirium

and in psychiatric disorders (mania). Pathological laughter and crying may occur as one component of pseudobulbar palsy ("pseudobulbar affect").

Reference
Heilman KM, Blonder LX, Bowers D, Valenstein E. Emotional disorders associated with neurological diseases. In: Heilman KM, Valenstein E, editors. Clinical neuropsychology. 4th ed. Oxford: Oxford University Press; 2003. p. 447–78.

Cross References
Delirium; Disinhibition; Frontal lobe syndromes; Moria; Pathological crying, Pathological laughter; Pseudobulbar palsy; *Witzelsucht*

Emprosthotonos

Emprosthotonos is an abnormal posture consisting of flexion of the head on the trunk and the trunk on the knees, sometimes with flexion of the limbs (*cf.* opisthotonos). Such attacks of "bowing" may be seen in infantile epilepsy syndromes such as West's syndrome, sometimes called salaam seizures or jack-knife spasms. Describing the tonic spasms of tetanus, Gowers noted that "Opisthotonic spasm is the rule, to which the exceptions are few. Rarely the trunk is bent forwards, from predominant cramp in the abdominal muscles and other flexors of the spine – "emprosthotonos". Still more rarely there is slight lateral flexion, "pleurotothonos", or the trunk and neck are rigid in a straight line, "orthotonos"."

Reference
Gowers WR. Manual of diseases of the nervous system, vol 2, 2nd ed. London: J&A Churchill; 1893. p. 682.

Cross References
Opisthotonos; Seizures; Spasm

Encephalopathy

Encephalopathy is a general term referring to any acute or chronic diffuse disturbance of brain function (literally "sick brain"). Characteristically it is used to describe an altered level of consciousness, which may range from drowsiness to a failure of selective attention, to hypervigilance; with or without: disordered perception, memory (*i.e.* cognitive deficits); epileptic seizures; headache; abnormal movements such as tremor, myoclonus, or asterixis; and focal neurological deficits (less common). Clearly these features overlap with those of delirium, sometimes itself denoted as "toxic-metabolic encephalopathy".

As with terms such as coma and stupor, it is probably better to give a description of the patient's clinical state rather than use a term that is open to variable interpretation.

Although the term encephalopathy is sometimes reserved for metabolic causes of diffuse brain dysfunction, this usage is not universal. Conditions which may be described as an encephalopathy include:

- Metabolic disorders: hypoxia/ischaemia, hypoglycaemia; organ failure, electrolyte disturbances, hypertension.
- Drug/toxin ingestion.
- Brain inflammation/infection (*e.g.* encephalitis).
- Miscellaneous conditions, *e.g.* Alzheimer's disease, Creutzfeldt-Jakob disease.

Cross References
Asterixis; Coma; Delirium; Myoclonus; Stupor; Tremor

En Garde Position
- see FENCER'S POSTURE, FENCING POSTURE

Enhanced Ptosis

Enhanced ptosis describes the increased drooping (*i.e.* worsening) of a ptotic eyelid when the contralateral eyelid is manually lifted. Enhanced ptosis may be explained by the action of Hering's law of equal innervation to paired yoked muscles (*i.e.* the eyelids). Recognised causes of enhanced ptosis include myasthenia gravis, Miller Fisher syndrome, botulism, and Lambert Eaton myasthenic syndrome

Reference
Gorelick PB, Rosenberg M, Pagano RJ. Enhanced ptosis in myasthenia gravis. *Arch Neurol.* 1981; **38**: 531.

Cross References
Curtainng; Ptosis

Enophthalmos
Enophthalmos is an inward displacement of the eyeball (sinking or withdrawal) into the eye socket (*cf.* exophthalmos). It is classically described as one of the cardinal features of Horner's syndrome (along with miosis, ptosis, and anhidrosis) but is seldom actually measured. Enophthalmos may also occur in dehydration (probably the most common cause), orbital trauma (*e.g.* orbital floor fracture), senile orbital fat atrophy, hemifacial atrophy (Parry-Romberg syndrome), and orbital tumour causing tethering and posterior traction on the eyeball.

Cross References
Anhidrosis; Exophthalmos; Horner's syndrome; Miosis; Parry-Romberg syndrome; Ptosis

Entomopia
Entomopia (literally "insect eye") is the name given to a grid-like pattern of multiple copies of the same visual image; hence, this is a type of polyopia. This phenomenon has been reported in migraine; its pathogenesis is uncertain.

References
Larner AJ. Entomopia. *Adv Clin Neurosci Rehabil.* 2006; **6**(4): 30.
Lopez JR, Adornato BT, Hoyt WF. "Entomopia": a remarkable case of cerebral polyopia. *Neurology.* 1993; **43**: 2145–6.

Cross Reference
Polyopia

Entrainment Test
An entrainment test has been advocated for the identification of psychogenic tremor, in which the examiner asks the patient to tap another limb at a different frequency to the tremor. Entrainment of tapping and tremor suggests that the latter is psychogenic.

Reference
Roper LS, Saifee TA, Parees I, Rickards H, Edwards MJ. How to use the entrainment test in the diagnosis of functional tremor. *Pract Neurol.* 2013; **13**: 396–8.

Cross Reference
Tremor

Environmental Dependency Syndrome
- see IMITATION BEHAVIOUR; UTILIZATION BEHAVIOUR

Environmental Tilt
Environmental tilt, also known as tortopia, is the sensation that visual space is tilted on its side or even upside down ("floor-on-ceiling" phenomenon, "upside-down" reversal of vision, *verkehrtsehen*). This may last seconds to minutes. The temptation to dismiss such bizarre symptoms as functional should be resisted, since environmental tilt is presumed to reflect damage to connections between cerebellar and central vestibular-otolith pathways causing cortical mismatch of visual and vestibular three-dimensional coordinate maps. It has been reported in the following situations:

- Posterior circulation ischaemia: lateral medullary syndrome of Wallenberg, transient ischaemic attacks in basilar artery territory.
- Demyelinating disease.

- Head injury.
- Encephalitis.
- Following third ventriculostomy for hydrocephalus.

Reference
Sierra-Hildago F, de Pablo-Fernandez E, Herrero-San Martin A et al. Clinical and imaging features of the room tilt illusion. *J Neurol.* 2012; **259**: 2555–64.
Cross References
Lateral medullary syndrome; Vertigo; Vestibulo-ocular reflexes

Epiphora
Epiphora is overflow of tears down the cheek. This may be due to a blocked nasolacrimal duct, or irritation to the cornea causing increased lacrimation, but it may also be neurological in origin, *e.g.* due to the sagging of the lower eyelid (ectropion) in a peripheral facial (VII) nerve (Bell's) palsy, or the "crocodile tears" following aberrant facial nerve regeneration. Lacrimation is also a feature of trigeminal autonomic cephalalgias such as cluster headache.
Cross References
Bell's palsy; Crocodile tears

Epley Manoeuvre
- see HALLPIKE MANEOUVRE, HALLPIKE TEST; VERTIGO

Erythropsia
This name has been given to a temporary distortion of colour vision in which objects take on an abnormal reddish hue. This has been characterized as a visual illusion. There are various causes, including drug use, visual diseases, and pseudophakia.
Cross References
Illusion; "Monochromatopsia"; Phantom chromatopsia

Esophoria
Esophoria is a variety of heterophoria in which there is a tendency for the visual axes to deviate inward (latent convergent strabismus). Clinically this may be observed using the cover-uncover test as an outward movement of the covered eye as it is uncovered. Esophoria may occur in individuals with hyperopia (long-sightedness).
Cross References
Cover tests; Exophoria; Heterophoria

Esotropia
Esotropia is a variety of heterotropia in which there is manifest inward turning of the visual axis of one eye; the term is synonymous with convergent strabismus. It may be demonstrated using the cover test as an outward movement of the eye which is forced to assume fixation by occlusion of the other eye.

Esotropia may be associated with congenital latent nystagmus (*i.e.* nystagmus appearing when one eye is covered) in the presence of amblyopia; the slow phase in the viewing eye is towards the nose.

With lateral rectus muscle paralysis, the eyes are esotropic or crossed on attempted lateral gaze towards the paralysed side, but the images are uncrossed. Acute esotropia has been described following contralateral thalamic infarction.
Cross References
Amblyopia; Cover tests; Diplopia; Exotropia; Heterotropia; Nystagmus

Eutonia
Kinnier Wilson used this term to describe an emotional lack of concern associated with the dementia of multiple sclerosis. It may perhaps reflect the cognitive anosognosia of a dementia syndrome.

Ewart Phenomenon
This is the elevation of ptotic eyelid on swallowing, a synkinetic movement. The mechanism is said to be aberrant regeneration of fibres from the facial (VII) nerve to the oculomotor (III) nerve innervating the levator palpebrae superioris muscle.
Cross References
Ptosis; Synkinesia, Synkinesis

Exophoria
Exophoria is a variety of heterophoria in which there is a tendency for the visual axes to deviate outward (latent divergent strabismus). Clinically this may be observed in the cover-uncover test as an inward movement as the covered eye is uncovered. Exophoria may occur in individuals with myopia, and may be physiological in many subjects because of the alignment of the orbits.
Cross References
Cover tests; Esophoria; Heterophoria

Exophthalmos
Exophthalmos is forward displacement of the eyeball. The definition and the causes overlap with proptosis. The most common cause is dysthyroid eye disease (Graves' disease).
Cross References
Lid retraction; Proptosis

Exosomaesthesia
The sensory disturbance associated with parietal lobe lesions may occasionally lead the patient to refer the source of a stimulus to some point outside the body, exosomaesthesia. A possible example occurs in Charles Dickens's novel *Hard Times* (1854) in which Mrs Gradgrind locates her pain as "somewhere in the room".

Exotropia
Exotropia is a variety of heterotropia in which there is manifest outward turning of the visual axis of an eye; the term is synonymous with divergent strabismus. It may be demonstrated using the cover test as an inward movement of the eye which is forced to assume fixation by occlusion of the other eye.
    When the medial rectus muscle is paralysed, the eyes are exotropic (wall-eyed) on attempted lateral gaze towards the paralysed side, and the images are crossed.
Cross References
Cover tests; Esotropia; Heterotropia

Extensor Posturing
- see DECEREBRATE RIGIDITY

External Malleolar Sign
- see CHADDOCK'S SIGN

External Ophthalmoplegia
- see OPHTHALMOPARESIS, OPHTHALMOPLEGIA

Extinction
The failure to sense a stimulus on one side when stimulation is simultaneously presented on both sides was described by Morris Bender as extinction to simultaneous stimulation. Extinction is the failure to respond to a novel or meaningful sensory stimulus on one side when a homologous stimulus is given simultaneously to the contralateral side (*i.e.* double simultaneous stimulation); it is sometimes called "suppression". The stimuli may be visual, auditory, or tactile, *e.g.* asking the patient to say which hand is touched when the eyes are shut. It is important to show that the patient responds appropriately to each hand being

touched individually, but then neglects one side when both are touched simultaneously. With repeated testing the phenomenon may break down: extinguishing of extinction.

More subtle defects may be tested using simultaneous bilateral heterologous (asymmetrical) stimuli, although it has been shown that some normal individuals may show extinction in this situation.

A motor form of extinction has been postulated, manifesting as increased limb akinesia when the contralateral limb is used simultaneously (hemiakinesia).

The presence of extinction is one of the behavioural manifestations of neglect, and most usually follows non-dominant (right) hemisphere (parietal lobe) lesions. There is evidence for physiological interhemispheric rivalry or competition in detecting visual stimuli from both hemifields, which may account for the emergence of extinction following brain injury.

Reference
Fink GR, Driver J, Rorden C, Baldeweg T, Dolan RJ. Neural consequences of competing stimuli in both visual hemifields: a physiological basis for visual extinction. *Ann Neurol.* 2000; **47**: 440–6.

Cross References
Akinesia; Hemiakinesia; Neglect; Visual extinction

Extrapyramidal Signs
- see PARKINSONISM

Eyelid Apraxia
Eyelid apraxia is an inability to open the eyelids at will, although they may open spontaneously at other times (*i.e.* there is voluntary-automatic dissociation). Eyelids may be opened manually or by a backwards head thrust. The term has been criticised on the grounds that this may not always be a true "apraxia", in which case the term "levator inhibition" may be preferred since the open eyelid position is normally maintained by tonic activity of the levator palpebrae superioris. Clinically there is no visible contraction of orbicularis oculi, which distinguishes eyelid apraxia from blepharospasm (however, perhaps paradoxically, the majority of cases of eyelid apraxia occur in association with blepharospasm). Neurophysiological studies do in fact show abnormal muscle contraction in the pre-tarsal portion of orbicularis oculi, which has prompted the suggestion that "focal eyelid dystonia" may be a more appropriate term. Although the phenomenon may occur in isolation, associations have been reported with:

- Progressive supranuclear palsy (Steele-Richardson-Olszewski syndrome).
- Parkinson's disease.
- Huntington's disease.
- Multiple system atrophy.
- MPTP intoxication.
- Motor neurone disease.
- Acute phase of nondominant hemisphere cerebrovascular event.
- Wilson's disease.
- Neuroacanthocytosis.

The precise neuroanatomical substrate is unknown but the association with basal ganglia disorders points to involvement of this region. The underlying mechanisms may be heterogeneous, including involuntary inhibition of levator palpebrae superioris. Botulinum toxin injections may be helpful in some patients.

References
Kanazawa M, Shimohata T, Sato M, Onodera O, Tanaka K, Nishizawa M. Botulinum toxin A injections improve apraxia of eyelid opening without overt blepharospasm associated with neurodegenerative diseases. *Mov Disord.* 2008; **22**: 597–8.
Kerty E, Eidal K. Apraxia of eyelid opening: clinical features and therapy. *Eur J Ophthalmol.* 2006; **16**: 204–8.
Cross References
Apraxia; Blepharospasm; Dystonia

Eyelid Retraction
- see LID RETRACTION

F

"Face-Hand Test"
- see "ARM DROP"

Facial Paresis, Facial Weakness

Facial paresis, or prosopoplegia, may result from:

- Central (upper motor neurone) lesions.
- Peripheral (lower motor neurone; facial (VII) nerve) lesions.
- Neuromuscular junction transmission disorders.
- Primary disease of muscle (*i.e.* myogenic).

Facial paresis is thus clinically heterogeneous: not all facial weakness is Bell's palsy.

- *Upper motor neurone facial weakness* ("central facial palsy"):

  The ability to raise the eyebrow is preserved due to the bilateral supranuclear connections to the frontalis muscle. A dissociation between volitional and emotional facial movements may also occur. Emotional facial palsy refers to the absence of emotional facial movement but with preserved volitional movements, as may be seen with frontal lobe (especially non-dominant hemisphere) precentral lesions (as in abulia, Fisher's sign) and in medial temporal lobe epilepsy with contralateral mesial temporal sclerosis. Conversely, volitional paresis without emotional paresis may occur when corticobulbar fibres are interrupted (precentral gyrus, internal capsule, cerebral peduncle, upper pons).

  Causes of upper motor neurone facial paresis include:

  Unilateral:

  Hemisphere infarct (with hemiparesis).
  Lacunar infarct (facio-brachial weakness, +/− dysphasia).
  Space occupying lesions: intrinsic tumour, metastasis, abscess.

  Bilateral:

  Motor neurone disease.
  Diffuse cerebrovascular disease.
  Pontine infarct (locked-in syndrome).

- *Lower motor neurone facial weakness* (peripheral origin):

  If this is due to facial (VII) nerve palsy, it results in ipsilateral weakness of frontalis (*cf.* upper motor neurone facial paresis), orbicularis oculi, buccinator, orbicularis oris and platysma. Clinically this produces:

  drooping of the side of the face with loss of the nasolabial fold.
  widening of the palpebral fissure with failure of lid closure (lagophthalmos).
  eversion of the lower lid (ectropion) with excessive tearing (epiphora).
  inability to raise the eyebrow, close the eye, frown, blow out the cheek, show the teeth, laugh, and whistle.
  +/− dribbling of saliva from the paretic side of the mouth.
  depression of the corneal reflex (efferent limb of reflex arc affected).
  speech alterations: softening of labials (p, b).

© Springer International Publishing Switzerland 2016

A.J. Larner, *A Dictionary of Neurological Signs,*
DOI 10.1007/978-3-319-29821-4_6

Depending on the precise location of the facial nerve injury, there may also be paralysis of the stapedius muscle in the middle ear, causing sounds to seem abnormally loud (especially low tones: hyperacusis), and impairment of taste sensation on the anterior two-thirds of the tongue if the chorda tympani is affected (ageusia, hypogeusia). Lesions within the facial canal distal to the meatal segment cause both hyperacusis and ageusia; lesions in the facial canal between the nerve to stapedius and the chorda tympani cause ageusia but no hyperacusis; lesions distal to the chorda tympani cause neither ageusia nor hyperacusis (*i.e.* facial motor paralysis only). Lesions of the cerebellopontine angle cause ipsilateral hearing impairment and corneal reflex depression (afferent limb of the corneal reflex arc affected) in addition to facial weakness. There is also a sensory branch to the posterior wall of the external auditory canal which may be affected resulting in local hypoaesthesia (Hitselberg sign).

Causes of lower motor neurone facial paresis include:

- Bell's palsy: idiopathic lower motor neurone facial weakness, assumed to result from a viral neuritis.
- Herpes zoster (Ramsey Hunt syndrome).
- Diabetes mellitus.
- Lyme disease (neuroborreliosis, Bannwarth's disease).
- Sarcoidosis.
- Leukaemic infiltration, lymphoma.
- HIV seroconversion.
- Neoplastic compression (*e.g.* cerebellopontine angle tumour; rare).
- Facial nerve neuroma.

These latter conditions may need to be differentiated from Bell's palsy.
In bilateral facial weakness, particular consideration should be given to the possibility of:

- Guillain-Barré syndrome.
- HIV.
- Lyme disease.
- Sarcoidosis.
- Malignant infiltration.
- Amyloidosis.

Causes of recurrent facial paresis of lower motor neurone type include:

- Diabetes mellitus.
- Lyme disease.
- Sarcoidosis.
- Leukaemia, lymphoma.

In myasthenia gravis, a disorder of neuromuscular transmission at the neuromuscular junction, there may be concurrent ptosis, diplopia, bulbar palsy and limb weakness, and evidence of fatigable weakness.

Myogenic facial paresis may be seen in facioscapulohumeral (FSH) dystrophy, myotonic dystrophy, and mitochondrial disorders. In primary disorders of muscle the pattern of weakness and family history may suggest the diagnosis.

References
Borod JC, Koff E, Lorch MP, Nicholas M, Welkowitz J. Emotional and non-emotional facial behaviour in patients with unilateral brain damage. *J Neurol Neurosurg Psychiatry.* 1988; **51**: 826–32.
Hopf HC, Muller-Forell W, Hopf NJ. Localization of emotional and volitional facial paresis. *Neurology*. 1992; **42**: 1918–23.

Jacob A, Cherian PJ, Radhakrishnan K, Sankara SP. Emotional facial paresis in temporal lobe epilepsy: its prevalence and lateralizing value. *Seizure*. 2003; **12**: 60–4.
Masterson L, Vallis M, Quinlivan R, Prinsley P. Assessment and management of facial nerve palsy. *BMJ*. 2015; **351**: h3725.

Cross References

Abulia; Ageusia; Bell's palsy; Bell's phenomenon, Bell's sign; *Bouche de tapir*; Cerebellopontine angle syndrome; Clapham's sign; Corneal reflex; Eight-and-a-half syndrome; Epiphora; Fisher's sign; Hitselberg sign; Hyperacusis; Lagophthalmos; Locked-in syndrome; Lower motor neurone (LMN) syndrome; Pseudobulbar palsy; Upper motor neurone (UMN) syndrome

Facilitation

Facilitation describes the increase in impulse transmission across the neuromuscular junction detected following repeated muscle contraction (*cf.* fatigue). Clinically, facilitation may be demonstrated by the brief appearance of tendon reflexes which are absent at rest following prolonged (*ca.* 10–30 s) forced maximal contraction against resistance, *e.g.* the biceps jerk after elbow flexion, knee jerk after knee extension; and by Lambert's sign (increased force of grip with sustained contraction; this increase in strength of affected muscles detected in the first few seconds of maximal voluntary contraction may also be known as augmentation) Increments in compound muscle action potentials are seen after exercise or high frequency repetitive nerve stimulation.

These phenomenona of post-tetanic potentiation are most commonly seen in the Lambert-Eaton myasthenic syndrome (LEMS), a disorder of neuromuscular junction transmission associated with the presence of autoantibodies directed against presynaptic voltage-gated calcium ion (Ca^{2+}) channels (VGCC). The mechanism is thought to be related to an increased build up of Ca^{2+} ions within the presynaptic terminal with the repetitive firing of axonal action potentials, partially overcoming the VGCC antibody-mediated ion channel blockade, and leading to release of increasing quanta of acetylcholine.

Cross References

Augmentation; Fatigue; Lambert's sign

"False-Localising Signs"

Neurological signs may be described as "false-localising" when their appearance reflects pathology distant from the expected anatomical locus. The classic example, and probably the most frequently observed, is abducens (VI) nerve palsy (unilateral or bilateral) in the context of raised intracranial pressure, presumed to result from stretching of the nerve over the ridge of the petrous temporal bone. Many false-localising signs occur in the clinical context of raised intracranial pressure, either idiopathic (idiopathic intracranial hypertension [IIH]) or symptomatic (secondary to tumour, haematoma, abscess). A brief topographical overview of false-localising signs, moving from central to peripheral, includes:

- Motor system:

    Amyotrophy of parietal lobe origin affecting the upper limb (Silverstein syndrome).
    Kernohan's notch syndrome: false-localising hemiparesis.
    Cerebellar syndrome with anterior cerebral artery territory infarction damaging frontocerebellar pathways.
    Brainstem compression causing diaphragm paralysis.
- Sensory system:

    Sensory level with parietal lobe lesion (with or without amyotrophy of upper limb muscles: Christiansen-Silverstein syndrome).
    Hemianopia due to raised intracranial pressure if temporal lobe herniation causes posterior cerebral artery compromise.
    Radicular symptoms (pseudoradicular syndrome) with thalamic lesion.

- Cranial nerves:

    Proptosis with middle cranial fossa tumour.

    Oculomotor (III) nerve palsy with contralateral supratentorial lesion.

    Divisional oculomotor nerve palsy with brainstem or subarachnoid space pathology.

    Trochlear nerve palsy with IIH.

    Trigeminal nerve palsy with IIH.

    Abducens nerve palsy with IIH.

    Facial nerve palsy with IIH.

    Vestibulocochlear nerve dysfunction with IIH.

- Spinal cord and roots:

    Foramen magnum/upper cervical cord lesion causing hand muscle wasting ("remote atrophy").

    Lower cervical/upper thoracic myelopathy producing mid-thoracic girdle sensation.

    Urinary retention with rostral spinal cord compression.

    Radiculopathy with IIH, may even mimic Guillain-Barré syndrome.

(More details may be found in specific entries.)

Of note, some of these so-called false localising signs may simply reflect incorrect diagnosis: for example, virtually all reported cases of Silverstein or Christiansen-Silverstein syndrome predate the advent of modern neuroimaging techniques.

References

Larner AJ. False localising signs. *J Neurol Neurosurg Psychiatry.* 2003; **74**: 415–18.

Larner AJ. A topographical anatomy of false-localising signs. *Adv Clin Neurosci Rehabil.* 2005; **5**(1): 20–1.

O'Connell JE. Trigeminal false localizing signs and their causation. *Brain.* 1978; **101**: 119–42.

Cross References

Abducens (VI) nerve palsy; Divisional palsy; "Dorsal guttering"; Girdle sensation; Kernohan's notch syndrome; Oculomotor (III) nerve palsy; Proptosis; Pseudoradicular syndrome; Urinary retention

Fan Sign (*Signe De L'éventail*)
- see BABINSKI'S SIGN (1)

Fasciculation

Fasciculation refers to rapid, flickering, twitching, involuntary movements within a muscle belly resulting from spontaneous activation of a bundle, or fasciculus, of muscle fibres (*i.e.* a motor unit), insufficient to produce movement around a joint. Fasciculation may also be induced by lightly tapping over a partially denervated muscle belly. The term was formerly used synonymously with fibrillation, but the latter term is now reserved for contraction of a single muscle fibre, or a group of fibres smaller than a motor unit. Fasciculation may need to be distinguished clinically and neurophysiologically from myokymia or neuromyotonia.

Brief and localized fasciculation can be a normal finding (*e.g.* in the intrinsic foot muscles, especially abductor hallucis, and gastrocnemius, but not tibialis anterior), particularly if unaccompanied by other neurological symptoms and signs (wasting, weakness, sensory disturbance, sphincter dysfunction). Such benign fasciculation may cause anxiety, particularly in clinicians.

Persistent fasciculation most usually reflects a pathological process involving the lower motor neurones in the anterior (ventral) horn of the spinal cord and/or in brainstem motor nuclei, typically motor neurone disease (in which cramps are an early associated symptom). Facial and perioral fasciculations are highly characteristic of spinal and bulbar muscular atrophy (Kennedy's disease). However, fasciculation is not pathognomonic of lower motor neurone pathology since it may on rare occasions be seen with upper motor neurone pathology.

The pathophysiological mechanism of fasciculation is thought to be spontaneous discharge from motor nerves, but the site of origin of this discharge is uncertain. Although ectopic neural discharge from anywhere along the lower motor neurone from cell body to nerve terminal could produce fasciculation, the commonly encountered assumption that this originates from the anterior horn cell body is not entirely supported by the available evidence, which points to an additional, more distal, origin in the motor axons. Denervation of muscle fibres may lead to nerve fibre sprouting (axonal and collateral) with subsequent enlargement of motor units which makes fasciculation more obvious clinically.

Fasciculation may be seen in:

- Motor neurone disease (amyotrophic lateral ascelrosis) with lower motor neurone involvement (*i.e.* progressive muscular atrophy, progressive bulbar atrophy, flail limb variants).
- Other motor neurone disorders: spinal muscular atrophy; spinal and bulbar muscular atrophy (Kennedy's disease, X-linked bulbospinal muscular atrophy), especially perioral: chin fasciculations may be pathognomonic for Kennedy's disease; facial onset sensory and motor neuronopathy (FOSMN).
- Cervical radiculopathy (restricted to myotomal distribution).
- Multifocal motor neuropathy with conduction block.
- Benign fasciculation syndrome: typically seen only after exercise and without associated muscle atrophy or weakness; cramp-fasciculation syndrome. Extensive longitudinal follow-up may be required to confirm the "benign" label.
- Almost any lower motor neurone disease, especially compression.
- Metabolic causes: thyrotoxicosis, tetany, after treatment with acetylcholinesterase inhibitors, anaesthetic muscle relaxants.

References
Desai J, Swash M. Fasciculations: what do we know of their significance? *J Neurol Sci.* 1997; **152**(suppl1): S43–8.
Kleine BU, Stegeman DF, Schelhaas HJ, Zwarts MJ. Firing pattern of fasciculations in ALS: evidence for axonal and neuronal origin. *Neurology.* 2008; **70**: 353–9.
Simon NG, Kiernan MC. Fasciculation anxiety syndrome in clinicians. *J Neurol.* 2013; **260**: 1743–7.
Singh V, Gibson J, McLean B, Boggild M, Silver N, White R. Fasciculations and cramps: how benign? Report of four cases progressing to ALS. *J Neurol.* 2011; **258**: 573–8.
Cross References
Calf hypertrophy; Cramp; Fibrillation; Flail arm; Lower motor neurone (LMN) syndrome; Myokymia; Neuromyotonia

Fast Micrographia
In "fast" micrographia, written letters are small from the outset of writing, sometimes approximating to a straight line, though produced at normal speed without fatigue. This pattern has been observed in progressive supranuclear palsy and with globus pallidus lesions, and contrasts with "slow" micrographia, writing which becomes progressively slower and smaller, as seen in idiopathic Parkinson's disease.

References
Meenakshisundaram U, Velmurugendran CU, Prabash PR. Fast micrographia: an unusual but distinctive sign. *Ann Indian Acad Neurol.* 2013; **16**: 172–3.
Quinn NP. Fast micrographia and pallidal pathology. *J Neurol Neurosurg Psychiatry.* 2002; **72**: 135. (abstract).

Cross Reference
Micrographia

Fatigue
The term fatigue may be used in different neurological contexts to refer to both a sign and a symptom.

The sign of fatigue, also known as peripheral fatigue, consists of a reduction in muscle strength or endurance with repeated muscular contraction. This most characteristically occurs in disorders of neuromuscular junction transmission (*e.g.* myasthenia gravis), but it may also be observed in disorders of muscle (*e.g.* myopathy, polymyositis) and neurogenic atrophy (*e.g.* motor neurone disease). In myasthenia gravis, fatigue may be elicited in the extraocular muscles by prolonged upgaze, causing eyelid drooping; in bulbar muscles by prolonged counting or speech, causing hypophonia; and in limb muscles by repeated contraction, especially of proximal muscles (*e.g.* shoulder abduction, "wing flaps"), leading to weakness in previously strong muscles. Fatigue in myasthenia gravis is thought to be caused by a decline in the amount of acetylcholine released from motor nerve terminals with successive neural impulses, along with a reduced number of functional acetylcholine receptors (AChR) at the motor end-plates, due to binding of AChR antibodies and/or complement mediated destruction of the postsynaptic folds. Decrements in compound muscle action potentials are seen after repetitive nerve stimulation.

Fatigue may also be used to describe a gradual decline in the amplitude and speed of initiation of voluntary movements, hypometria and hypokinesia, as seen in disorders of the basal ganglia, especially Parkinson's disease, *e.g.* "slow" micrographia may be ascribed to "fatigue". Progressive supranuclear palsy is notable for lack of such fatigue.

Fatigue as a symptom, or central fatigue, is an enhanced perception of effort and limited endurance in sustained physical and mental activities. This may occur in multiple sclerosis (MS), post-polio syndrome, post-stroke syndromes, and chronic fatigue syndrome (CFS). In MS and CFS, fatigue may be a prominent and disabling complaint even though neurological examination reveals little or no clinical deficit. Fatigue may be evaluated with various instruments, such as the Krupp Fatigue Severity Score. This type of fatigue is ill-understood: in MS, frequency-dependent conduction block in demyelinated axons has been suggested, as has hypothalamic pathology. Current treatment is symptomatic (amantadine, modafanil, 3,4-diaminopyridine) and rehabilitative (graded exercise).

References
Chaudhuri A, Behan PO. Fatigue in neurological disorders. *Lancet*. 2004; **363**: 978–88.
Induruwa I, Constantinescu CS, Gran B. Fatigue in multiple sclerosis – a brief review. *J Neurol Sci.* 2012; **323**: 9–15.
Cross References
Dystonia; Hypokinesia; Hypometria; Micrographia; Weakness

Fehlleistungen
- see PARAPRAXIA, PARAPRAXIS

Femoral Nerve Stretch Test
The femoral nerve stretch test (FNST), or reverse straight leg raising test, consists of extension of the hip with the knee straight with the patient lying prone, a manoeuvre which exerts traction on the femoral nerve or L3 root and may exacerbate pain in a femoral neuropathy or L3 radiculopathy, perhaps caused by a retroperitoneal haemorrhage. Crossed FNST is reported to be sensitive for high lumbar radiculopathy.

Typical ipsilateral sciatic pain induced by the performing FNST may be indicative of a L4/L5 intervertebral disc protrusion.

References
Christodoulides AN. Ipsilateral sciatica on femoral nerve stretch test is pathognomonic of an L4/5 disc protrusion. *J Bone Joint Surg Br.* 1989; **71**: 88–9.

Nadler SF, Malanga GA, Stitik TP, Keswani R, Foye PM. The crossed femoral nerve stretch test to improve diagnostic sensitivity for the high lumbar radiculopathy: 2 case reports. *Arch Phys Med Rehabil*. 2001; **82**: 522–3.
Cross Reference
Lasègue's sign

Fencer's Posture, Fencing Posture
Epileptic seizures arising in or involving the supplementary motor area may lead to adversial head and eye deviation, abduction and external rotation of the contralateral arm, flexion at the elbows, and posturing of the legs, with maintained consciousness, a phenomenon christened by Penfield the "fencing posture" because of its resemblance to the *en garde* position adopted by fencers. These seizures may also be known as "salutatory seizures".
Cross Reference
Seizures

Festinant Gait, Festination
Festinant gait or festination is a gait disorder characterized by rapid short steps (Latin: *festinare*, to hurry, hasten, accelerate) due to inadequate maintenance of the body's centre of gravity over the legs. To avoid falling and to maintain balance the patient must "chase" the centre of gravity, leading to an increasing speed of gait and a tendency to fall forward when walking (propulsion). A similar phenomenon may be observed if the patient is pulled backwards (retropulsion). Festination may also be associated with freezing of gait.

Festination is common in idiopathic Parkinson's disease; it is associated with longer duration of disease and higher Hoehn & Yahr stage of disease. Festination may be related to the flexed posture and impaired postural reflexes commonly seen in these patients. It is less common in symptomatic causes of parkinsonism, but has been reported, for example in aqueduct stenosis.
References
Giladi N, Shabtai H, Rozenberg E, Shabtai E. Gait festination in Parkinson's disease. *Parkinsonism Relat Disord*. 2001; **7**: 135–8.
Leheta O, Boschert J, Krauss JK, Whittle IR. Festination as the leading symptom of late onset idiopathic aqueduct stenosis. *J Neurol Neurosurg Psychiatry*. 2002; **73**: 599–600.
Morris ME, Iansek R, Galna B. Gait festination and freezing in Parkinson's disease: pathogenesis and rehabilitation. *Mov Disord*. 2008; **23**(Suppl2): S451–60. [Erratum *Mov Disord*. 2008; **23**: 1639–40].
Cross References
Freezing of gait; Parkinsonism; Postural reflexes

Fibrillation
Fibrillation was previously synonymous with fasciculation, but the term is now reserved for the spontaneous contraction of a single muscle fibre, or a group of fibres smaller than a motor unit, hence this is more appropriately regarded as a sign detected on neurophysiological testing (fibrillation potential) without clinical correlate.
Cross Reference
Fasciculation

Finger Agnosia
Finger agnosia is a type of tactile agnosia, in which there is inability to identify which finger has been touched when the eyes are closed, despite knowing that a finger has been touched; or inability to point to or move a finger when it is named; or inability to name the fingers (patient's own fingers or those of another person). This is a disorder of body schema, and may be regarded as a partial form of autotopagnosia.

Finger agnosia is most commonly observed with lesions of the dominant parietal lobe. It may occur in association with acalculia, agraphia, and right-left disorientation, with or without alexia and difficulty spelling words, hence as one feature of Gerstmann syndrome. It may be more common in indivduals with synaesthesia. Isolated cases of finger agnosia in association with left corticosubcortical posterior parietal infarction have been reported. Since this causes no functional deficit, it may be more common than reported. It may be found in Alzheimer's disease.

References
Davis AS, Trotter JS, Hertza J, Bell CD, Dean RS. Finger agnosia and cognitive deficits in patients with Alzheimer's disease. *App Neuropsychol Adult.* 2012; **19**: 116–20.
Della Sala S, Spinnler H. Finger agnosia: fiction or reality? *Arch Neurol.* 1994; **51**: 448–50.
Cross References
Agnosia; Autotopagnosia; Gerstmann syndrome; Synaesthesia

"Finger Chase"
- see ATAXIA; CEREBELLAR SYNDROMES

Finger Drop
- see WRIST DROP

Finger-Floor Distance
In patients with leg (+/− low back) pain suspected of having lumbosacral nerve root compression, a finger-floor distance of > 25 cm when the patient bends forward and attempts to touch the floor with the fingers has been found to be an independent predictor of radiological (MR imaging) compression. This was not the case for the straight leg raising test.
Reference
Vroomen PCAJ, de Krom MCTFM, Wilmink JT, Kester ADM, Knottnerus JA. Diagnostic value of history and physical examination in patients suspected of lumbosacral nerve root compression. *J Neurol Neurosurg Psychiatry.* 2002; **72**: 630–4.
Cross Reference
Lasègue's sign

"Finger-to-Nose Test"
- see ATAXIA; CEREBELLAR SYNDROMES

Fisher's Sign
Fisher's sign is the paucity of facial expression conveying emotional states or attitudes (emotional facial paresis). It follows nondominant (right) hemisphere lesions and may accompany emotional dysprosody of speech.
Cross References
Abulia; Aprosodia, Aprosody; Facial paresis, Facial weakness

Fist-Edge-Palm Test
In the fist-edge-palm test, sometimes known as the Luria test or three step motor sequence, the patient is requested to place the hand successively in three positions, imitating movements made by the examiner and then doing them alone: fist, vertical palm, palm resting flat on table. Copying motor sequences assesses motor programming ability. Defects in this programming, such as lack of kinetic melody, loss of sequence, or repetition of previous pose or position, are especially conspicuous with anterior cortical lesions. This test is incorporated into the Frontal Assessment Battery.
References
Dubois B, Slachevsky A, Litvan I, Pillon B. The FAB: a frontal assessment battery at bedside. *Neurol.* 2000; **55**: 1621–6.
Luria AR. Higher cortical functions in man. 2nd ed. New York: Basic Books; 1980. p. 423–4.
Cross Reference
Frontal lobe syndromes

Flaccidity
Flaccidity refers to floppiness, which implies a loss of normal muscular tone (hypotonia). This may occur transiently after acute lesions of the corticospinal tracts (flaccid paraparesis), before the development of spasticity, or as a result of lower motor neurone syndromes. It is sometimes difficult to separate the change in tone from concurrent weakness.
Cross References
Hypotonia, Hypotonus; Lower motor neurone (LMN) syndrome

Flail Foot
- see CAUDA EQUINA SYNDROME; FOOT DROP

Flail Limb
Flail limb (flail arm, flail leg) refers to severe and symmetrical limb wasting and weakness without significant functional involvement of other regions. These are variant forms of motor neurone disease (amyotrophic lateral sclerosis), the "flail arm syndrome" having previously been described as Vulpian-Bernhart's form. Alternative designations for flail arm syndrome include amyotrophic brachial diplegia, dangling arm syndrome, and neurogenic man-in-a-barrel syndrome.

Men are reported to be much more frequently affected than women, and this group as a whole shows improved survival compared to other motor neurone disease patients. Cognition may be relatively well preserved, as for other isolated lower motor neurone forms of motor neurone disease.
References
Larner AJ. Neuropsychological neurology. The neurocognitive impairments of neurological disorders. Cambridge: Cambridge University Press; 2008. p. 68.
Wijesekera LC, Mathers S, Talman P, et al. Natural history and clinical features of the flail arm and flail leg ALS variants. *Neurology*. 2009; **72**: 1087–94.
Cross References
Amyotrophy; "Man-in-the-barrel"

Flap, Flapping Tremor
- see ASTERIXIS

Flexibilitas Cerea **(Waxy Flexibility)**
- see CATATONIA

Flexion-Adduction Sign
Neuralgic amyotrophy (Parsonage-Turner syndrome) may cause arm pain, which may be prevented by holding the arm flexed at the elbow and adducted at the shoulder.
Reference
Waxman SG. The flexion-adduction sign in neuralgic amyotrophy. *Neurology*. 1979; **29**: 1301–4.

Flexor Posturing
- see DECORTICATE RIGIDITY

Flexor Spasms
- see SPASM

"Flick Sign"
A flicking, shaking movement of the hands made by patients with carpal tunnel syndrome to try to relieve the paraesthesia and pain caused by the condition, typically noted on waking at night, may be described as the "flick sign". This may be the most sensitive and specific of the various signs described in carpal tunnel syndrome.

References
D'Arcy CA, McGee S. Does this patient have carpal tunnel syndrome? *JAMA*. 2000; **283**: 3110–7.
Hi ACF, Wong S, Griffith J. Carpal tunnel syndrome. *Pract Neurol*. 2005; **5**: 210–7.
Cross References
Phalen's sign; Tinel's sign

Floccillation
- see CARPHOLOGIA, CARPHOLOGY

Flycatcher Tongue
- see TROMBONE TONGUE

Flynn Phenomenon
The Flynn phenomenon is paradoxical constriction of the pupils in darkness. This has been documented in various conditions including congenital achromatopsia, following optic neuritis, and in autosomal dominant optic atrophy.

Reference
Frank JW, Kushner BJ, France TD. Paradoxic pupillary phenomena: a review of patients with pupillary constriction to darkness. *Arch Ophthalmol*. 1988; **106**: 1564–6.
Cross Reference
Pupillary reflexes

"*Folles Larmes Prodromiques*"
- see *FOU RIRE PRODROMIQUE*

"Fonzarelli" Sign
This name has been given to focal thumb dystonia in Parkinson's disease, a movement reminiscent of the "thumbs up" gesture associated with the character of Arthur "Fonzie" Fonzarelli in the US TV sitcom *Happy Days* broadcast in the 1970s and 1980s.

Reference
Turner MR, Matthews L, Ebers GC. Teaching video NeuroImage: the "Fonzarelli" sign: focal thumb dystonia as an early manifestation of Parkinson disease. *Neurology*. 2008; **71**: e11.
Cross Reference
Dystonia

Foot Drop
Foot drop, often manifest as the foot dragging during the swing phase of the gait, causing tripping and/or falls, may be due to upper or lower motor neurone lesions, which may be distinguished clinically.

- *Stiff foot drop, with upper motor neurone lesions*:

    leads to a circumducting gait; it may be possible to see or hear the foot dragging or scuffing along the floor, and this may cause excessive wear on the point of the shoe. There will be other upper motor neurone signs (hemiparesis; spasticity, clonus, hyperreflexia, Babinski's sign).

    Causes of stiff foot drop include:

    - Cerebral infarct.
    - Motor neurone disease.
- *Floppy foot drop, with lower motor neurone lesions*:

    leads to a stepping gait (steppage) to try to lift the foot clear of the floor in the swing phase, and a slapping sound on planting the foot. At worst, there is a flail foot in which both the dorsiflexors and the plantar flexors of the foot are weak (*e.g.* in high sciatic nerve or sacral plexus lesions). Other lower motor neurone signs may be present (hypotonia, areflexia or hyporeflexia).

Causes of floppy foot drop include:

- Isolated common peroneal nerve palsy: the most common cause, usually due to compression of the nerve at the head of the fibula, causing painless weakness in foot dorsiflexion and eversion, sensory loss on the anterolateral leg and dorsum of the foot, with normal reflexes; may have a Tinel sign on tapping the nerve over the fibular head.
- Sciatic neuropathy (rare).
- Lumbosacral plexopathy (rare; may be painful).
- L4/L5 radiculopathy: may also have hip abduction weakness, and sensory loss conforming to dermatomal boundaries; may be painful.
- Motor or sensorimotor polyneuropathy (*e.g.* hereditary motor and sensory neuropathy).
- Motor neuronopathy (anterior horn cell disease: look for fasciculation).
- Mononeuropathy multiplex (may be painful).

These may be distinguished on clinical and/or neurophysiological grounds. Foot drop may also occur with myopathies and muscular dystrophies.
Reference
Stevens F, Weerkamp NJ, Cals JWL. Foot drop. *BMJ*. 2015; **350**: h1736.
Cross References
Cauda equina syndrome; Dermatomal sensory loss; Hemiparesis; Lower motor neurone (LMN) syndrome; Neuropathy; Steppage, Stepping gait; Upper motor neurone (UMN) syndrome

Foot Grasping
- see GRASP REFLEX

Forced Ductions
Forced ductions, performed by grasping the anaesthetised sclera with forceps and then moving the eye through its range of motions, may be used to determine whether restricted eye movement is mechanical, due to a lesion within the orbit, such as thyroid ophthalmopathy or superior oblique tendon sheath (Brown's) syndrome.

Forced Grasping
- see GRASP REFLEX

Forced Groping
Forced groping describes involuntary movements of a hand, as if searching for an object or item which has touched or brushed against it; the hand may follow the object around if it moves ("magnetic movements"). There may be an accompanying grasp reflex. This type of behaviour may be displayed by an alien hand, most usually in the context of corticobasal degeneration. Forced groping may be conceptualised as an exploratory reflex which is "released" from frontal lobe control by a pathological process, as in utilization behaviour.
Reference
Adie WS, Critchley M. Forced grasping and groping. *Brain*. 1927; **50**: 142–70.
Cross References
Alien hand, Alien limb; Grasp reflex; Magnetic movements; Utilization behaviour

Forced Laughter and Crying
- see EMOTIONALISM, EMOTIONAL LABILITY; PATHOLOGICAL CRYING, PATHOLOGICAL LAUGHTER

Forced Upgaze

Forced upgaze describes tonic upward gaze deviation, which may be seen in coma after diffuse hypoxic-ischaemic brain injury with relative sparing of the brainstem. Forced upgaze may also be psychogenic, in which case it is overcome by cold caloric stimulation of the ear drums. Forced upgaze must be differentiated clinically from oculogyric crisis.

Cross References
Caloric testing; Coma; Oculogyric crisis

Forearm and Finger Rolling

The forearm and finger rolling tests detect subtle upper motor neurone lesions with high specificity and modest sensitivity. Either the forearms or the index fingers are rapidly rotated around each other in front of the torso for about 5 s, then the direction is reversed. Normally the appearance is symmetrical but with a unilateral upper motor neurone lesion one arm or finger remains relatively stationary, with the normal rotating around the abnormal limb. Thumb rolling may also be a sensitive test for subtle upper motor neurone pathology.

Reference
Anderson NE. The forearm and finger rolling tests. *Pract Neurol*. 2010; **10**: 39–42.

Cross References
Bed cycling test; Pronator drift; Thumb rolling test; Upper motor neurone (UMN) syndrome

Foreign Accent Syndrome

The foreign accent syndrome is a rare phonological disorder, such that speech production includes non-native vowels or consonants and hence sounds as though it is foreign, or different from the speaker's native intonation. There is no language disorder since comprehension of spoken and written language is preserved; hence it is qualitatively different from Broca's aphasia. This syndrome probably overlaps with other disorders of speech production, labelled as phonetic disintegration, pure anarthria, aphemia, apraxic dysarthria, verbal or speech apraxia, and cortical dysarthria. Case heterogeneity is noted; some cases may be non-organic.

References
Kurowski KM, Blumstein SE, Alexander M. The foreign accent syndrome: a reconsideration. *Brain Lang*. 1996; **54**: 1–25.
Monrad-Krohn GH. Dysprosody or altered "melody" of language. *Brain*. 1947; **70**: 405–15.
Ryalls J, Miller N. Foreign accent syndromes: the stories people have to tell. Hove: Psychology Press; 2014.

Cross References
Aphasia; Aphemia; Aprosodia, Aprosody

Formication

Formication is a tactile or haptic visceral hallucination, as of ants crawling over the skin. It may occur in isolation, perhaps reflecting spontaneous neuronal firing from cutaneous afferents reaching conscious threshold, or in the context of Ekbom's syndrome (delusional parasitosis).

Cross References
Ekbom's syndrome; Hallucination; Paraesthesia; Tinel's sign

Fortification Spectra

Fortification spectra, also known as teichopsia, are visual hallucinations which occur as an aura, either in isolation (migraine aura without headache) or prior to an attack of migraine (migraine with aura; "classical migraine"). The appearance is a radial array likened to the design of medieval castles, not simply of battlements. Hence these are more complex visual phenomena than simple flashes of light (photopsia) or scintillations. They are thought to result from spreading depression, of possible ischaemic origin, in the occipital cortex. The term was first used by John Fothergill (1712–1780) in his 1778 publication on "Sick Head-Ach" (sic), from which he himself suffered. The visions of Hildegard von Bingen (1098–1179), illustrated in the 12th century, are thought possibly to reflect migrainous fortification spectra.

References
Fothergill J. Remarks on that complaint commonly known under the name of the Sick-Head-ach. *Med Obs Inq.* 1778; **3**: 219–43.
Plant GT. The fortification spectra of migraine. *BMJ.* 1986; **293**: 1613–7.
Singer C. The visions of Hildegard of Bingen. In: From magic to science. Essays on the scientific twilight. London: Ernest Benn; 1928.p. 199–239.

Cross References
Aura; Hallucination; Photopsia; Teichopsia

Foster Kennedy Syndrome
The Foster Kennedy syndrome consists of optic atrophy in one eye with optic disc oedema in the other eye. Anosmia ipsilateral to the optic atrophy may also be found.

This syndrome is classically due to a tumour, typically an olfactory groove meningioma, which compresses the ipsilateral optic nerve to cause atrophy, and also causes raised intracranial pressure with consequent contralateral papilloedema.

Similar clinical appearances have been reported in other conditions, sometimes called a pseudo-Foster Kennedy syndrome, such as sequential anterior ischaemic optic neuropathy and idiopathic intracranial hypertension.

Reference
Kennedy F. Retrobulbar neuritis as an exact diagnostic sign of certain tumors and abscesses in the frontal lobe. *Am J Med Sci.* 1911; **142**: 355–68.

Cross References
Disc swelling; Optic atrophy; Papilloedema

Fou Rire Prodromique
Fou rire prodromique, or laughing madness, was first described by Féré in 1903. It consists of pathological (mood incongruent) laughter which heralds the development of stroke, typically in the brainstem as a consequence of basilar artery occlusion but sometimes in the capsular genu.

Pathological crying as a prodrome of brainstem stroke has also been described (*"folles larmes prodromiques"*).

References
Coelho M, Ferro JM. Fou rire prodromique. Case report and systematic review of the literature. *Cerebrovasc Dis.* 2003; **16**: 101–4.
Larner AJ. Basilar artery occlusion associated with pathological crying: "folles larmes prodromiques"? *Neurology.* 1998; **51**: 916–7.
Larner AJ. Charles Féré (1852-1907). *J Neurol.* 2011; **258**: 524–5.

Cross Reference
Pathological crying, Pathological laughter

Freezing of Gait
Freezing of gait is defined as a brief episodic absence or a marked reduction of forward progression of the feet despite the intention to walk. This occurs in Parkinson's disease and other forms of parkinsonism (progressive supranucelar palsy, vascular parkinsonism). Various clinical patterns are reported, including trembling in place, shuffling forward, and complete akinesia.

This is one of the unpredictable motor fluctuations in late Parkinson's disease, associated with longer duration of disease and treatment, which may lead to falls, usually forward onto the knees, and injury. It may occur at gait initiaition, in confined spaces (*e.g.* doorways), when trying to turn, or when trying to do two things at once. Freezing of gait may occur either during an off period or wearing off period, or randomly, *i.e.* unrelated to drug dosage or timing.

There are no clear treatment protocols for freezing of gait. Strategies include use of dopaminergic agents and, anecdotally, L-threodops, but these agents are not reliably helpful, particularly in random freezing. Methylphenidate has also been tried. Use of visual targets (real or imagined) may help, *e.g.* stepping over a line.

References
Lewis SJ, Barker RA. A pathophysiological model of freezing of gait in Parkinson's disease. *Parkinsonism Relat Disord.* 2009; **15**: 333–8.
Nonnekes J, Snijders AH, Nutt JG, Deuschl G, Giladi N, Bloem BR. Freezing of gait: a practical approach to management. *Lancet Neurol.* 2015; **14**: 768–78.
Okuma Y. Practical approach to freezing of gait in Parkinson's disease. *Pract Neurol.* 2014; **14**: 222–30.

Cross Reference
Parkinsonism

Fregoli Syndrome
- see DELUSION

Frey's Syndrome
- see GUSTATORY SWEATING

Froment's Sign
Jules Froment has two eponymous signs:

- Activated rigidity or synkinesis; sometimes known as Froment's manoeuvre.
- In an ulnar nerve lesion, flexion of the distal phalanx of the thumb (flexor pollicis longus, innervated by the median nerve) is seen when attempting to squeeze a sheet of paper between the thumb and the index finger, as a compensation for the weakness of thumb adduction (adductor pollicis, innervated by the ulnar nerve), also known as Froment's prehensile thumb sign, or the *signe du journal* or newspaper sign The term is also sometimes used for weakness of little finger adduction (palmar interossei), evident when trying to grip a piece of paper between the ring and little finger.

Reference
Broussolle E, Rethy MP, Thobois S. Jules Froment (1878-1946). *J Neurol.* 2009; **256**: 1581–2.

Cross References
Rigidity; Synkinesia, Synkinesis; Wartenberg's sign (1)

Frontal Ataxia
- see ATAXIA

Frontal Lobe Syndromes
The frontal lobes of the brain have enlarged greatly during phylogeny; their diverse connections with the basal ganglia, basal forebrain, and cerebellum, as well as other cortical areas, reflect their multiple motor and behavioural functions. Damage to the frontal lobes may produce a variety of clinical signs, most frequently changes in behaviour. Such changes may easily be overlooked with the traditional neurological examination, although complained of by patient's relatives, and hence specific bedside tests of frontal lobe function should be utilized, for example:

- Verbal fluency: e.g. letter/phonemic (F, A, S) probably a more specific test than category/semantic (animals, foods).
- Proverb interpretation: *e.g.* "Make hay while the sun shines"; "Too many cooks spoil the broth"; interpretation tends to be concrete in frontal lobe disorders.

- Cognitive estimates: *e.g.* height of the Post Office Tower in London, length of a man's spine, distance from London to Edinburgh; may be grossly abnormal or inappropriate.
- Copying motor sequences, to assess motor programming ability: *e.g.* Luria fist-edge-palm test (three step motor sequence with hand).
- Alternating sequence tests: *e.g.* alternating finger flexion/extension out of phase in two hands, or repeatedly writing m n m n m n (also used as tests of praxis, which may be affected with frontal lobe pathology); swapping a coin from hand to hand behind back in a predictable pattern and asking the patient which hand the coin is in.
- Set-shifting or go/no go tests, in which an alternating pattern is suddenly changed, *e.g.* changing the previously predictable (left/right) pattern of coin hidden in clenched hand swapped over behind back; rhythmic tapping with pen on a surface (I tap once, you tap twice; I tap twice, you tap once); tests of response inhibition (ask patient to clap three times, s/he does so multiple times, the applause sign).

A useful clinico-anatomical classification of frontal lobe syndromes which reflects the functional subdivisions of the frontal lobes is as follows:

- *Orbitofrontal syndrome* ("disinhibited"):
  disinhibited behaviour (including sexual disinhibition), impulsivity.
  inappropriate affect, *witzelsucht*, euphoria.
  emotional lability (moria).
  lack of judgment, insight.
  distractibility, lack of sustained attention; hypermetamorphosis.
  motor perseverations are not a striking feature.
- *Medial prefrontal syndrome* ("apathetic, akinetic"):
  little spontaneous movement, bradykinesia, hypokinesia.
  sparse verbal output (akinetic mutism).
  urinary incontinence.
  sensorimotor signs in lower limbs.
  indifference to pain.
- *Frontal convexity or dorsolateral prefrontal syndrome* ("dysexecutive"):
  apathy; abulia, indifference.
  motor perseveration.
  difficulty planning, adapting to changing environmental demands, set-shifting; stimulus boundedness.
  reduced verbal fluency.
  deficient motor programming, *e.g.* three step hand sequence, rhythmical tapping (go/no-go test).

Overlap between these regional syndromes may occur.

These frontal lobe syndromes may be accompanied by various neurological signs (frontal release signs or primitive reflexes). Other phenomena associated with frontal lobe pathology include imitation behaviours (echophenomena) and, less frequently, utilization behaviour, features of the environmental dependency syndrome.

Frontal lobe syndromes may occur as a consequence of various pathologies:

- Neurodegenerative diseases: especially behavioural variant frontotemporal lobar degeneration; occasionally in Alzheimer's disease.
- Structural lesion: tumour (intrinsic, extrinsic), normal pressure hydrocephalus.
- Cerebrovascular event.
- Head injury.
- Inflammatory metabolic disease: multiple sclerosis, X-linked adrenoleukodystrophy.

References
Damasio AR, Anderson SW. The frontal lobes. In: Heilman KM, Valenstein E, editors.
Clinical neuropsychology. 4th ed. Oxford: Oxford University Press; 2003. p. 404–46.
Rosen HJ, Allison SC, Schauer GF, Gorno-Tempini ML, Weiner MW, Miller
BL. Neuroanatomical correlates of behavioural disorders in dementia. *Brain*. 2005; **128**:
2612–25.
Cross References
Abulia; Akinesia; Akinetic mutism; Alternating fist closure test; Apathy; Applause sign;
Attention; Disinhibition; Dysexecutive syndrome; Emotionalism, Emotional lability;
Fist-edge-palm test; Frontal release signs; Hypermetamorphosis; Hyperorality;
Hyperphagia; Hypersexuality; Perseveration; Urinary incontinence; Utilization behav-
iour; *Witzelsucht*

Frontal Release Signs
Frontal release signs are so named because of the belief that they are released from frontal
inhibition by diffuse pathology within the frontal lobes (usually vascular or neurodegenerative) with which they are often associated, although they may be a feature of normal ageing.
Some of these responses are present during infancy but disappear during childhood, hence
the terms "primitive reflexes" or "developmental signs" are also used (Babinski's sign may
therefore fall into this category). The term "psychomotor signs" has also been used since
there is often accompanying change in mental status. The frontal release signs may be categorised as:

- *Prehensile*:

  Sucking reflex (tactile, visual).
  Grasp reflex: hand, foot.
  Rooting reflex (turning of the head towards a tactile stimulus on the face).
- *Nociceptive*:

  Snout reflex.
  Pout reflex.
  Glabellar (blink) reflex.
  Palmomental reflex.

The corneomandibular and nuchocephalic reflexes may also be categorised as "frontal
release" signs. (More details may be found in specific entries.)
Some of these signs are of little clinical value (*e.g.* palmomental reflex). Concurrent clinical findings may include dementia, gait disorder (frontal gait, *marche à petit pas*), urinary
incontinence, akinetic mutism and *gegenhalten*. Common causes of these findings are diffuse
cerebrovascular disease and motor neurone disease, and they may be more common in
dementia with Lewy bodies than other causes of an extrapyramidal syndrome. All increase
with age in normal individuals.
References
Borroni B, Broli M, Constanzi C, et al. Primitive reflex evaluation in the clinical assessment
of extrapyramidal syndromes. *Eur J Neurol*. 2006; **13**: 1026–8.
Franssen EH. Neurologic signs in ageing and dementia. In: Burns A, editor. Ageing and
dementia: a methodological approach. London: Edward Arnold; 1993. p. 144–74.
Van Boxtel MP, Bosma H, Jolles J, Vreeling FW. Prevalence of primitive reflexes and the
relationship with cognitive change in healthy adults: a report from the Maastricht Aging
Study. *J Neurol*. 2006; **253**: 935–41.
Cross References
Age-related signs; Babinski's sign (1); Corneomandibular reflex; *Gegenhalten*; Grasp reflex;
Marche à petit pas; Palmomental reflex; Pout reflex; Rooting reflex; Sucking reflex

Fugue

Fugue, and fugue-like state, are used to refer to a syndrome characterized by loss of personal memory (hence the alternative name of "twilight state"), automatic and sometimes repetitive behaviours, and wandering or driving away from normal surroundings. Fugue may be:

- Psychogenic: associated with depression (sometimes with suicide); alcoholism, amnesia; "hysteria".
- Epileptic: complex partial seizures.
- Narcoleptic.

Some patients with frontotemporal dementia may spend the day walking long distances, and may be found a long way from home, unable to give an account of themselves, and aggressive if challenged; generally they are able to find their way home (spared topographical memory) despite their other cognitive deficits.

Cross References

Amnesia; Automatism; Dementia; Poriomania; Seizures

Functional Weakness and Sensory Disturbance

Various signs have been deemed useful indicators of functional or "non-organic" neurological illness, including:

- Collapsing or "give way" weakness.
- Hoover's sign.
- Babinski's trunk-thigh test.
- "Arm drop".
- *Belle indifférence.*
- Sternocleidomastoid sign.
- Midline splitting sensory loss.
- Functional postures, gaits:
    - monoplegic "dragging".
    - fluctuation of impairment.
    - excessive slowness, hesitation.
    - "psychogenic Romberg" sign.
    - "walking on ice".
    - uneconomic posture, waste of muscle energy, excessive effort.
    - sudden knee buckling.

Although such signs may be suggestive, their diagnostic utility has never been formally investigated in prospective studies, and many, if not all, have been reported with "organic" illness. Hence it is unwise to rely on them as diagnostic indicators.

References

Lempert T, Brandt T, Dieterich M, et al. How to identify psychogenic disorders of stance and gait: a video study in 37 patients. *J Neurol.* 1991; **238**: 140–6.

Stone J, Warlow C, Sharpe M. The symptom of functional weakness: a controlled study of 107 patients. *Brain.* 2010; **133**: 1537–51.

Cross References

"Arm drop"; Babinski's trunk-thigh test; *Belle indifférence*; Collapsing weakness; Harvey's sign; Hoover's sign; Sternocleidomastoid test; "Wrestler's sign"

Funnel Vision

- see "TUNNEL VISION"

G

Gag Reflex

The gag reflex is elicited by touching the posterior pharyngeal wall, tonsillar area, or the base of the tongue, with the tip of a thin wooden ("orange") stick. Depressing the tongue with a wooden spatula, and the use of a torch for illumination of the posterior pharynx, may be required to get a good view. There is a palatal response (palatal reflex), consisting of upward movement of the soft palate with ipsilateral deviation of the uvula; and a pharyngeal response (pharyngeal reflex or gag reflex) consisting of visible contraction of the pharyngeal wall. Lesser responses include medial movement, tensing, or corrugation of the pharyngeal wall. In addition there may be head withdrawal, eye watering, coughing, and retching. Hence there is variability of response in different individuals. Some studies claim the reflex is absent in many normal individuals, especially with increasing age, without evident functional impairment; whereas others find it in all healthy individuals, although variable stimulus intensity is required to elicit it.

The afferent limb of the reflex arc is the glossopharyngeal (IX) nerve, the efferent limb in the glossopharyngeal and vagus (X) nerves. Hence individual or combined lesions of the glossopharyngeal and vagus nerves depress the gag reflex, as in neurogenic bulbar palsy.

Dysphagia is common after a stroke, and the gag reflex is often performed to assess the integrity of swallowing. Some argue that absence of the reflex does not predict aspiration and is of little diagnostic value, since this may be a normal finding in elderly individuals, whereas pharyngeal sensation (feeling the stimulus at the back of the pharynx) is rarely absent in normals and is a better predictor of the absence of aspiration. Others find that even a brisk pharyngeal response in motor neurone disease may be associated with impaired swallowing. Hence the value of the gag reflex remains debatable. A videoswallow study may be a better technique to assess the integrity of swallowing.

References
Davies AE, Kidd D, Stone SP, MacMahon J. Pharyngeal sensation and gag reflex in healthy subjects. *Lancet*. 1995; **345**: 487–8.
Hughes TAT, Wiles CM. Palatal and pharyngeal reflexes in health and motor neuron disease. *J Neurol Neurosurg Psychiatry*. 1996; **61**: 96–8.
Cross References
Bulbar palsy; Dysphagia

Gait Apraxia

Gait apraxia is a name that has been given to an inability to walk despite intact motor systems and sensorium. Patients with gait apraxia are often hesitant, seemingly unable to lift their feet from the floor or put one foot in front of the other ("magnetic gait", "gait ignition failure"). Arms may be held out at the sides to balance for fear of falling; fear may be so great that the patient sits in a chair gripping its sides. These phenomena may be observed with lesions of the frontal lobe and white matter connections, with or without basal ganglia involvement, for example in diffuse cerebrovascular disease and normal pressure hydrocephalus. A syndrome of isolated gait apraxia has been described with focal degeneration of the medial frontal lobes. Key neuroanatomical correlates include the supplementary motor area, parasagittal convexity premotor cortex, and subjacent white matter. In modern classifications of gait disorders, gait apraxia is subsumed into the categories of frontal gait disorder, frontal disequilibrium, and isolated gait ignition failure.

© Springer International Publishing Switzerland 2016
A.J. Larner, *A Dictionary of Neurological Signs*,
DOI 10.1007/978-3-319-29821-4_7

Gait apraxia is an important diagnosis to establish since those afflicted generally respond poorly, if at all, to physiotherapy; moreover, because both patient and therapist often become frustrated because of lack of progress, this form of treatment is often best avoided.

References
Elble RJ. Gait and dementia: moving beyond the notion of gait apraxia. *J Neural Transm.* 2007; **114**: 1253–8.
Nadeau SE. Gait apraxia: further clues to localization. *Eur Neurol.* 2007; **58**: 142–5.
Nutt JG, Marsden CD, Thompson PD. Human walking and higher-level gait disorders, particularly in the elderly. *Neurology.* 1993; **43**: 268–79.

Cross Reference
Apraxia

Gambling
Gambling may be characterised as an executive function task, amenable to testing with instruments such as the Iowa Gambling Task (IGT) and the Cambridge Gamble Task. The neuroanatomical substrates of such decision making are believed to encompass the prefrontal cortex and the amygdala.

Gambling may be defined as pathological when greater risks are taken and potential losses are correspondingly greater; this may be classified as an impulse control disorder. Pathological gambling may occur in patients with Parkinson's disease treated with various dopamine agonists, and in behavioural variant frontotemporal dementia patients who display risky decision-making, sometimes even in the early stages of disease and without evidence of behavioural disinhibition or impulsiveness.

References
Larner AJ. Gambling. *Adv Clin Neurosci Rehabil.* 2007; **7**(1): 26.
Manes FF, Torralva T, Roca M, Gleichgerrcht E, Bekinschtein TA, Hodges JR Frontotemporal dementia presenting as pathological gambling. *Nat Rev Neurol.* 2010; **6**: 347–52.
Siri C, Cilia R, De Gaspari D, et al. Cognitive status of patients with Parkinson's disease and pathological gambling. *J Neurol.* 2010; **257**: 247–52.

Cross Reference
Punding

Ganglionopathy
- see NEURONOPATHY

Ganser Phenomenon, Ganser Syndrome
The Ganser phenomenon consists of giving approximate answers to questions which can at times verge on the absurd (Q: "How many legs does a cow have?"; A: "Three"), also known as paralogia or *vorbereiden*. This may occur in psychiatric disease such as depression, schizophrenia, and malingering, and sometimes in neurological disease (head injury, epilepsy).

A Ganser syndrome of hallucinations, conversion disorder, cognitive disorientation and approximate answers is also described, but of uncertain nosology.

References
Dwyer J, Reid S. Ganser's syndrome. *Lancet.* 2004; **364**: 471–3.
Enoch MD, Ball HN. Uncommon psychiatric syndromes, 4th edn. London: Arnold; 2001, p. 74–94.
Jimenez-Gomez B, Quintero J. Ganser syndrome: review and case report. *Actas Espanolas de Psiquiatria* 2012; **40**: 161–4.

Gaping
Gaping, or involuntary opening of the mouth, may occur as a focal dystonia of the motor trigeminal nerve, also known as Brueghel syndrome after that artist's painting *De Gaper* ("Yawning man", *ca.* 1558) which is said to illustrate a typical case. Afflicted individuals may

also demonstrate paroxysmal hyperpnoea and upbeating nystagmus, suggesting a brainstem (possibly pontine) localization of pathology. The condition should be distinguished from other cranial dystonias with blepharospasm (Meige syndrome).

Reference
Gilbert GJ. Brueghel syndrome: its distinction from Meige syndrome. *Neurology*. 1996; **46**: 1767–9.
Cross References
Blepharospasm; Brueghel's syndrome; Dystonia; Nystagmus

Gaslight Phenomenon, Gaslight Syndrome
This describes a scenario in which one partner attempts to have the other labeled as insane or mentally ill, probably reflecting psychiatric illness (*e.g.* morbid jealousy) in the initiating partner. The name is taken from a 1938 play, *Gas Light*, by Patrick Hamilton, which dramatized this psychological phenomenon.
Reference
Kutcher SP. The gaslight syndrome. *Can J Psychiatry*. 1982; **27**: 224–7.

Gaze-Evoked Phenomena
A variety of symptoms have been reported to be evoked, on occasion, by alteration of the direction of gaze:

- Amaurosis: associated with a lesion, usually intraorbital, compressing the central retinal artery.
- Laughter.
- Nystagmus: usually indicative of a cerebellar lesion; may occur as a side-effect of medications; also convergence-retraction nystagmus on upgaze in dorsal midbrain (Parinaud's) syndrome.
- Phosphenes: increased mechanosensitivity in demyelinated optic nerve.
- Segmental constriction of the pupil (Czarnecki's sign) following aberrant regeneration of the oculomotor (III) nerve to the iris sphincter.
- Tinnitus: may develop after resection of cerebellopontine angle tumours, may be due to abnormal interaction between vestibular and cochlear nuclei.
- Vertigo.

Reference
Leopold NA. Gaze-induced laughter. *J Neurol Neurosurg Psychiatry*. 1977; **40**: 815–7.
Cross References
Amaurosis; Czarnecki's sign; Nystagmus; Parinaud's syndrome; Phosphene; Vertigo

Gaze Palsy
Gaze palsy is a general term for any impairment or limitation in conjugate (yoked) eye movements. This may be supranuclear, nuclear, or infranuclear in origin. Preservation of the vestibulo-ocular reflexes may help differentiate supranuclear gaze palsies from nuclear/ infranucelar causes.
Cross References
Locked-in syndrome; Ophthalmoparesis, Ophthalmoplegia; Supranuclear gaze palsy; Vestibulo-ocular reflexes

Gegenhalten
- see PARATONIA

Geophagia, Geophagy
Geophagia or geophagy describes earth or clay eating, reports of which dating back to Hippocratic times have been found. This behaviour may also fall under the rubric of pica, or pagophagia, a morbid craving for unusual or unsuitable food. It apparently occurs most

frequently in children and pregnant women and in tropical areas. Besides the obvious risk of infection from ingesting potentially contaminated material, geophagia may be associated with neurological complications. Cases of flaccid quadriparesis and of proximal myopathy associated with profound hypokalaemia in the context of geophagia have been reported, which may lead to walking difficulty.

References
Larner AJ. Neurological signs: geophagia (geophagy) and pica (pagophagia). *Adv Clin Neurosci Rehabil.* 2009; **9**(4): 20.
Woywodt A, Kiss A. Geophagia: the history of earth-eating. *J R Soc Med.* 2002; **95**: 143–6.
Young SL, Sherman PW, Lucks JB, Pelto GH. Why on earth? Evaluating hypotheses about the physiological functions of human geophagy. *Q Rev Biol.* 2011; **86**: 97–120.

Cross Reference
Pica

Gerstmann Syndrome
The Gerstmann syndrome, or angular gyrus syndrome, consists of a constellation of clinical features including acalculia, agraphia (of central type), finger agnosia, and right-left disorientation; there may in addition be alexia and difficulty spelling words but these are not necessary parts of the syndrome.

Gerstmann syndrome occurs with lesions of the angular gyrus and supramarginal gyrus in the posterior parietotemporal region of the dominant (usually left) hemisphere, for example infarction in the territory of the middle cerebral artery. Very occasional cases of "crossed Gerstmann syndrome" have been reported (*i.e.* right-sided lesion in a right-handed patient).

All the signs comprising Gerstmann syndrome do fractionate or dissociate, *i.e.* they are not causally related, or representative of a unitary neuropsychological function, as was once suggested. Hence this may be an example of a disconnection syndrome. Nonetheless the Gerstmann syndrome remains useful for the purposes of clinical localisation.

References
Rusconi E, Pinel P, Dehaene S, Kleinschmidt A. The enigma of Gerstmann's syndrome: a telling tale of the vicissitudes of neuropsychology. *Brain.* 2010; **133**: 320–32.
Rusconi E, Pinel P, Eger E, et al. A disconnection account of Gerstmann syndrome: functional neuroanatomy evidence. *Ann Neurol.* 2009; **66**: 654–62 [Erratum: *Ann Neurol.* 2009; **66**: 869].
Triarhou LC. Josef Gerstmann (1887–1969). *J Neurol.* 2008; **255**: 614–5.

Cross References
Acalculia; Agraphia; Alexia; Finger agnosia; Right-left disorientation

Geschwind Syndrome
The Geschwind, or Gastaut-Geschwind, syndrome comprises hypergraphia, hyperreligiosity, and hyposexuality. It may occur as part of an interictal psychosis in patients with complex partial seizures of temporal lobe origin, particularly with a non-dominant focus. This clinical picture has also been described in the context of frontotemporal dementia.

References
Postiglione A, Milan G, Pappata S, et al. Fronto-temporal dementia presenting as Geschwind's syndrome. *Neurocase.* 2008; **14**: 264–70.
Sandrone S. Norman Geschwind (1926–1984). *J Neurol.* 2013; **260**: 3197–8.
Trimble MR. The Gastaut-Geschwind syndrome. In: Trimble MR, Bolwig TG, editors. The temporal lobes and the limbic system. Petersfield: Wrightson Biomedical; 1992, p. 137–47.
Waxman SG, Geschwind N. The interictal behavior syndrome of temporal lobe epilepsy. *Arch Gen Psychiatry.* 1975; **32**: 1580–6.

Cross References
Hypergraphia; Hyperreligiosity; Hyposexuality

Geste Antagoniste
- see SENSORY TRICKS

Gibbus
Gibbus is an angulation of the spine due to vertebral collapse, which may be due to osteoporosis, metastatic disease, or spinal tuberculosis. There may be associated myelopathy if the spinal cord is compromised. Camptocormia (bent spine syndrome) enters the differential diagnosis.
Cross References
Camptocormia; Myelopathy

Girdle Sensation
Compressive lower cervical or upper thoracic myelopathy may produce spastic paraparesis with a false-localising mid-thoracic sensory level or "girdle sensation" (*cf.* cuirasse). The pathophysiology is uncertain, but ischaemia of the thoracic watershed zone of the anterior spinal artery from compression at the cervical level has been suggested. "Girdle-like tightening sensation" has also been described as a consequence of thoracic polyradiculopathy in sarcoidosis.
References
Ochiai H, Yamakawa Y, Minato S, Nakahara K, Nakano S, Wakisaka S. Clinical features of the localized girdle sensation of mid-trunk (false localizing sign) appeared [*sic*] in cervical compressive myelopathy patients. *J Neurol*. 2002; **249**: 549–53.
Yakushiji Y, Yamada K, Nagatsuka K, Hashimoto Y, Miyashita K, Naritomi H. "A girdle-like tightening sensation" misapprehended as abdominal splanchnopathy in a sarcoidosis patient. *Intern Med*. 2005; **44**: 647–52.
Cross References
"False-localising signs"; Paraparesis; Suspended sensory loss

"Give-Way" Weakness
- see COLLAPSING WEAKNESS; FUNCTIONAL WEAKNESS AND SENSORY DISTURBANCE

Glabellar Tap Reflex
The glabellar tap reflex, also known as Myerson's sign or the nasopalpebral reflex, is elicited by repeated gentle tapping with a finger on the forehead whilst observing the eyelids blink (*i.e.* blink reflex). Tapping is preferably done with irregular cadence, and in such as way that the patient cannot see the approaching finger (to avoid blinking due to the threat or menace reflex),
   Usually, reflexive blinking in response to tapping habituates quickly, but in extrapyramidal disorders it may not do so. This sign was once thought useful for the diagnosis of idiopathic Parkinson's disease but in fact it is fairly non-specific, occurring in many akinetic-rigid disorders.
References
Brodsky H, Vuong KD, Thomas M, Jankovic J. Glabellar and palmomental reflexes in parkinsonian disorders. *Neurology*. 2004; **63**: 1096–8.
Schott JM, Rossor MN. The grasp and other primitive reflexes. *J Neurol Neurosurg Psychiatry*. 2003; **74**: 558–60.
Cross References
Blink reflex; Parkinsonism

Glossolalia
Glossolalia, or speaking in tongues, may be considered a normal phenomenon in certain Christian denominations, as divinely inspired, since it is mentioned in the Bible (1 Corinthians, 14:27–33, although St Paul speaks here of the importance of an interpreter, since "God is not the author of confusion"), but it is not confined to adherents of Christianity or even overtly religious environments.
   Glossolalia may be conceptualised as a form of automatic speech, usually of a pseudolanguage which may be mistaken for a foreign tongue. Such happenings may occur in trance-like states, or in pathological states such as schizophrenia, possibly related to abnormal temporal lobe discharges. Some examples may in fact be jargon aphasia.

References
Enoch MD, Ball HN. Uncommon psychiatric syndromes, 4th edn. London: Arnold; 2001, p. 237–40.
Reeves RR, Kose S, Abubakr A. Temporal lobe discharges and glossolalia. *Neurocase*. 2014; **20**: 236–40.
Cross Reference
Jargon aphasia

"Glove And Stocking" Sensory Loss
Sensory loss, to all or selected modalities, confined to the distal parts of the limbs, the so-called "glove and stocking" distribution, implies the presence of a peripheral sensory neuropathy. If the neuropathy involves both sensory and motor fibres, motor signs (distal weakness, reflex diminution or loss) may also be present.
Cross References
Acroparaesthesia; Neuropathy

Goosebumps
- see ANSERINA

Gordon's Sign
Gordon's sign is an extensor plantar response in response to squeezing the calf muscles, also called the paradoxical flexor response. As with Chaddock's sign and Oppenheim's sign, this reflects an expansion of the receptive field of the reflex.
Cross References
Babinski's sign (1); Plantar response

Gowers' Manoeuvre, Gowers' Sign
Gowers' sign is a characteristic manoeuvre used by patients with proximal lower limb and trunk weakness to rise from the ground. From the lying position, the patient rolls to the kneeling position, pushes on the ground with extended forearms to lift the hips and straighten the legs, so forming a triangle with the hips at the apex with hands and feet on the floor forming the base (known in North America as the "butt-first manoeuvre"). The hands are then used to push on the knees and so lift up the trunk ("climbing up oneself").

This sign was originally described by Gowers in the context of Duchenne muscular dystrophy (or pseduohypertrophic muscular dystrophy, as Gowers called it) but it may be seen in other causes of proximal leg and trunk weakness, *e.g.* Becker muscular dystrophy, spinal muscular atrophy. Gowers was not the first to describe the sign; Bell had reported it almost 50 years before Gowers' account.

Gowers' name is also associated with a manoeuvre to stretch the sciatic nerve and hence exacerbate sciatic symptoms.
References
Pearce JMS. Gowers' sign. In: Fragments of neurological history. London: Imperial College Press; 2003, p. 378–80.
Tyler KL. William Richard Gowers (1845–1915). *J Neurol*. 2003; **250**: 1012–3.

Graefe's Sign
- see VON GRAEFE'S SIGN

"Grandchild Sign"
This sign is said to be present if the child of an individual with dementia answers in the negative when asked if they would allow the patient to drive their own children (*i.e.* the patient's grandchildren). It is said to be an indicator that the demented patient should no longer be driving.

Reference
Rabins PV, Lyketsos CG, Steele CD. Practical dementia care, 2nd edn. Oxford: Oxford University Press; 2006, p. 193

Graphaesthesia
- see AGRAPHAESTHESIA

Graphanaesthesia
- see AGRAPHAESTHESIA

Graphospasm
- see WRITER'S CRAMP

Grasp Reflex
The grasp reflex consists of progressive forced closure of the hand (contraction of flexor and adductor muscles) when tactile stimulation (*e.g.* the examiner's hand) is moved slowly, exerting pressure, across the patient's palm in an upward direction. Once established, the patient is unable to release the grip (forced grasping), allowing the examiner to draw the arm away from the patient's body. There may also be accompanying groping movements of the hand, once touched, in search of the examiner's hand or clothing (forced groping, magnetic movement). Although categorized as a reflex, it may sometimes be accessible to modification by will (so-called alien grasp reflex). It is usually bilateral, even with unilateral pathology. Foot grasping or plantar grasp reflex (*i.e.* flexion and adduction of the toes and curling of the sole of the foot in response to pressure on the sole), may coexist, as may other frontal release signs (*e.g.* pout reflex, palmomental reflex, *gegenhalten*).

The grasp reflex may be categorized as a frontal release sign (or primitive reflex) of prehensile type, since it is most commonly associated with lesion(s) in the frontal lobes or deep nuclei and subcortical white matter. Clinicoradiological correlations suggest the cingulate gyrus is the structure most commonly involved, followed by the supplementary motor area. Luria maintained that forced grasping resulted from extensive lesions of premotor region, disturbing normal relationships with the basal ganglia.

References
De Renzi E, Barbieri C. The incidence of the grasp reflex following hemispheric lesion and its relation to frontal damage. *Brain*. 1992; **115**: 293–313.
Luria AR. Higher cortical functions in man, 2nd edn. New York: Basic Books; 1980, p. 223.
Mestre T, Lang AE. The grasp reflex: a symptom in need of treatment. *Mov Disord*. 2010; **25**: 2479–85.
Schott JM, Rossor MN. The grasp and other primitive reflexes. *J Neurol Neurosurg Psychiatry*. 2003; **74**: 558–60.
Cross References
Akinetic mutism; Alien grasp reflex; Frontal release signs

Groucho Marx Manoeuvre
Named for the American comic actor Julius Henry "Groucho" Marx (1890–1977), this manoeuvre requires the forehead to be wrinkled quickly two or three times, so testing the frontalis muscle innervated by the facial nerve.
Reference
Ross RT. How to examine the nervous system, 4th edn. Totawa, New Jersey: Humana Press; 2006, p. 98.
Cross Reference
Facial paresis, Facial weakness

Gustatory Epiphora
- see CROCODILE TEARS

Gustatory Sweating
Gustatory sweating, or Frey's syndrome, is perspiration of the cheek, jaw, temple and neck when eating. This is an autonomic synkinesis, following the aberrant regeneration of damaged autonomic fibres travelling in the glossopharyngeal and vagus nerves, for example following neck dissection. If severe, it may be treated with botulinum toxin injections.
Cross Reference
Synkinesia, Synkinesis

Guttmann's Sign
Guttmann's sign is facial vasodilatation associated with nasal congestion, hypertension, bradycardia, sweating, mydriasis and piloerection, due to autonomic overactivity occurring as a feature of the acute phase of high spinal cord lesions.

Gynaecomastia
Gynaecomastia is inappropriate breast development in males. It is most often benign and of cosmetic rather than clinical importance, but may be pathological, as in chronic liver disease and certain neurological diseases:

- Excessive pituitary prolactin release secondary to impaired dopamine release from the hypothalamus due to local tumour or treatment with dopaminergic antagonist drugs (*e.g.* antipsychotic medications).
- Spinal and bulbar muscular atrophy (Kennedy's syndrome, X-linked).
- Klinefelter's syndrome (47,XYY).
- POEMS syndrome.

Reference
Narula HS, Carlson HE. Gynaecomastia – pathophysiology, diagnosis and treatment. *Nat Rev Endocrinol.* 2014; **10**: 684–98.

H

Habit Spasm
- see SPASM; TIC

"Half Moon" Syndrome
- see TEMPORAL CRESCENT SYNDROME

Hallpike Manoeuvre, Hallpike Test
The Hallpike manoeuvre (Nylen-Bárány manoeuvre, positioning manoeuvre, Dix-Hallpike positioning test) is a test used in the investigation of vertigo to induce (or to modify) nystagmus by stimulating the otolith organs of the inner ear.

It is most usually performed by briskly tilting the patient's head backwards to 30–45° below the horizontal ("head hanging position") and then turning it 45° to one side or the other, thus stimulating the posterior semicircular canal. Prior to performing the manoeuvre, the examiner should warn the patient that s/he may feel "giddy" or vertiginous, and to keep their eyes open throughout, since the development of nystagmus with the symptoms of vertigo is the observation of interest to the examiner.

With a peripheral lesion (*e.g.* benign paroxysmal positional vertigo, diseases of the labyrinth), nausea, vomiting and rotational-vertical nystagmus occur several seconds after the manoeuvre and then rapidly fatigue (usually <30 s), only to recur when the patient is returned to the upright position, with the nystagmus now in the opposite direction. Repetition of the manoeuvre (if the patient can be persuaded to undergo it) causes less severe symptoms (habituation). This is the diagnostic test for benign paroxysmal positional vertigo (BPPV). Central lesions (disorders of the vestibular connections) tend to produce isolated nystagmus which does not fatigue or habituate with repetition.

Variants of the Hallpike manoeuvre are described for BPPV of anterior or horizontal semicircular canal origin. Caloric testing may be required to elicit the causes of dizziness if the Hallpike manoeuvre is uninformative.

References
Bronstein AM. Vestibular reflexes and positional manoeuvres. *J Neurol Neurosurg Psychiatry*. 2003; **74**: 289–93.
Dix MR, Hallpike CS. The pathology, symptomatology and diagnosis of certain common disorders of the vestibular system. *Proc R Soc Med*. 1952; **45**: 341–54.
Lanska DJ, Remler B. Benign paroxysmal positioning vertigo: classic descriptions, origins of the provocative positioning technique, and conceptual developments. *Neurology*. 1997; **48**: 1167–77.

Cross References
Caloric testing; Nystagmus; Vertigo; Vestibulo-ocular reflexes

Hallucination
An hallucination is a perception in the absence of adequate peripheral stimulus (*cf.* illusion, although there may be some overlap). Such perceptions are substantial, constant, occur in objective space, and are usually not accompanied by insight (*cf.* pseudohallucination). They most usually occur in the visual and auditory domains.

© Springer International Publishing Switzerland 2016
A.J. Larner, *A Dictionary of Neurological Signs*,
DOI 10.1007/978-3-319-29821-4_8

Visual hallucinations may vary in complexity. They may be "simple", such as spots or flashes of light (photopsia, photism, scintillation), or "complex", ranging from patterns (fortification spectra, epileptic aura) to fully formed objects or individuals. They may be transient, such as brief visions of a person or animal (passage hallucinations, for example in Parkinson's disease) or long lasting. Visual hallucinations are not necessarily pathological, for example if experienced when falling asleep or waking (hypnagogic, hypnopompic). There are many other associations including both psychiatric and neurological disease, including:

- Delirium: especially hyperalert/agitated subtype.
- Withdrawal states: *e.g.* delirium tremens; hypnotics, anxiolytics.
- Drug overdose: *e.g.* anticholinergic drugs.
- Neurodegenerative disorders: dementia with Lewy bodies (a diagnostic criterion) more often than Alzheimer's disease: these may be associated with cholinergic depletion, and improved with cholinesterase inhibitor drugs; idiopathic Parkinson's disease (with or without treatment).
- Narcolepsy-cataplexy.
- Peduncular hallucinosis.
- Migraine aura: usually visual or somaesthetic; less often auditory or olfactory.
- Charles Bonnet syndrome (visual hallucinations in the visually impaired).
- Schizophrenia.
- Epilepsy: complex partial seizures.
- "Alice in Wonderland" syndrome.

Different mechanisms may account for visual hallucinations in different conditions: defective visual input and processing may occur in visual pathway lesions, whereas epilepsy may have a direct irritative effect on brain function; visual hallucinations associated with brainstem lesions may result from neurotransmitter abnormalities (cholinergic, serotonergic).

Auditory hallucinations may be simple sounds (acoasms: such as ringing or knocking) or complex sounds (voices, music) and may be associated with focal pathology in the temporal cortex. Third person hallucinations, commenting on a person's actions, are one of the first rank symptoms of schizophrenia.

Visceral hallucinations may be characterised as superficial, kinaesthetic (felt in muscles or joints), or visceral (stretching, heaviness, or pain in inner organs, *e.g.* the epigastric or visceral aura of complex partial seizures). Superficial visceral hallucinations may be further characterised as thermic (abnormal perception of heat or cold), haptic (sensation of touch, including formication), and hygric (perception of fluid running over the skin).

References

Burghaus L, Eggers C, Timmermann L, Fink GR, Diederich NJ. Hallucinations in neurodegenerative diseases. *CNS Neurosci Ther.* 2012; **18**: 149–59.

Ffytche D. Visual hallucination and illusion disorders: a clinical guide. *Adv Clin Neurosci Rehabil.* 2004; **4**(2): 16–8.

Kathirvel N, Mortimer A. Causes, diagnosis and treatment of visceral hallucinations. *Prog Neurol Psychiatry.* 2013; **17**(1): 6–10.

Manford M, Andermann F. Complex visual hallucinations. Clinical and neurobiological insights. *Brain.* 1998; **121**: 1819–40.

Tekin S, Cummings JL. Hallucinations and related conditions. In: Heilman KM, Valenstein E, editos. Clinical neuropsychology. 4th ed. Oxford: Oxford University Press; 2003. p. 479–94.

Cross References

"Alice in Wonderland" syndrome; Anwesenheit; Charles Bonnet syndrome; Delirium; Formication; Fortification spectra; Illusion; Parosmia; Photism; Photopsia; Pseudohallucination

Hammer Toes
Hammer toes are a feature of hereditary neuropathies, *e.g.* Charcot-Marie-Tooth disease, some cases of hereditary neuropathy with liability to pressure palsies, and Friedreich's ataxia. There may be associated pes cavus.
Cross Reference
Pes cavus

Hand Elevation Test
This is one of the provocative tests for carpal tunnel syndrome: it is said to be positive if paraesthesia develops in the distribution of the median nerve after raising the hand over the head for up to 2 min.
References
D'Arcy CA, McGee S. Does this patient have carpal tunnel syndrome? *JAMA*. 2000; **283**: 3110–7.
Hi ACF, Wong S, Griffith J. Carpal tunnel syndrome. *Pract Neurol*. 2005; **5**: 210–7.
Cross References
Phalen's sign; Tinel's sign

Harlequin Phenomenon, Harlequin Sign, Harlequin Syndrome
The harlequin phenomenon, sign or syndrome refers to asymmetrical facial flushing (erythrosis) with sweating (hyperhidrosis) after exercise. That it reflects localised autonomic dysfunction may be indicated by its associations with congenital Horner's syndrome, and as one element in the spectrum of Holmes-Adie syndrome and Ross's syndrome, although it can occur in isolation (about half of described cases). Harlequin sign has on occasion been described in association with multiple sclerosis and superior mediastinal neurinoma.
References
Guilloton L, Demarquay G, Quesnel L, De Charry F, Drouet A, Zagnoli F. Dysautonomic syndrome of the face with Harlequin sign and syndrome: three new cases and a review of the literature [in French]. *Rev Neurol (Paris)*. 2013; **169**: 884–91.
Lance JW. Harlequin syndrome. *Pract Neurol*. 2005; **5**: 176–7.
Cross References
Holmes-Adie pupil, Holmes-Adie syndrome; Horner's syndrome

Harvey's Sign
A high frequency tuning fork (440–1024 Hz) applied to the mucosa overlying the nasal septum produces a painful stimulus which has been advocated as useful in differentiating true from simulated coma, or status epilepticus from pseudostatus.
Reference
Harvey P. Harvey's 1 and 2. *Pract Neurol*. 2004; **4**: 178–9.
Cross Reference
Functional weakness and sensory disturbance

Head Droop, Head Drop
- see DROPPED HEAD SYNDROME

Head Impulse Test
The head impulse test, also known as the head thrust test, assesses the vestibulo-ocular reflex. It consists of a rapid turning of the patient's head to one side by the examiner, by about 15°, sufficiently rapid to ensure that smooth pursuit eye movements do not compensate for head turning. The examiner observes the ability of the subject to maintain fixation on a distant target. If the vestibulo-ocular reflex is intact fixation is maintained. If the vestibulo-ocular reflex is impaired, then an easily visible saccade back to the target occurs at the end of the movement. Tilting the head down by 20° and moving the head unpredictably may optimise testing.

This test is recommended in patients suffering a first attack of acute spontaneous vertigo. Sensitivity and specificity of around 80% for detecting a peripheral vestibular lesion such as acute unilateral vestibular neuritis has been reported. To avoid false negatives, it has been suggested that the test should be performed with high acceleration, five to ten times. If the test is normal in suspected vestibular neuritis, this implies a normal vestibulo-ocular reflex and that vertigo does not originate in the peripheral vestibular system, and hence a central cause for vertigo such as cerebellar infarction needs to be excluded.

References
Halmagyi GM, Curthoys IS. A clinical sign of canal paresis. *Arch Neurol*. 1988; **45**: 737–9.
Newman-Toker DE, Kattah JC, Alverina JE, Wang DZ. Normal head impulse test differentiates acute cerebellar strokes from vestibular neuritis. *Neurology*. 2008; **70**: 2378–85.
Schubert MC, Das VE, Tusa RJ, Herdman SJ. Optimizing the sensitivity of the head thrust test for diagnosing vestibular hypofunction. *Neurology*. 2002; **58(Suppl 3)**: A439. (Abstract P06.031).
Weber KP, Aw ST, Todd MJ, McGarvie LA, Curthoys IS, Halmagyi GM. Head impulse test in unilateral vestibular loss: vestibulo-ocular reflex and catch-up saccades. *Neurology*. 2008; **70**: 454–63.

Cross References
Vertigo; Vestibulo-ocular reflexes

Head Retraction Sign
- see HYPEREKPLEXIA

Head Snap
Head snap denotes a jerking movement of the head which occurs when affected patients perform the "finger-to-nose test", evident just as the finger reaches the nose. It occurs in patients with essential tremor, and is distinguished from head tremor because it does not have an oscillatory quality, comprising a single unidirectional jerking motion.

Reference
Sternberg EJ, Alcalay RN, Levy OA, Louis ED. The "head snap": a subtle clinical feature during the finger-nose-finger maneuver in essential tremor. *Tremor Other Hyperkinet Mov (N Y)*. 2013; **3**. pii: tre-03-159-3719-1.

Head Thrust
- see EYELID APRAXIA; OCULAR APRAXIA

Head Thrust Test
- see HEAD IMPULSE TEST

Head Tilt
Head tilt may be observed with:

- Diplopia, cranial nerve palsies (IV, VI); skew deviation.
- Neck dystonia (laterocollis, retrocollis).
- Incipient tonsillar herniation with cerebellar tumours, sometimes associated with neck stiffness and limitation of neck movement.

The term has also been used as equivalent to "head turning".

Cross References
Bielschowsky's sign, Bielschowsky's test; Diplopia; "Head turning sign"; Laterocollis; Ocular tilt reaction

Head Tremor
Head tremor may be characterized as "yes-yes" (nodding, *tremblement affirmatif*) when predominantly in the vertical plane, or "no-no" (side-to-side, *tremblement negatif*) when predominantly in the horizontal plane. A combination of both may be observed in dystonic head tremors.

Head tremor may occur in isolation or with evidence of tremor elsewhere (*e.g.* postural limb tremor, vocal tremor, in essential tremor), or dystonia (*e.g.* torticollis). In essential tremor the head movements are often intermittent, "yes-yes", and of frequency about 7 Hz. Dystonic head tremor is often jerky and disorganized, with a frequency of less than 5 Hz. Cerebellum and brainstem disease, such as multiple sclerosis, can also produce head tremor (or titubation). Head tremor is an exceptionally rare symptom of Parkinson's disease. It may also be seen as a consequence of aortic valve regurgitation (De Musset's sign).

Treatment of head tremor varies with cause. Possible treatments, of variable efficacy, include:

- essential tremor: propranolol, topiramate, primidone, nicardipine, gabapentin.
- dystonic tremor: levodopa, anticholinergics, propranolol, botulinum toxin injections.
- cerebellar tremor: isoniazid, carbamazepine, ondansetron.

Cross References
Dystonia; Tremor

"Head Turning Sign"
It is often observed that patients who are cognitively impaired turn their head towards their spouse, partner, or carer to seek assistance when asked to give a history of their problems, or during tests of neuropsychological function. This "head turning sign" (it has also been described as a "positive head tilt") is an easily observed and categorised clinical sign. Pragmatic studies of unselected new outpatient clinic cohorts suggest that it has good specificity, *i.e.* is reliably absent in those without cognitive impairment. It may therefore be a useful screening observation, its presence indicating the need for further investigation of cognitive function.

"Head turning" has also been used to describe a symptom observed in focal onset epileptic seizures, but without apparent lateralizing or localizing significance.

References
Larner AJ. Head turning sign: pragmatic utility in clinical diagnosis of cognitive impairment. *J Neurol Neurosurg Psychiatry*. 2012; **83**: 852–3.
Lipton AM, Marshall CD. The common sense guide to dementia for clinicians and caregivers. New York: Springer; 2013. p. 46.
Ochs R, Gloor P, Quesney F, Ives J, Olivier A. Does head-turning during a seizure have lateralizing or localizing significance? *Neurology*. 1984; **34**: 884–90.

Cross Reference
Dementia

Heautoscopy
This term was coined to denote seeing oneself, encountering ones alter ego or *doppelgänger*. Hence unlike the situation in autoscopy, there are two selves, a reduplicated body rather than a mirror image; egocentric and body-centred perspectives do not coincide. According to Critchley, the condition used to be called "specular hallucinosis", and the Swedish naturalist Linnaeus (1707–1788) apparently had episodes, seeing himself sitting in his study, or gazing at a flower and plucking it. A polyopic form (*i.e.* more than one double) is also described.

References
Brugger P. Reflective mirrors: perspective taking in autoscopic phenomena. *Cogn Neuropsychiatry*. 2002; **7**: 179–94.
Brugger P, Blanke O, Regard M, Bradford DT, Landis T. Polyopic heautoscopy: case report and review of the literature. *Cortex*. 2006; **42**: 666–74.
Critchley M. The divine banquet of the brain and other essays. New York: Raven Press; 1979. p. 11, 101.

Cross References
Autoscopy; Hallucination

Heel-Knee-Shin Test, Heel-Shin Test
A frequently used test of co-ordination in which the patient, sitting on the examination couch, is asked to lift the heel onto the contralateral knee, then run it smoothly down the shin bone towards the foot. Jerky performance, or a tendency for the heel to slide off the shin, may be seen in an ataxic limb. Performance is difficult to interpret if there is limb weakness or dystonia.
Cross References
Ataxia; Cerebellar syndromes; Shin-tapping

Heel-Toe Walking
- see TANDEM WALKING

Hemeralopia
Hemeralopia, or day blindness, is worsening of vision in bright light (*cf.* nyctalopia). This phenomenon may reflect severe impairment of blood flow to the eye, such that photostressing the macula by exposure to bright light is followed by only slow regeneration of the bleached photopigments. If due to retinal ischaemia, hemeralopia may be accompanied by neovascularization of the retina. Impoverished perfusion pressure may be demonstrated by pressing on the eyeball (*e.g.* with the thumb) during ophthalmoscopy ("digital ophthalmodynamometry") and observing the collapse of retinal arteries: thumb pressure greater than diastolic retinal artery pressure causes intermittent collapse; thumb pressure greater than systolic pressure leads to a cessation of pulsation.

Hemeralopia may also occur in retinal diseases such as cone-rod dystrophies, and with cataract.

The words hemeralopia and nyctalopia have apparently been used in an opposite sense by many non-English-speaking doctors. Hence, the terms "day blindness" and "night blindness" may be preferred to avoid any ambiguity.
References
Furlan AJ, Whisnant JP, Kearns TP. Unilateral visual loss in bright light: an unusual symptom of carotid artery occlusive disease. *Arch Neurol.* 1979; **36**: 675–6.
Ohba N, Ohba A. Nyctalopia and hemeralopia: the current usage trend in the literature. *Br J Ophthalmol.* 2006; **90**: 1548–9.
Cross Reference
Nyctalopia

Hemiachromatopsia
- see ACHROMATOPSIA; ALEXIA

Hemiakinesia
Hemiakinesia is akinesia or hypokinesia (inability or difficulty initiating movement) confined to one side of the body. Although hemiakinesia is the norm at the onset of idiopathic Parkinson's disease ("hemiparkinsonism"), persistent hemiakinesia should prompt a re-evaluation of this diagnosis. Corticobasal degeneration often remains unilateral; a search for structural lesions of the basal ganglia should also be undertaken. Hemiakinesia may also indicate motor neglect, usually with right-sided lesions. Lesions of the basal ganglia, ventral ("motor") thalamus, limbic system, and frontal lobes may cause hemiakinesia.
Cross References
Akinesia; Extinction; Hemiparkinsonism; Hypokinesia; Neglect; Parkinsonism

Hemialexia
This is the inability to read words in the visual left half-field in the absence of hemianopia. It may occur after callosotomy (complete, or partial involving only the splenium), and represents a visual disconnection syndrome.

Reference
Zaidel E, Iacobini M, Zaidel DW, Bogen JE. The callosal syndromes. In: Heilman KM, Valenstein E, editors. Clinical neuropsychology. 4th ed. Oxford: Oxford University Press; 2003. p. 347–403.
Cross References
Alexia; Hemianomia

Hemianomia
This is the absence of verbal report of stimuli presented in the visual left half-field in the absence of hemianopia. It may occur after callosotomy (complete, or partial involving only the splenium), and represents a visual disconnection syndrome.
Reference
Zaidel E, Iacobini M, Zaidel DW, Bogen JE. The callosal syndromes. In: Heilman KM, Valenstein E, editors. Clinical neuropsychology. 4th ed. Oxford: Oxford University Press; 2003. p. 347–403.
Cross References
Anomia; Hemialexia

Hemianopia
Hemianopia (or hemianopsia) is a defect of one half of the visual field: this may be vertical, or horizontal (= altitudinal field defect). Hemianopic defects may be congruent (homonymous) or non-congruent (heteronymous), and may be detected by standard confrontational testing of the visual fields or by automated means (*e.g.* Goldman perimetry). These tests of the visual fields are an extension of the tests for visual acuity which assess areas away from the fovea. Because of the strict topographic arrangement of neural pathways within the visual system, particular abnormalities of the visual fields give a very precise indication of the likely site of pathology.

- *Homonymous hemianopia*:

    Reflects a post-chiasmal lesion. It is important to assess whether the vertical meridian of a homonymous hemianopia cuts through the macula (macula splitting), implying a lesion of the optic radiation; or spares the macula (macula sparing), suggesting an occipital cortical lesion. Incongruous defects may be found with lesions of the optic tract. Commonly, homonymous hemianopias result from cerebrovascular disease causing occipital lobe infarction, or intraparnechymal tumour, but they may be "false-localising" due to raised intracranial pressure if temporal lobe herniation causes posterior cerebral artery compromise. Ictal hemianopia is also described, in association with epileptic seizures of occipital lobe origin.

- *Heteronymous hemianopia*:

    Reflects a chiasmal lesion. The most common of these is a bitemporal hemianopia due to chiasmal compression, for example by a pituitary lesion or craniopharyngioma. Tilted optic discs may also be associated with bitemporal field loss but this extends to the blind spot and not the vertical meridian as in chiasmal pathology ("pseudobitemporal hemianopia"). Binasal defects are rare, suggesting lateral compression of the chiasm, for example from bilateral carotid artery aneurysms; binasal hemianopia is also described with optic nerve head lesions, or as a normal variant. Unilateral (monocular) temporal hemianopia may result from a lesion anterior to the chiasm which selectively affects only the ipsilateral crossing nasal fibres (junctional scotoma of Traquair).

Unawareness of visual field loss, or anosognosic hemianopia, occurs principally with right-sided brain lesions.

Bilateral homonymous hemianopia or double hemianopia may result in cortical blindness.

Reference
Zhang X, Kedar S, Lynn MJ, Newman NJ, Biousse V. Natural history of homonymous hemianopia. *Neurology*. 2006; **66**: 901–5.
Cross References
Alexia; Altitudinal field defect; Anosognosia; Binasal hemianopia; Bitemporal hemianopia; Cortical blindness; "False-localising signs"; Macula sparing, Macula splitting; Quadrantanopia; Scotoma; Visual field defects

Hemiataxia

Hemiataxia is ataxia confined to one half of the body. The vast majority of isolated hemiataxic syndromes reflect a lesion of the ipsilateral cerebellar hemisphere, but on occasion supratentorial lesions may cause hemiataxia (posterior limb of the internal capsule, thalamus). However, in almost all of these cases hemiataxia coexists with ipsilateral hemiparesis (ataxic hemiparesis), hemisensory disturbance (hemiataxia-hypesthesia), or both. Cerebellar diaschisis is the mechanism usually invoked to explain hemiataxia when there is no associated cerebellar pathlology.

Reference
Kishi M, Sakakibara R, Nagao T, Terada H, Ogawa E. Isolated hemiataxia and cerebellar diaschisis after a small dorsolateral medullary infarct. *Case Rep Neurol*. 2009; **1**: 41–6.
Cross References
Ataxia; Ataxic hemiparesis; Cerebellar syndromes; Cerebellopontine angle syndrome; Lateral medullary syndrome

Hemiballismus

Hemiballismus is unilateral ballismus, an involuntary hyperkinetic movement disorder in which there are large amplitude, vigorous ("flinging") irregular movements. Hemiballismus overlaps clinically with hemichorea ("violent chorea"); the term *hemiballismus-hemichorea* is sometimes used to reflect this overlap. Hemiballismic limbs may show a loss of normal muscular tone (hypotonia).

Neuroanatomically, hemiballismus is most often associated with lesions of the contralateral subthalamic nucleus of Luys or its efferent pathways, although there are occasional reports of its occurrence with lesions of the caudate nucleus, putamen, globus pallidus, lentiform nucleus, thalamus, and precentral gyrus; and even with ipsilateral lesions. Neuropathologically, vascular events (ischaemia, haemorrhage) are the most common association but hemiballismus has also been reported with space-occupying lesions (tumour, arteriovenous malformation), inflammation (encephalitis, systemic lupus erythematosus, post-streptococcal infection), demyelination, metabolic causes (hyperosmolal non-ketotic hyperglycaemia), infection (toxoplasmosis in AIDS), drugs (oral contraceptives, phenytoin, levodopa, neuroleptics) and head trauma.

Pathophysiologically, hemiballismus is thought to result from reduced conduction through the direct pathway within the basal ganglia-thalamo-cortical motor circuit (as are other hyperkinetic involuntary movements, such as choreoathetosis). Removal of excitation from the globus pallidus following damage to the efferent subthalamic-pallidal pathways disinhibits the ventral anterior and ventral lateral thalamic nuclei which receive pallidal projections and which in turn project to the motor cortex.

Hemiballismus of vascular origin usually improves spontaneously, but drug treatment with neuroleptics (haloperidol, pimozide, sulpiride) may be helpful. Other drugs which are sometimes helpful include tetrabenazine, reserpine, clonazepam, clozapine, and sodium valproate.

References
Albin RL, Young AB, Penney JB. The functional anatomy of basal ganglia disorders. *Trends Neurosci*. 1989; **12**: 366–75.
Lee MS, Marsden CD. Movement disorders following lesions of the thalamus or subthalamic region. *Mov Disord*. 1994; **9**: 493–507.

Martin JP. Hemichorea resulting from a local lesion of the brain. (The syndrome of the body of Luys.). *Brain*. 1927; **50**: 637–51.
Postuma RB, Lang AE. Hemiballism: revisiting a classic disorder. *Lancet Neurol*. 2003; **2**; 661–8.
Cross References
Ballism, Ballismus; Chorea, Choreoathetosis; Hemichorea; Hypotonia, Hypotonus

Hemichorea
Hemichorea is unilateral chorea, an involuntary movement disorder which overlaps with hemiballismus, and with which it shares a similar pathophysiology and aetiology. It may replace hemiballismus during recovery from a contralateral subthalamic lesion.
Cross References
Chorea, Choreoathetosis; Hemiballismus

Hemidystonia
Hemidystonia is dystonia affecting the whole of one side of the body, a pattern which mandates structural brain imaging because of the chance of finding a causative structural lesion (vascular, neoplastic), which is greater than with other patterns of dystonia (focal, segmental, multifocal, generalized). Such a lesion most often affects the contralateral putamen or its afferent or efferent connections.
Reference
Marsden CD, Obeso JA, Zaranz JJ, Lang AE. The anatomical basis of symptomatic hemidystonia. *Brain*. 1985; **108**: 461–83.
Cross Reference
Dystonia

Hemifacial Atrophy
- see PARRY-ROMBERG SYNDROME

Hemifacial Spasm
Hemifacial spasm is an involuntary dyskinetic (not dystonic) movement disorder consisting of painless contractions of muscles on one side of the face, sometimes triggered by eating or speaking, and exacerbated by fatigue or emotion. The movements give a twitching appearance to the eye or side of the mouth, sometimes described as a pulling sensation. Patients often find this embarrassing because it attracts the attention of others. The movements may continue during sleep. Paradoxical elevation of the eyebrow as orbicularis oris contracts and the eye closes may be seen (Babinski's "other sign"). Only very rarely may such movements be bilateral, indeed this finding may call the diagnosis of hemifacial spasm into question.

Hemifacial spasm may be idiopathic, or associated with neurovascular compression of the facial (VII) nerve, usually at the root entry zone, often by a tortuous anterior or posterior inferior cerebellar artery. Other causes include intrapontine lesions (*e.g.* demyelination), following a Bell's palsy, and mass lesions (tumour, arteriovenous malformation) located anywhere from the facial nucleus to the stylomastoid foramen. Very rarely, contralateral (false-localising) posterior fossa lesions have been associated with hemifacial spasm, suggesting that kinking or distortion of the nerve, rather than direct compression, may be of pathogenetic importance.

Structural lesions may be amenable to surgical resection. For idiopathic hemifacial spasm, or patients declining surgery, botulinum toxin injections are the treatment of choice.
References
Chaudhry N, Srivastava A, Joshi L. Hemifacial spasm: the past, present and future. *J Neurol Sci*. 2015; **356**: 27–31.
Evidente VGH, Adler CH. Hemifacial spasm and other craniofacial movement disorders. *Mayo Clin Proc*. 1998; **73**: 67–71.
Cross References
Babinski's sign (2); Bell's palsy; Dyskinesia; "False-localising signs"; *Tic convulsif*

Hemi-inattention
– see NEGLECT

Hemimicropsia
- see MICROPSIA

Hemineglect
- see NEGLECT

Hemiparalexia
- see ALEXIA

Hemiparaplegia
- see MONOPARESIS, MONOPLEGIA

Hemiparesis
Hemiparesis is a weakness affecting one side of the body, less severe than a hemiplegia. Characteristically this affects the extensor muscles of the upper limb more than flexors, and the flexors of the leg more than extensors ("pyramidal" distribution of weakness), producing the classic hemiparetic/hemiplegic posture with flexed arm and extended leg, the latter permitting standing and a circumducting gait.

Hemiparesis results from damage (most usually vascular) to the corticospinal pathways anywhere from motor cortex to the cervical spine. Accompanying signs may give clues as to localisation, the main possibilities being hemisphere, brainstem, or cervical cord.

Hemisphere lesions may also cause hemisensory impairment, hemianopia, aphasia, agnosia or apraxia; headache, and unilateral partial ptosis, may sometimes feature. Spatial neglect, with or without anosognosia, may also occur, particularly with right-sided lesions producing a left hemiparesis. Pure motor hemiparesis may be seen with lesions of the internal capsule, corona radiata, and basal pons (lacunar/small deep infarct), in which case the face and arm are affected more than the leg; such facio-brachial predominance may also be seen with cortico-subcortical lesions laterally placed on the contralateral hemisphere. Crural predominance suggests a contralateral paracentral cortical lesion or one of the lacunar syndromes.

Brainstem lesions may produce diplopia, ophthalmoplegia, nystagmus, ataxia, and crossed facial sensory loss or weakness in addition to hemiparesis ("alternating hemiplegia").

Spinal lesions are more likely to show bilateral long tract signs (*e.g.* bilateral Babinksi's sign) and may have accompanying spinal or root pain, sphincter disturbance, and a sensory or motor level.

Hemiparesis is most usually a consequence of a vascular event (cerebral infarction). Tumour may cause a progressive hemiparesis (although meningiomas may on occasion produce transient "stroke-like" events). Hemiparetic multiple sclerosis is rare but well described. Transient hemiparesis may be observed as an ictal phenomenon (Todd's paresis), or in familial hemiplegic migraine which is associated with mutations in voltage-gated ion channel genes. Mills syndrome is an ascending or descending hemiplegia which may represent a unilateral form of motor neurone disease or primary lateral sclerosis.

Cross References
Agnosia; Anosognosia; Aphasia; Apraxia; Babinski's sign (1); "False-localising signs"; Hemianopia; Hemiplegia; Myelopathy; Neglect; Ptosis; Upper motor neurone (UMN) syndrome; Weakness

Hemiparkinsonism
Hemiparkinsonism describes the finding of parkinsonian signs restricted to one side of the body, most usually akinesia, in which case the term hemiakinesia may be used. Idiopathic Parkinson's disease may present with exclusively or predominantly unilateral features

(indeed, lack of asymmetry at onset may argue against this diagnosis) but persistent hemiparkinsonism, particularly if unresponsive to adequate doses of levodopa, should alert the clinician to other possible diagnoses, including corticobasal degeneration or structural lesions.
Cross References
Hemiakinesia; Parkinsonism

Hemiplegia
Hemiplegia is a complete weakness affecting one side of the body, *i.e.* clinically a more severe picture than hemiparesis.
Cross References
Hemiparesis; Weakness

Hemiplegia Cruciata
Cervicomedullary junction lesions at the level where the pyramidal tract decussates may result in paresis of the contralateral upper extremity and ipsilateral lower extremity: hemiplegia cruciata. There may be concurrent facial sensory loss with onion skin pattern, respiratory insufficiency, bladder dysfunction and cranial nerve palsies. Such cases of isolated damage to the pyramidal decussation are very rare.
Cross Reference
Onion peel, Onion skin; Pyramidal decussation syndrome

Hemiprosopometamorphopsia
This term has been used to describe changed perception limited to one half of the face (appearing deformed, longer), associated with a contralateral corpus callosum lesion.
Reference
Tabuas-Pereira M, Parra J, Duro D, Maduro AMC, Santana MIJ. Hemiprosopometamorphopsia as the presenting symptom of Marchiafava-Bignami disease. *Eur J Neurol*. 2015; **22**(Suppl 1): 337.
Cross Reference
Metamorphopsia

Hennebert's Sign
Hennebert's sign is the induction of vertigo and nystagmus by pressure changes in the external auditory canal, such as when using pneumatic otoscopy or simply with tragal pressure. These findings are highly suggestive of the presence of a bony labyrinthine fistula. There may be a history of chronic otitis media.
Cross References
Nystagmus; Vertigo

Henry and Woodruff Sign
This refers to deviation of the eyes towards the ground with the patient lying on each side, which has been proposed as a diagnostic sign for psychogenic states resembling coma and in differentiating pseudoseizures from epileptic seizures.
References
Henry JA, Woodruff GH. A diagnostic sign in states of apparent unconsciousness. *Lancet*. 1978; **ii**: 920–1.
Mellers JDC. The approach to patients with "non-epileptic seizures". *Postgrad Med J*. 2005; **81**: 498–504.

Hertwig-Magendie Sign
- see SKEW DEVIATION

Heterochromia Iridis
Different colour of the irides may be seen in congenital Horner's syndrome, and in Waardenburg syndrome of nerve deafness, white forelock, abnormal skin pigmentation, and synophrys.
Cross Reference
Horner's syndrome

Heterophoria
Heterophoria is a generic term for a latent tendency to imbalance of the ocular axes (latent strabismus; *cf.* heterotropia). This may be clinically demonstrated using the cover-uncover test: if there is movement of the covered eye as it is uncovered and takes up fixation, this reflects a phoria. Phorias may be in the horizontal (esophoria, exophoria) or vertical plane (hyperphoria, hypophoria).
Reference
Shaunak S, O'Sullivan E, Kennard C. Eye movements. In: Hughes RAC, editor. Neurological investigations. London: BMJ Publishing; 1997. p. 253–82.
Cross References
Cover tests; Esophoria; Exophoria; Heterotropia; Hyperphoria; Hypophoria

Heterotropia
Heterotropia is a generic term for manifest deviation of the eyes (manifest strabismus; *cf.* heterophoria), synonymous with squint. This may be obvious: an amblyopic eye, with poor visual acuity and fixation, may become deviated. Sometimes it may be more subtle, coming to attention only with the patient's complaint of diplopia.

Using the alternate cover (cross cover) test, in which binocular fixation is not permitted, an imbalance in the visual axes may be demonstrated, but this will not distinguish between heterotropia and heterophoria. To make this distinction the cover test is required: if the uncovered eye moves to adopt fixation then heterotropia is confirmed. Tropias may be in the horizontal (esotropia, exotropia) or vertical plane (hypertropia, hypotropia).
Reference
Shaunak S, O'Sullivan E, Kennard C. Eye movements. In: Hughes RAC, editor. Neurological Investigations. London: BMJ Publishing; 1997. p. 253–82.
Cross References
Amblyopia; Cover tests; Esotropia; Exotropia; Heterophoria; Hypertropia; Hypotropia

Hiccups
A hiccup (or hiccough) is a brief burst of inspiratory activity involving the diaphragm and the inspiratory intercostal muscles with reciprocal inhibition of expiratory intercostal muscles. The sound ("hic") and discomfort result from glottic closure immediately after the onset of diaphragmatic contraction, *i.e.* the latter is insufficient or asynchronous. Hiccups may be characterized as a physiological form of myoclonus (or singultus).

Most episodes of hiccups are self-limited, but prolonged or intractable hiccuping (*hoc-quet diabolique*) should prompt a search for a structural or functional cause, either gastroen-terological or neurological (a possible example is described in Somerset Maugham's short story *P&O*).

Hiccuping is seldom the only abnormality if the cause is neurological since it usually reflects pathology within the medulla or affecting the afferent and efferent nerves of the respiratory muscles. Medullary causes include:

- Infarction (posterior inferior cerebellar artery territory; lateral medullary syndrome, especially middle level and dorsolateral lesion locations).
- Tumour.
- Abscess.

- Tuberculoma.
- Syrinx.
- Haematoma.
- Demyelination.
- CNS infection, *e.g.* viral encephalitis.

Hiccup with exclusively supratentorial lesion has been described.

Treatment of hiccups should be aimed at the underlying cause. If none is identified, physical measures to stop the hiccups such as rebreathing may then be tried. There is no compelling evidence base for any of the many various pharmacotherapies tried.

References

Moretto EN, Wee B, Wiffen PJ, Murchison AG. Interventions for treating persistent and intractable hiccups in adults. *Cochrane Database Sys Rev.* 2013; **1**: CD008768.

Park MH, Kim BJ, Koh SB, Park MK, Park KW, Lee DH. Lesional location of lateral medullary infarction presenting hiccups (singultus). *J Neurol Neurosurg Psychiatry.* 2005; **76**: 95–8.

Tiedt HO, Wenzel R. Persistent hiccups as sole manifestation of right cortical infarction without apparent brainstem lesion. *J Neurol.* 2013; **260**: 1913–4.

Cross References

Lateral medullary syndrome; Myoclonus

High-Stepping Gait

- see STEPPAGE, STEPPING GAIT

Hip Abduction Sign

The hip abduction sign refers to abduction of the thighs when attempting to rise from the ground, due to relative weakness of hip adductors with preserved strength in hip abductors. The sign was first described in patients with sarcoglycanopathies, a group of autosomal recessive limb-girdle muscular dystrophies, and is reported to have a sensitivity of 76 % and a specificity of 98 % for this diagnosis. It may perhaps be envisaged as the equivalent to Gowers' sign but with hip adductor, rather than gluteal, weakness.

Reference

Khadilkar SV, Singh RK. Hip abduction sign: a new clinical sign in sarcoglycanopathies. *J Clin Neuromuscul Dis.* 2001; **3**: 13–5.

Cross Reference

Gowers' sign

Hippus

Hippus is excessive pupillary unrest, *i.e.* rhythmic, oscillatory, contraction and dilatation of the pupil. It may reflect an imbalance between afferent pupillary sympathetic and parasympathetic autonomic activity. Hippus may be a normal phenomenon; it may be observed during recovery from an oculomotor (III) nerve palsy, but otherwise is of no localizing significance.

Hitselberg Sign

Hypoaesthesia of the posterior wall of the external auditory canal may be seen in facial paresis since the facial (VII) nerve sends a sensory branch to innervate this territory; this has been termed Hitselberg sign.

Cross Reference

Facial paresis, Facial weakness

Hocquet Diabolique

- see HICCUPS

Hoffmann's Sign
Hoffmann's sign or reflex is a digital reflex consisting of flexion of the thumb and index finger in response to snapping or flicking the distal phalanx of the middle finger, causing a sudden extension of the joint. Although sometimes a normal finding, for example in the presence of generalised hyperreflexia (anxiety, hyperthyroidism), it may be indicative of a corticospinal tract lesion above C5 or C6, particularly if present unilaterally.

References
Cook C, Cleland J, Huijbregts P. Creation and critique of studies of diagnostic accuracy: use of the STARD and QUADAS methodological quality assessment tools. *J Man Manip Ther*. 2007; **15**: 93–102. [at 96].
Mahmoudi Nezhad GS, Dalfardi B. Johann Hoffmann (1857–1919). *J Neurol*. 2014; **261**: 1848–9.

Cross References
Trömner's sign; Upper motor neurone (UMN) syndrome

Hoffmann-Tinel Sign
- see TINEL'S SIGN

Holmes-Adie Pupil, Holmes-Adie Syndrome
The Holmes-Adie, or tonic, pupil is an enlarged pupil which, in a darkened environment, is unresponsive to a phasic light stimulus, but may respond slowly to a tonic light stimulus. Reaction to accommodation is preserved (*i.e.* there is partial iridoplegia), hence this is one of the causes of light-near pupillary dissociation. A Holmes-Adie pupil is usually unilateral, and hence a cause of anisocoria.

Holmes-Adie pupil may be associated with other neurological features (the Holmes-Adie syndrome). These include loss of lower limb tendon reflexes (especially ankle jerks); impaired corneal sensation; chronic cough; and localised or generalised anhidrosis, sometimes with hyperhidrosis (Ross's syndrome). Holmes-Adie syndrome is much more common in women than men.

Pathophysiologically Holmes-Adie pupil results from a peripheral lesion of the parasympathetic autonomic nervous system and shows denervation supersensitivity, constricting with application of dilute (0.2%) pilocarpine (*cf.* pseudo-Argyll Robertson pupil).

References
Kawasaki A. Approach to the patient with abnormal pupils. In: Biller J, editor. Practical neurology. 2nd ed. Philadelphia: Lippincott Williams & Wilkins; 2002. p. 135–46.
Martinelli P. Holmes-Adie syndrome. *Lancet*. 2000; **356**: 1760–1.
Pearce JMS. The Holmes-Adie tonic pupil and Hughlings Jackson. In: Fragments of neurological history. London: Imperial College Press; 2003. p. 249–51.

Cross References
Anhidrosis; Anisocoria; Hyperhidrosis; Light-near pupillary dissociation; Pseudo-Argyll Robertson pupil

Holmes' Tremor
Holmes' tremor, also known as rubral tremor, or midbrain tremor, has been defined as a rest and intention tremor, of frequency <4.5 Hz. The rest tremor may resemble parkinsonian tremor, and is exacerbated by sustained postures and voluntary movements. Hence there are features of rest, postural and kinetic (intention) tremor. Once attributed to lesions of the red nucleus (hence "rubral"), the anatomical substrate is now thought to be interruption of fibres of the superior cerebellar peduncle (hence "midbrain") carrying cerebellothalamic and/or cerebello-olivary projections; lesions of the ipsilateral cerebellar dentate nucleus may produce a similar clinical picture. Recognised causes include multiple sclerosis, head injury and stroke. Hypertrophic olivary degeneration may be seen on brain imaging. If a causative lesion is defined, there is typically a delay before tremor appearance (4 weeks to 2 years).

References
Alusi SH, Worthington J, Glickman S, Bain PG. A study of tremor in multiple sclerosis. *Brain*. 2001; **124**: 720–30.
Deuschl G, Bain P, Brin M and an Ad Hoc Scientific Committee. Consensus statement of the Movement Disorder Society on tremor. *Mov Disord*. 1998; **13**(Suppl 3): 2–23.
Cross Reference
Tremor

Hoover's Sign
Hoover's sign describes the finding of apparent weakness of voluntary hip flexion with normal involuntary hip extension during contralateral hip flexion against resistance. When a recumbent patient attempts to lift one leg, downward pressure is felt under the heel of the other leg because concurrent hip extension is a normal synergistic or synkinetic movement. The finding of this synkinetic movement, detected when the heel of the supposedly paralysed leg presses down on the examiner's palm, constitutes Hoover's sign: no increase in pressure is felt beneath the heel of a paralysed leg in an organic hemiplegia. Hence the finding of Hoover's sign may be used to help differentiate organic from functional hemiplegia or monoplegia.

In addition, the synkinetic hip extension movement is accentuated when attempting to raise a contralateral paretic leg, whereas in functional weakness it is abolished.

In a cohort of patients with suspected stroke, Hoover's sign was moderately sensitive (0.63) and very specific (1.00) for a diagnosis of functional weakness.
Reference
McWhirter L, Stone J, Sandercock P, Whiteley W. Hoover's sign for the diagnosis of functional weakness: a prospective unblinded cohort study in patients with suspected stroke. *J Psychosom Res*. 2011; **71**: 384–6.
Cross References
"Arm drop"; Babinski's trunk-thigh test; Functional weakness and sensory disturbance; Synkinesia, Synkinesis

Horner's Syndrome
Horner's syndrome, or Bernard-Horner syndrome, is defined by a constellation of clinical findings, most usually occurring unilaterally, *viz.*:

- partial ptosis, due to weakness of Müller's muscle.
- miosis, due to the unopposed action of the sphincter pupillae muscle, innervated by the parasympathetic nervous system; this is most obvious in a dimly lit room.
- anhidrosis, a loss of sweating (if the lesion is distal to the superior cervical ganglion).
- enophthalmos, retraction of the eyeball (though this is seldom measured).

The first two mentioned signs are usually the most evident and bring the patient to medical attention; the latter two are usually less evident or absent. Additional features which may be seen include:

- heterochromia iridis, different colour of the iris (if the lesion is congenital).
- elevation of the inferior eyelid due to a weak inferior tarsal muscle ("reverse ptosis", or "upside-down ptosis").

Horner's syndrome results from impairment of ocular sympathetic innervation. The sympathetic innervation of the eye consists of a long, three-neurone, pathway, extending from the diencephalon down to the cervicothoracic spinal cord, then back up to the eye via the superior cervical ganglion and the internal carotid artery, and the ophthalmic division of the trigeminal (V) nerve. A wide variety of pathological processes, spread across a large area, may cause a Horner's syndrome, although many examples remain idiopathic despite intensive investigation. Hence Horner's syndrome is a good lateralizing but a poor localizing sign. Recognised causes include:

- brainstem/cervical cord disease (vascular, demyelination, syringomyelia).
- Pancoast tumour.
- malignant cervical lymph nodes.
- carotid aneurysm, carotid artery dissection.
- involvement of T1 fibres, *e.g* in T1 radiculopathy, or lower trunk brachial plexopathy.
- cluster headache.
- congenital.

Determining whether the lesion causing a Horner's syndrome is pre- or postganglionic may be done by applying to the eye 1% hydroxyamphetamine hydrobromide, which releases noradrenaline into the synaptic cleft, which dilates the pupil if Horner's syndrome results from a preganglionic lesion. However, this is not particularly helpful in determining cause, whereas accompanying neurological features are: contralateral hemiparesis would mandate investigation for carotid dissection (MRI, angiography), and this is probably sensible for any painful Horner's syndrome of acute onset. Arm symptoms and signs in a smoker mandate a chest radiograph for Pancoast tumour. Associated ipsilateral abducens (VI) nerve palsy (Parkinson's syndrome) suggests cavernous sinus disease. If the Horner's syndrome is isolated and painless, then no investigation may be required. In this situation, a symptomatic cause is seldom identified despite investigation. Syringomyelia presenting with isolated Horner's syndrome has been reported.

Unilateral miosis may be mistaken for contralateral mydriasis if ptosis is subtle, leading to suspicion of partial oculomotor nerve palsy on the "mydriatic" side. Observation of anisocoria in the dark will help here, since increased anisocoria indicates a sympathetic defect (normal pupil dilates) whereas less anisocoria suggests a parasympathetic lesion. Applying to the eye 10% cocaine solution will also diagnose a Horner's syndrome if the pupil fails to dilate after 45 min in the dark (normal pupil dilates).

Reference
Van der Wiel HL. Johann Friedrich Horner. *J Neurol*. 2002; **249**: 636–7.

Cross References
Anhidrosis; Anisocoria; Enophthalmos; Miosis; Plexopathy; Pourfour du Petit syndrome; Ptosis; Radiculopathy

Horologagnosia
This term has been proposed for a (transient) syndrome characterized by inability to tell the time observing a clock or watch but with preserved ability for clock setting or giving verbally the position of the hands.

Reference
Kartsounis LD, Crewes H. Horologagnosia: an impairment of the ability to tell the time. *J Neurol Neurosurg Psychiatry*. 1994; **57**: 384–5.

Cross Reference
Agnosia

Howship-Romberg Sign
This is neuralgic pain in the inner thigh as a consequence of obturator neuropathy or obturator hernia (more often with anterior than posterior branch type).

References
Karasaki T, Nakagawa T, Tanaka N. Obturator hernia: the relationship between anatomical classification and the Howship-Romberg sign. *Hernia*. 2014; **18**: 413–6.
Schiffter R. Moritz Heinrich Romberg (1795–1873). *J Neurol*. 2010; **257**: 1409–10.

Hoyt-Spencer Sign
This name is given to the triad of findings characteristic of chronic optic nerve compression, especially due to spheno-orbital optic nerve sheath meningiomas:

- Optociliary shunt vessels.
- Disc pallor.
- Visual loss.

Reference
Hollenhorst RW Jr, Hollenhorst RW Sr, MacCarthy CS. Visual prognosis of optic nerve sheath meningiomas producing shunt vessels on the optic disk: the Hoyt-Spencer syndrome. *Trans Am Ophthalmol Soc.* 1977; **75**: 141–63.

"Hung-Up" Reflexes
- see WOLTMAN'S SIGN

Hutchinson's Pupil
Hutchinson's pupil is unilateral pupillary dilatation ipsilateral to a supratentorial (usually extrinsic) space-occupying lesion, which may be the earliest sign of raised intracranial pressure. It reflects involvement of peripheral pupilloconstrictor fibres in the oculomotor (III) nerve, perhaps due to compression on the margin of the tentorium.
Cross References
Anisocoria; Mydriasis; Oculomotor (III) nerve palsy

Hyperacusis
Hyperacusis is an abnormal loudness of sounds, especially low tones, due to paralysis of the stapedius muscle, whose normal reflex function is to damp conduction across the ossicular chain of the middle ear. This most commonly occurs with lower motor neurone facial (VII) nerve (Bell's) palsy, located proximal to the nerve to stapedius. Ageusia may also be present if the chorda tympani branch of the facial nerve is involved. Hyperacusis may occasionally occur with central (brainstem) lesions.
    Reduction or absence of the stapedius reflex may be tested using the stethoscope loudness imbalance test: with a stethoscope placed in the patients ears, a vibrating tuning fork is placed on the bell. Normally the perception of sound is symmetrical, but sound lateralizes to the side of facial paresis if the attenuating effect of the stapedius reflex is lost.
Cross References
Ageusia; Bell's palsy; Facial paresis, Facial weakness

Hyperaesthesia
Hyperaesthesia describes an increased sensitivity to sensory stimulation of any modality, *e.g.* pain (hyperalgesia), touch.
Cross References
Anaesthesia; Hyperalgesia

Hyperalgesia
Hyperalgesia describes the exaggerated perception of pain from a stimulus which is normally painful (*cf.* allodynia). This may result from sensitization of nociceptors (paradoxically this may sometimes be induced by morphine) or abnormal ephaptic cross-excitation between primary afferent fibres.
Cross References
Allodynia; Dysaesthesia; Hyperpathia

Hyperekplexia

Hyperekplexia (literally, to jump excessively) is an involuntary movement disorder in which there is a pathologically exaggerated startle response, usually to sudden unexpected auditory stimuli, but sometimes also to tactile (especially trigeminal) and visual stimuli.

The startle response is a sudden shock-like movement which consists of eye blink, grimace, abduction of the arms, and flexion of the neck, trunk, elbows, hips, and knees. The head retraction sign, in response to finger tapping the centre of the face, glabella, bridge of the nose, upper lip or chin, is a characteristic sign, characterized as a facial withdrawal reflex.

The muscular jerk of startle satisfies the definition of myoclonus. Ideally for hyperekplexia to be diagnosed there should be a physiological demonstration of exaggerated startle response, but this criterion is seldom adequately fulfilled. Hyperekplexia syndromes may be classified as:

- *Idiopathic*: the majority.
- *Hereditary/familial*:

  An autosomal dominant disorder with muscular hypertonia in infancy, leg jerks and gait disorder. Familial cases have been associated with mutations in the α_1 subunit of the inhibitory glycine receptor gene.

- *Symptomatic*:

  perinatal ischaemic-hypoxic encephalopathy.
  brainstem lesions (encephalitis, haemorrhage).
  thalamic lesions (inflammation, vascular).
  drugs (cocaine, amphetamines).
  Tourette syndrome.

Attacks may respond to the GABA agonist clonazepam.

References

Matsumoto J, Hallett M. Startle syndromes. In: Marsden CD, Fahn S, editors. Movement disorders 3. Boston: Butterworth; 1994. p. 418–33.

Meinck HM. Cramps, spasms, startles and related symptoms. In: Schmitz B, Tettenborn B, Schomer DL, editors. The paroxysmal disorders. Cambridge: Cambridge University Press; 2010. p. 130–44.

Cross References

Myoclonus; Urinary incontinence

Hypergraphia

Hypergraphia is a form of increased writing activity. It has been suggested that it should refer specifically to all transient increased writing activity with a non-iterative appearance at the syntactic or lexicographemic level (*cf.* automatic writing behaviour).

Hypergraphia may be seen as part of the interictal psychosis which sometimes develops in patients with complex partial seizures from a temporal lobe (especially non-dominant hemisphere) focus, or with other non-dominant temporal lobe lesions (vascular, neoplastic, demyelinative, neurodegenerative), or psychiatric disorders (schizophrenia). Hypergraphia is a feature of Geschwind's syndrome, along with hyperreligiosity and hyposexuality.

Reference

Van Vugt P, Paquier P, Kees L, Cras P. Increased writing activity in neurological conditions: a review and clinical study. *J Neurol Neurosurg Psychiatry*. 1996; **61**: 510–4.

Cross References

Automatic writing behaviour; Hyperreligiosity; Hyposexuality

Hyperhidrosis

Hyperhidrosis is excessive (unphysiological) sweating. This may be "essential" (*i.e.* without obvious cause), or seen as a feature of acromegaly, Parkinson's disease, or occurring in a band above a spinal cord injury. Localised hyperhidrosis caused by food (gustatory sweating) may result from aberrant connections between nerve fibres supplying sweat glands and salivary glands. Other causes of hyperhidrosis include mercury poisoning, phaeochromocytoma, and tetanus. Transient hyperhidrosis contralateral to a large cerebral infarct in the absence of autonomic dysfunction has also been described. Regional syndromes of hyperhidrosis (hands, feet, axillae) are also described.

Treatment is difficult. Symptoms may be helped (but not abolished) by low dose anticholinergic drugs, clonidine or propantheline. For focal syndromes, botulinum toxin injections or sympathectomy may be helpful.

References
Labar DR, Mohr JP, Nichols FT, Tatemichi TK. Unilateral hyperhidrosis after cerebral infarction. *Neurology*. 1988; **38**: 1679–82.
Naumann M, Mathias CJ. Treatment of hyperhidrosis. In: Mathias CJ, Bannister R, editors. Autonomic failure. A textbook of clinical disorders of the autonomic nervous system. 5th ed. Oxford: Oxford University Press; 2013. p. 404–9.
Cross References
Anhidrosis; Diaphoresis; Gustatory sweating; Holmes-Adie pupil, Holmes-Adie syndrome

Hyperkinesia

Hyperkinesia indicates an involuntary movement disorder characterized by excessive amplitude of movement, such as ballism, or chorea, or the speech disorders occurring with them.
Cross References
Ballism, Ballismus; Chorea, Choreoathetosis; Dysarthria

Hyperlexia

Hyperlexia has been used to refer to the ability to read easily and fluently (*i.e.* decode printed text to sound) without necessarily comprehending the meaning of the text which has been read, not an infrequent finding in patients with autism.

Hypermetamorphosis

Hypermetamorphosis is an overattention to external stimuli. Patients with hypermetamorphosis may explore compulsively and touch everything in their environment. This excessive tendency to take notice of and to attend and react to every visual stimulus is one element of the environmental dependency syndrome and may be associated with other forms of utilization behaviour, imitation behaviour (echolalia, echopraxia) and frontal release signs such as the grasp reflex. It occurs with severe frontal lobe damage and may be observed following recovery from herpes simplex encephalitis and in frontal lobe dementias including Pick's disease. Bitemporal lobectomy may also result in hypermetamorphosis, as a feature of the Klüver-Bucy syndrome.

Reference
Danek A. "Hypermetamorphosis". Heinrich Neumann's (1814–1884) legacy [in German]. *Nervenarzt*. 2007; **78**: 342–6.
Cross References
Attention; Echolalia; Echopraxia; Frontal release signs; Grasp reflex; Imitation behaviour; Klüver-Bucy syndrome; Utilization behaviour

Hypermetria
- see DYSMETRIA

Hypermnesia
- see EIDETIC MEMORY; SYNAESTHESIA

Hyperorality
Hyperorality is a neurobehavioural abnormality consisting of drinking more than usual, eating excessively, eating anything in sight, and putting objects inappropriately into the mouth. It is a feature of frontal lobe pathology. It is one element of the Klüver-Bucy syndrome, along with hypersexuality.
Cross References
Geophagia, Geophagy; Klüver-Bucy syndrome

Hyperpathia
Hyperpathia is an unpleasant sensation, often a burning pain, associated with elevated threshold for cutaneous sensory stimuli such as light touch or hot and cold stimuli, especially repetitive stimuli. Even light stimuli may produce pain. Clinical features of hyperpathia may include summation (pain perception increases with repeated stimulation) and aftersensations (pain continues after stimulation has ceased). The term thus overlaps to some extent with hyperalgesia (although the initial stimulus need not be painful itself) and dysaesthesia. There is an accompanying diminution of sensibility due to a raising of the sensory threshold (*cf.* allodynia), and the pain is not stimulus-bound (*i.e.* spreads beyond the area of stimulation).

Hyperpathia is a feature of thalamic lesions, and hence tends to involve the whole of one side of the body following a unilateral lesion such as a cerebral haemorrhage or thrombosis. Generalized hyperpathia may also be seen in variant Creutzfeldt-Jakob disease, in which posterior thalamic (pulvinar) lesions are said to be a characteristic neuroradiological finding.
Cross References
Allodynia; Dysaesthesia; Hyperalgesia

Hyperphagia
Hyperphagia is increased or excessive eating. Binge eating, particularly of sweet things, is one of the neurobehavioural disturbances seen in behavioural variant frontotemporal dementia. Hyperphagia may be one feature of a more general tendency to put things in the mouth (hyperorality), for example in the Klüver-Bucy syndrome.
Cross References
Hyperorality; Klüver-Bucy syndrome

Hyperphoria
Hyperphoria is a variety of heterophoria in which there is a latent upward deviation of the visual axis of one eye. Using the cover-uncover test, this may be observed clinically as the downward movement of the eye as it is uncovered.
Cross References
Cover tests; Heterophoria; Hypophoria

Hyperpilaphesie
This name is given to the augmentation of some sensory faculties in response to other sensory deprivation, for example touch sensation in the blind. This is presumably a reflection of compensatory enhancement as a consequence of cross-modal plasticity within the brain, as seen for example in some Braille readers.

Hyperpronation
- see CHOREA, CHOREOATHETOSIS; DECEREBRATE RIGIDITY

Hyperreflexia
Hyperreflexia is an exaggerated briskness of the tendon reflexes. This may be physiological in an anxious patient (reflexes often denoted ++), or pathological in the context of corticospinal pathway pathology (upper motor neurone syndrome, often denoted +++). It is sometimes difficult to distinguish normally brisk reflexes from pathologically brisk reflexes. Hyperreflexia (including a jaw jerk) in isolation cannot be used to diagnose an upper motor neurone syndrome, and asymmetry of reflexes is a soft sign. On the other hand, upgoing plantar responses are a hard sign of upper motor neurone pathology; other accompanying signs (weakness, sustained clonus, absent abdominal reflexes) also indicate abnormality.

Hyperreflexia reflects an increased gain in the stretch reflex. This may be due to impaired descending inhibitory inputs to the monosynaptic reflex arc. Rarely pathological hyperreflexia may occur in the absence of spasticity, suggesting different neuroanatomical substrates underlying these phenomena.

"Hyperreflexia" of the bladder detrusor muscle may be a cause of urinary urge incontinence.

Reference
Sherman SJ, Koshland GF, Laguna JF. Hyper-reflexia without spasticity after unilateral infarct of the medullary pyramid. *J Neurol Sci*. 2000; **175**: 145–55.

Cross References
Abdominal reflexes; Clonus; Jaw jerk; Reflexes; Spasticity; Urinary incontinence; Upper motor neurone (UMN) syndrome; Weakness

Hyperreligiosity
Hyperreligiosity (or religiosity) is a neurobehavioural symptom, manifest as sudden religious conversion, or increased and unswerving orthodoxy in devotion to religious rituals. It may be encountered along with hypergraphia and hyposexuality as a feature of Geschwind's syndrome in patients with temporal lobe epilepsy. It has also been observed in some patients with frontotemporal dementia. The finding is cross-cultural, having been described in Christians, Moslems, and Sikhs. In the context of refractory epilepsy, it has been associated with reduced volume of the right hippocampus, but not right amygdala.

References
Trimble MR, Freeman A. An investigation of religiosity and the Gastaut-Geschwind syndrome in patients with temporal lobe epilepsy. *Epilepsy Behav*. 2006; **9**: 407–14.
Wuerfel J, Krishnamoorthy ES, Brown RJ et al. Religiosity is associated with hippocampal but not amygdala volumes in patients with refractory epilepsy. *J Neurol Neurosurg Psychiatry*. 2004; **75**: 640–2.

Cross References
Hypergraphia; Hyposexuality

Hypersexuality
Hypersexuality is a pathological increase in sexual drive and activity. Recognised causes include bilateral temporal lobe damage, as in the Klüver-Bucy syndrome, septal damage, hypothalamic disease (rare) with or without subjective increase in libido, and dopaminergic drug treatment in Parkinson's disease. Hypersexuality is also a feature of the Kleine-Levin syndrome. Sexual disinhibition may be a feature of frontal lobe syndromes, particularly of the orbitofrontal cortex.

Reference
Devinsky J, Sacks O, Devinsky O. Kluver-Bucy syndrome, hypersexuality, and the law. *Neurocase*. 2010; **16**: 140–5.

Cross References
Disinhibition; Frontal lobe syndromes; Klüver-Bucy syndrome; Punding

Hypersomnolence

Hypersomnolence is characterized by excessive daytime sleepiness, with a tendency to fall asleep at inappropriate times and places, for example during meals, telephone conversations, at the wheel of a car. Causes of hypersomnolence include:

- Narcolepsy or the narcoleptic syndrome: may be accompanied by other features such as sleep paralysis, hypnagogic hallucinations, cataplexy.
- Midbrain lesions.
- Idiopathic CNS hypersomnia.
- Kleine-Levin syndrome.
- Nocturnal hypoventilation, due to:
    Obstructive sleep apnoea-hypopnoea syndrome (OSAHS; Pickwickian syndrome). Chest wall anomalies.
    Neuromuscular and myopathic disorders affecting the respiratory muscles, especially the diaphragm, for example:
        motor neurone disease.
        myotonic dystrophy.
        metabolic myopathies, *e.g.* acid maltase deficiency.
        mitochondrial disorders.
- Drugs: benzodiazepines, ergot-derivative dopamine agonists.
- Post-stroke sleep-related disorders.

Nocturnal hypoventilation as a consequence of obstructed breathing, often manifest as snoring, causes arterial oxygen desaturation as a consequence of hypopnoea/apnoea which may lead to disturbed sleep, repeated arousals associated with tachycardia and hypertension. Clinical signs may include a bounding hyperdynamic circulation and sometimes papilloedema, as well as features of any underlying neuromuscular disease. OSAHS may present in the neurology clinic with loss of consciousness (sleep secondary to hypersomnolence), stroke, morning headaches, and cognitive impairment (slowing). Investigations may reveal a raised haematocrit and early morning hypoxia. Sleep studies (polysomnography, pulse oximetry) confirm nocturnal hypoventilation with dips in arterial oxygen saturation. Treatment is with nocturnal continuous positive airway pressure (CPAP) ventilation. Modafinil is also licensed for this indication.

Cross References
Asterixis; Cataplexy; Papilloedema; Paradoxical breathing; Snoring

Hyperthermia

Body temperature is usually regulated within narrow limits through the co-ordinating actions of a centre for temperature control ("thermostat"), located in the hypothalamus (anterior-preoptic area), and effector mechanisms (shivering, sweating, panting, vasoconstriction, vasodilation), controlled by pathways located in or running through the posterior hypothalamus and peripherally in the autonomic nervous system. Lesions of the anterior hypothalamus (*e.g.* trauma, ischaemia, inflammation, tumour) may result in hyperthermia (*cf.* hypothermia). Other recognised causes of hyperthermia include:

- Infection: bacteria, viruses (pyrogens, *e.g.* interleukin-1).
- Malignant hyperthermia.
- Neuroleptic malignant syndrome (hyperthermia, rigidity, autonomic dysfunction).
- Heatstroke.
- Hyperthyroidism.
- Phaeochromocytoma crisis.

Cross Reference
Hypothermia

Hypertonia, Hypertonus
Hypertonia or hypertonus is an exaggeration of normal muscular tone, manifest as resistance to passive movement. It usually implies spasticity of corticospinal (pyramidal) pathway origin, rather than (leadpipe) rigidity of extrapyramidal origin.
Cross References
Clasp-knife phenomenon; Hyperreflexia; Paratonia; Rigidity; Spasiticity; Upper motor neurone (UMN) syndrome

Hypertrophy
- see MUSCLE HYPERTROPHY

Hypertropia
Hypertropia is a variety of heterotropia in which there is manifest upward vertical deviation of the visual axis of one eye. Using the cover test, this manifests as downward movement of the uncovered eye. Depending on the affected eye, this finding is often described as a "left-over right" or "right-over left". Asymptomatic hypertropia on lateral gaze is often congenital or physiological.
Cross References
Bielschowsky's sign, Bielschowsky's test; Cover tests; Heterotropia; Hypotropia

Hypoaesthesia
Hypoaesthesia (hypaesthesia, hypesthesia) is decreased sensitivity to, or diminution of, sensory perception in any modality, most frequently used to describe reduced sensitivity to pain (hypoalgesia) or touch.
Cross Reference
Anaesthesia

Hypoalgesia
Hypoalgesia is a decreased sensitivity to, or diminution of, pain perception in response to a normally painful stimulus.
Cross Reference
Analgesia

Hypogeusia
- see AGEUSIA

Hypohidrosis
- see ANHIDROSIS

Hypokinesia
Hypokinesia is a reduction in the speed of initiation of voluntary movements, which at worst may progress to an inability to initiate voluntary movement (akinesia). Repeated apposition of finger and thumb or foot tapping may be useful in demonstrating hypokinesia of gradual onset ("fatigue"). It may often coexist with bradykinesia and hypometria, and is a feature of disorders of the basal ganglia (akinetic-rigid or parkinsonian syndromes), for example:

● Parkinson's disease.
● Multiple system atrophy.
● Progressive supranuclear palsy (Steele-Richardson-Olszewski syndrome).
● Some variants of prion disease.

Some dysarthrias may also be described as hypokinetic.
Cross References
Akinesia; Bradykinesia; Dysarthria; Fatigue; Parkinsonism

Hypometria

Hypometria is a reduction in the amplitude of voluntary movements. It may be demonstrated by asking a patient to make repeated, large amplitude, opposition movements of thumb and forefinger, or tapping movements of the foot on the floor. A gradual decline in amplitude (which may be referred to as fatiguability; *cf.* fatigue) denotes hypometria. Voluntary saccadic eye movements may also show a "step", as a correcting additional saccade compensates for the undershoot (hypometria) of the original movement. Hypometria is a feature of parkinsonian syndromes such as idiopathic Parkinson's disease.

Cross References
Akinesia; Bradykinesia; Dysmetria; Fatigue; Hypokinesia; Parkinsonism; Saccades

Hypomimia

Hypomimia, or amimia, is a deficit or absence of expression by gesture or mimicry. This is usually most obvious as a lack of facial expressive mobility ("mask-like facies"). This is a feature of frontal-subcortical disease, *e.g.* basal ganglia disease producing akinetic-rigid or parkinsonian syndromes, and frontal lobe lesions (especially of the non-dominant hemisphere).

Cross References
Facial paresis, Facial weakness; Fisher's sign; Parkinsonism

Hypophonia

Hypophonia is a quiet voice, as in hypokinetic dysarthria. It is often a feature of parkinsonian syndromes (*e.g.* idiopathic Parkinson's disease, multiple system atrophy), and may occur early in progressive supranuclear palsy. In isolation, other causes of dysphonia may need to be considered.

Cross References
Dysarthria; Dysphonia; Parkinsonism

Hypophoria

Hypophoria is a variety of heterophoria in which there is a latent downward deviation of the visual axis of one eye. Using the cover-uncover test, this may be observed clinically as the upward movement of the eye as it is uncovered.

Cross References
Cover tests; Heterophoria; Hypophoria

Hyporeflexia

Hyporeflexia is a diminution of tendon reflexes, short of their total absence (areflexia). This may be physiological, as with the diminution of the ankle jerks with normal ageing; or pathological, most usually as a feature of peripheral lesions such as radiculopathy or neuropathy. The latter may be axonal or demyelinating, in the latter the blunting of the reflex may be out of proportion to associated weakness or sensory loss.

Although frequently characterized as a feature of the lower motor neurone syndrome, the pathology underlying hyporeflexia may occur anywhere along the monosynaptic reflex arc, including the sensory afferent fibre and dorsal root ganglion as well as the motor efferent fibre, and/or the spinal cord synapse.

Hyporeflexia may also accompany central lesions, particularly with involvement of the mesencephalic and upper pontine reticular formation. Hyporeflexia is an accompaniment of hemiballismus, and may also be noted in brainstem encephalitis (Bickerstaff's encephalitis), in which the presence of a peripheral nerve disorder is debated.

Hyporeflexia is not a feature of myasthenia gravis but may occur in Lambert-Eaton myasthenic syndrome (*cf.* facilitation); it is not seen in most muscle diseases unless they are advanced.

Cross References
Age-related signs; Areflexia; Facilitation; Lower motor neurone (LMN) syndrome; Reflexes

Hyposexuality

Hyposexuality describes a lack of sexual drive, interest, or activity. It may be associated with many diseases, physical or psychiatric, and/or medications which affect the central nervous system. Along with hypergraphia and hyperreligiosity, hyposexuality is one of the defining features of Geschwind syndrome.

References
Benson DF. The Geschwind syndrome. *Adv Neurol.* 1991; **55**: 411–21.
Pritchard PB. Hyposexuality: a complication of complex partial epilepsy. *Trans Am Neurol Assoc.* 1980; **105**: 193–5.

Cross References
Hypergraphia; Hyperreligiosity

Hypothermia

Hypothalamic damage, particularly in the posterior region, can lead to hypothermia (*cf.* hyperthermia) or poikilothermia (body temperature varying with ambient temperature, as in reptiles). There are many reported pathological causes, including tumour, trauma, infarct, haemorrhage, neurosarcoidosis, Wernicke's encephalopathy, fat embolism, histiocytosis X, and multiple sclerosis (rare). A rare syndrome of paroxysmal or periodic hypothermia has been described, and labelled as diencephalic epilepsy. Non-neurological causes of hypothermia are more common, including hypothyroidism, hypopituitarism, hypoglycaemia, and drug overdose.

Reference
Thomas DJ, Green ID. Periodic hypothermia. *BMJ.* 1973; **2**: 696–7.

Cross Reference
Hyperthermia

Hypotonia, Hypotonus

Hypotonia (hypotonus) is a diminution or loss of normal muscular tone, causing floppiness of the limbs. This is particularly associated with peripheral nerve or muscle pathology, as well as lesions of the cerebellum and certain basal ganglia disorders such as hemiballismus-hemichorea. Weakness preventing voluntary activity, rather than a reduction in stretch reflex activity, appears to be the mechanism underlying hypotonia.

Reference
Van der Meche FG, van Gijn J. Hypotonia: an erroneous clinical concept. *Brain.* 1986; **109**: 1169–78.

Cross References
Ataxia; Flaccidity; Hemiballismus; Hypertonia, Hypertonus

Hypotropia

Hypotropia is a variety of heterotropia in which there is manifest downward vertical deviation of the visual axis of one eye. Using the cover test, this manifests as upward movement of the uncovered eye. Depending on the affected eye, this finding is often described as a "left-over-right" or "right-over-left".

Cross References
Cover tests; "Double elevator palsy"; Heterotropia; Hypertropia

I

Ice Pack Test

The ice pack test, or ice-on-eyes test, is performed by holding an ice cube, wrapped in a towel or a surgical glove, over the levator palpebrae superioris muscle of a ptotic eye for 2–10 min. Improvement of ptosis is said to be specific for myasthenia gravis, perhaps because cold improves transmission at the neuromuscular junction (myasthenic patients often improve in cold as opposed to hot weather). This phenomenon is generally not observed in other causes of ptosis, although it has been reported in Miller Fisher syndrome. A pooled analysis of several studies gave a test sensitivity of 89% and specificity of 100% with correspondingly high positive and negative likelihood ratios. The test is easy to perform and without side effects (*cf*. tensilon test). Whether the ice pack test is also applicable to myasthenic diplopia has yet to be determined: false positives have been documented.

References
Larner AJ. The place of the ice pack test in the diagnosis of myasthenia gravis. *Int J Clin Pract*. 2004; **58**: 887–8.
Larner AJ, Thomas DJ. Can myasthenia gravis be diagnosed with the "ice pack test"? A cautionary note. *Postgrad Med J*. 2000; **76**: 162–3.
Reddy AR, Backhouse OC. "Ice-on-eyes", a simple test for myasthenia gravis presenting with ocular symptoms. *Pract Neurol*. 2007; **7**: 109–11.

Cross References
Diplopia; Fatigue; Ptosis

Ideational Apraxia
- see APRAXIA

Ideomotor Apraxia
- see APRAXIA

Idiomuscular Response
- see TIBIALIS ANTERIOR RESPONSE

Illusion

An illusion is a misinterpretation of a perception (*cf*. delusion, hallucination). Illusions occur in normal people when they are tired, inattentive, in conditions of poor illumination, or if there is sensory impairment. They also occur in disease states such as delirium, and psychiatric disorders (affective disorders, schizophrenia). Examples of phenomena which may be labelled illusory include:

- Visual: illusory visual spread, metamorphopsia, palinopsia, polyopia, teliopsia, Pulfrich phenomenon, visual alloaesthesia, visual perseveration.
- Auditory: palinacusis.
- Vestibular: vertigo.

Reference
Tekin S, Cummings JL. Hallucinations and related conditions. In: Heilman KM, Valenstein E, editors. Clinical neuropsychology. 4th ed. Oxford: Oxford University Press; 2003. p. 479–94.

Cross References
Delirium; Delusion; Hallucination

© Springer International Publishing Switzerland 2016   171
A.J. Larner, *A Dictionary of Neurological Signs*,
DOI 10.1007/978-3-319-29821-4_9

Illusory Visual Spread
- see VISUAL PERSEVERATION

Imitation Behaviour
Imitation behaviour is the reproduction by the patient of gestures (echopraxia) and/or utterances (echolalia) made by the examiner in front of the patient; these "echophenomena" are made by the patient without preliminary instructions to do so. They are consistent and have a compulsive quality to them, perhaps triggered by the equivocal nature of the situation. There may be accompanying primitive reflexes, particularly the grasp reflex, and sometimes utilization behaviour.

Imitation behaviour occurs with frontal lobe damage; originally mediobasal disease was thought to be the anatomical correlate, but more recent studies suggest upper medial and lateral frontal cortex. Certainly imitation behaviour never occurs with retrorolandic cortical lesions.

A distinction has been drawn between "naïve" imitation behaviour, which ceases after a direct instruction from the examiner not to imitate his/her gestures, which may be seen in some normal individuals; and "obstinate" imitation behaviour which continues despite an instruction to stop; the latter is said to be exclusive to frontotemporal dementia. In a study of imitation behaviour in dementia, it was not observed in patients with Alzheimer's disease.

References
De Renzi E, Cavalleri F, Facchini S. Imitation and utilisation behaviour. *J Neurol Neurosurg Psychiatry*. 1996; **61**: 396–400.
Ghosh A, Dutt A, Bhargava P, Snowden J. Environmental dependency behaviours in fronto-temporal dementia: have we been underrating them? *J Neurol*. 2013; **260**: 861–8.
Lhermitte F, Pillon B, Serdaru M. Human autonomy and the frontal lobes. Part I: imitation and utilization behaviour: a neuropsychological study of 75 patients. *Ann Neurol*. 1986; **19**: 326–34.
Shimomura T, Mori E. Obstinate imitation behaviour in differentiation of frontotemporal dementia from Alzheimer's disease. *Lancet*. 1998; **352**: 623–4.

Cross References
Echolalia; Echopraxia; Grasp reflex; Utilization behaviour

Imitation Synkinesis
– see MIRROR MOVEMENTS

Impersistence
Impersistence may be used to describe an inability to sustain simple motor acts, such as conjugate gaze, eye closure, protrusion of the tongue, or keeping the mouth open. It is most commonly seen with lesions affecting the right hemisphere, especially central and frontal mesial regions, and may occur in association with left hemiplegia, neglect, anosognosia, hemianopia, and sensory loss. These patients may also manifest perseveration, echolalia and echopraxia. A cognitive form of impersistence has also been suggested.

Impersistence is most often observed following cerebrovascular events but may also be seen in Alzheimer's disease and frontal lobe dementias, and metabolic encephalopathies. Impersistence of tongue protrusion and hand grip may be seen in Huntington's disease. Neuropsychologically, impersistence may be related to mechanisms of directed attention which are needed to sustain motor activity.

References
Fisher M. Left hemiplegia and motor impersistence. *J Nerv Ment Dis*. 1956; **123**: 201–18.
Heilman KM. Matter of mind. A neurologist's view of brain-behavior relationships. Oxford: Oxford University Press; 2002. p. 210.
Kertesz A, Nicholson I, Cancelliere A, Kassa K, Black SE. Motor impersistence: a right-hemisphere syndrome. *Neurology*. 1985; **35**: 662–6.

Cross References
Anosognosia, Echolalia; Echopraxia; Hemianopia; Milkmaid's grip; Neglect; Perseveration; Trombone tongue

Inattention
- see NEGLECT

Incontinence
- see URINARY INCONTINENCE

Intention Myoclonus
- see MYOCLONUS

Intermanual Conflict
Intermanual conflict is a behaviour exhibited by an alien hand (*le main étranger*) in which it reaches across involuntarily to interfere with the voluntary activities of the contralateral (normal) hand. "Diagonistic dyspraxia" probably refers to the same phenomenon. The hand acts at cross purposes to the other following voluntary activity. A "compulsive grasping hand" syndrome has been described which may be related to intermanual conflict, the difference being grasping of the contralateral hand in response to voluntary movement.

Intermanual conflict is more characteristic of the callosal, rather than the frontal, subtype of anterior or motor alien hand. It is most often seen in patients with corticobasal degeneration, but may also occur in association with callosal infarcts or tumours or following callosotomy.
Cross References
Alien hand, Alien limb; "Compulsive grasping hand"; Diagonistic dyspraxia

Intermetamorphosis
Intermetamorphosis describes a form of delusional misidentification in which people known to the patient are believed to exchange identities with each other (*cf.* Fregoli syndrome, in which one person can assume different physical appearance).
Reference
Ellis HD, Whitley J, Luaute JP. Delusional misidentification. The three original papers on the Capgras, Frégoli and intermetamorphosis delusions. (Classic Text No. 17). *Hist Psychiatry*. 1994; **5**: 117–46.
Cross Reference
Delusion

Internal Ophthalmoplegia
- see OPHTHALMOPARESIS, OPHTHALMOPLEGIA

Internuclear Ophthalmoplegia (INO)
Internuclear ophthalmoplegia (INO) is the term coined by Lhermitte in 1921 to describe ipsilateral weakness of eye adduction with contralateral nystagmus of the abducting eye (ataxic or dissociated nystagmus), but with preserved convergence. This may be obvious with pursuit eye movements, but is often better seen when testing reflexive saccades or optokinetic responses when the adducting eye is seen to "lag" behind the abducting eye. INO may be asymptomatic or, rarely, may cause diplopia, oscillopsia, or a skew deviation. INO may be unilateral or bilateral. The eyes are generally aligned in primary gaze, but if there is associated exotropia this may be labelled wall-eyed monocular or bilateral internuclear ophthalmoplegia (WEMINO, WEBINO syndromes).

The pathoanatomical substrate of INO is pathology affecting the medial longitudinal fasciculus (hence the alternative name of medial longitudinal fasciculus syndrome), a pathway linking the nuclei of the cranial ocular motor nerves (III, IV, VI). By far the most common cause of INO is demyelination, particularly in young patients, but other causes include infarction (particularly in older patients), Wernicke-Korsakoff syndrome, infection, trauma, tentorial herniation, haemorrhage, vasculitis, and paraneoplasia.

A similar clinical picture may be observed with pathology elsewhere, hence a "false-localising" sign and referred to as a pseudo-internuclear ophthalmoplegia, especially in myasthenia gravis.

References
Keane JR Internuclear ophthalmoplegia: unusual causes in 114 of 410 patients. *Arch Neurol.* 2005; **62**: 714–7.
Zee DS. Internuclear ophthalmoplegia: pathophysiology and diagnosis. In: Büttner U, Brandt TH, editors. Ocular motor disorders of the brain stem. London: Baillière Tindall; 1992. p. 455–70.

Cross References
Diplopia; "False-localising signs"; One-and-a-half syndrome; Optokinetic nystagmus, Optokinetic response; Oscillopsia; Pseudo-internuclear ophthalmoplegia; Saccades; Skew deviation

Intrusion
An intrusion is an inappropriate recurrence of a response (verbal, motor) to a preceding test or procedure after intervening stimuli. Schnider characterizes intrusions as a form of confabulation. Intrusions are thought to reflect inattention, and may be seen in dementing disorders or delirium. These phenomena overlap to some extent with the recurrent type of perseveration.

The term intrusion is also used to describe inappropriate saccadic eye movements which interfere with macular fixation during pursuit eye movements.

References
Fuld PA, Katzman R, Davies P, Terry RD. Intrusions as a sign of Alzheimer dementia: chemical and pathological verification. *Ann Neurol.* 1982; **11**: 155–9.
Schnider A. The confabulating mind. How the brain creates reality. Oxford: Oxford University Press; 2008.

Cross References
Confabulation; Delirium; Dementia; Perseveration; Saccadic intrusion, Saccadic pursuit

Inverse Horner's Syndrome
– see POURFOUR DU PETIT SYNDROME

Inverse Marcus Gunn Phenomenon
– see JAW WINKING; PTOSIS

Inverse Ocular Bobbing
– see OCULAR BOBBING

Inverse Uhthoff Sign
– see UHTHOFF'S PHENOMENON

Inverted Beevor's Sign
– see BEEVOR'S SIGN

Inverted Reflexes
A phasic tendon stretch reflex may be said to be inverted when:

- a distal reflex is present despite absence of a more proximal reflex, *e.g.* tapping the styloid process of the radius produces finger flexion without supinator (brachioradialis) response = "inverted brachioradialis reflex";
- the movement elicited is opposite to that normally seen, *e.g.* extension of the elbow rather than flexion when eliciting the supinator jerk; flexion of the forearm when tapping the triceps tendon (paradoxical triceps reflex); or flexion (hamstring contraction) rather than extension of the knee when tapping the patellar tendon.

The finding of inverted reflexes may reflect dual pathology, but more usually reflects a single lesion which simultaneously affects a root or roots, interrupting the local reflex arc, and the spinal cord, damaging corticospinal (pyramidal tract) pathways which supply segments below the reflex arc. Hence, an inverted supinator jerk is indicative of a lesion at C5/6, paradoxical triceps reflex occurs with C7 lesions; and an inverted knee jerk indicates interruption of the L2/3/4 reflex arcs, with concurrent damage to pathways descending to levels below these segments.

References
Boyle RS, Shakir RA, Weir AI, McInnes A. Inverted knee jerk: a neglected localising sign in spinal cord disease. *J Neurol Neurosurg Psychiatry*. 1979; **42**: 1005–7.
Wartenberg R. The examination of reflexes. A simplification. Chicago: Year Book Publishers; 1945.
Cross Reference
Reflexes

Ipsipulsion
– see LATEROPULSION

Iridoplegia
Iridoplegia is paralysis of the iris, with loss of the pupillary reflexes. This may be partial, as in Argyll Robertson pupil or Holmes-Adie pupil, or complete as in the internal ophthalmoplegia of an oculomotor (III) nerve palsy.
Cross References
Argyll Robertson pupil; Holmes-Adie pupil, Holmes-Adie syndome; Oculomotor (III) nerve palsy; Ophthalmoparesis, Ophthalmoplegia; Pupillary reflexes

Itch
– see PRURITUS

J

Jacksonian March

Jacksonian march is the sequential spread of a simple partial seizure to involve other body parts, for example jerking may spread from one hand up the arm, to the ipsilateral side of the face. It may culminate in a secondary generalised seizure. The pathophysiological implication is of electrical disturbance spreading through the homunculus of the motor cortex. A sensory equivalent occurs but is rare.

References

Jackson JH. A study of convulsions. *Trans St Andrews Med Grad Assoc*. 1870; **3**: 162–204.
Jefferson G. Jacksonian epilepsy. *Postgrad Med J*. 1935; **11**: 150–62.

Cross Reference

Seizures

Jactitation

Jactitation is literally "throwing about", but the term may also imply motor restlessness. The term has been used in various ways: to refer to jerking or convulsion of epileptic origin; or jerking of choreic origin; or of myoclonic origin, such as "hypnagogic jactitation" (physiological myoclonus associated with falling to sleep). It may also be used to refer to the restlessness seen in acute illness, high fever, and exhaustion, though differing from the restlessness implied by akathisia. Hence, it is essentially a non-specific term.

Cross References

Akathisia; Myoclonus; Seizures

Jamais Entendu

A sensation of unfamiliarity akin to *jamais vu* but referring to auditory experiences.

Cross Reference

Jamais vu

Jamais Vécu

- see *JAMAIS VU*

Jamais Vu

Jamais vu (literally "never seen") and *jamais vécu* ("never lived") are complex auras of focal onset epilepsy in which there is a sensation of strangeness or unfamiliarity about visual stimuli that have in fact been previously experienced (*cf. déjà vu*). This is suggestive of seizure onset in the limbic system, but is not lateralising (*cf. déjà vu*).

Cross References

Aura; *Déjà vu*

Jargon Aphasia

Jargon aphasia, a term coined by Hughlings Jackson, refers to a fluent aphasia characterized by a jumbled, unintelligible and meaningless (to the listener) output, with multiple paraphasias and neologisms, and sometimes echolalia (as in transcortical sensory aphasia). There may be a pressure of speech (logorrhoea).

There is debate as to whether jargon aphasia is simply a primary Wernicke/posterior/sensory type of aphasia with failure to self-monitor speech output, or whether additional deficits (*e.g.* pure word deafness, intellectual impairment) are also required. Others suggest

© Springer International Publishing Switzerland 2016
A.J. Larner, *A Dictionary of Neurological Signs*,
DOI 10.1007/978-3-319-29821-4_10

that jargon aphasia represents aphasia and anosognosia, leading to confabulation and reduplicative paramnesia.

References
Hillis AE, Boatman DB, Hart J, Gordon B. Making sense out of jargon. A neurolinguistic and computational account of jargon aphasia. *Neurology*. 1999; **53**: 1813–24.
Kinsbourne M, Warrington EK. Jargon aphasia. *Neuropsychologia*. 1963; **1**: 27–37.
Cross References
Anosognosia; Aphasia; Confabulation; Echolalia; Glossolalia; Logorrhoea; Neologism; Pure word deafness; Reduplicative paramnesia; Transcortical aphasias; Wernicke's aphasia

Jaw Claudication
Jaw claudication, or masticatory claudication, pain on chewing, is a classical symptom of giant cell (temporal) arteritis, but it may also be encountered in temporomandibular joint disease such as rheumatoid arthritis. External carotid artery stenosis proximal to the origins of the facial and maxillary branches has also been associated with jaw claudication, with improvement after carotid endarterectomy or stenting.

Reference
Goodman BW Jr, Shepard FA. Jaw claudication: its value as a diagnostic clue. *Postgrad Med*. 1983; **73**: 177–83.

Jaw Jerk
The jaw jerk, or masseter reflex, is contraction of the masseter and temporalis muscles in response to a tap on the jaw with the mouth held slightly open. Both the afferent and efferent limbs of the arc run in the mandibular division of the trigeminal (V) nerve, connecting centrally with the mesencephalic (motor) nucleus of the trigeminal nerve. The reflex is highly reproducible; there is a linear correlation between age and reflex latency, and a negative correlation between age and reflex amplitude.

Interruption of the reflex arc leads to a diminished or absent jaw jerk as in bulbar palsy (although an absent jaw jerk may be a normal finding, particularly in the elderly). Bilateral supranuclear lesions cause a brisk jaw jerk, as in pseudobulbar palsy (*e.g.* in motor neurone disease).

Reference
Pearce JM. The jaw jerk: an instance of misattribution. *J Neurol Neurosurg Psychiatry*. 2011; **82**: 351–2.
Cross References
Age-related signs; Bulbar palsy; Pseudobulbar palsy; Reflexes

Jaw Winking
Jaw winking, also known as the Marcus Gunn phenomenon, is widening of a congenital ptosis when a patient is chewing, swallowing, or opening the jaw (*i.e.* a trigemino-oculomotor synkinesis). It is believed to result from aberrant innervation of the pterygoid muscles and levator palpebrae superioris.

Eyelid closure on jaw movement or opening of the mouth, the inverse Marcus Gunn phenomenon, is also described, as the Marin-Amat syndrome, thought to be due to aberrant facial (VII) nerve regeneration.

References
Rana PVS, Wadia RS. The Marin-Amat syndrome: an unusual facial synkinesia. *J Neurol Neurosurg Psychiatry*. 1985; **48**: 939–41.
Sundareswaran S, Nipun CA, Kumar V. Jaw-winking phenomenon: report of a case with review of literature. *Indian J Dent Res*. 2015; **26**: 320–3.
Cross References
Ptosis; Synkinesia, Synkinesis

Jendrassik's Manoeuvre
Jendrassik's manoeuvre is used to enhance, or "bring out", absent or depressed tendon (phasic stretch) reflexes by isometric contraction of distant muscle groups, *e.g.* clenching teeth, or making a fist, interlocking fingers and pulling the hands against one another. If previously absent reflexes are then elicited, this may be denoted ±. Co-contraction increases the gain in the monosynaptic reflex arc, as distinct from facilitation or post-tetanic potentiation which is seen in Lambert-Eaton myasthenic syndrome following tetanic contraction of muscles involved in the reflex. Jendrassik's manoeuvre is not useful for cutaneous reflexes such as the plantar response.

References
Delwaide P, Toulouse P. Facilitation of monosynaptic reflexes by voluntary contractions of muscle in remote parts of the body. Mechanisms involved in the Jendrassik manoeuvre. *Brain*. 1981; **104**: 701–9.
Jendrassik E. Ueber allgemeine Localisation der Reflexe. *Deutsche Archiv fur Klinische Medicin*. 1894; **52**: 569–600.
Pasztor E. Erno Jendrassik (1851–1921). *J Neurol*. 2004; **251**: 366–7.

Cross References
Augmentation; Facilitation; Reflexes

Jerk Nystagmus
- see NYSTAGMUS

Jitteriness
Jitteriness implies an exaggerated startle response, reflecting CNS overactivity. This may be confused in neonates with clonic seizures, but in the former there is stimulus sensitivity and an absence of associated ocular movements. However, both may occur in hypoxic-ischaemic or metabolic encephalopathies or with drug withdrawal.

Cross Reference
Seizures

Joint Position Sense
- see PROPRIOCEPTION

Jugular Foramen Syndrome
The glossopharyngeal (IX), vagus (X), and accessory (XI) cranial nerves may be damaged by lesions at or around the jugular foramen, producing a jugular foramen (or Vernet's) syndrome. This produces:

- Dysphagia, dysphonia, palatal droop, impaired gag reflex; ipsilateral reduced taste sensation on the posterior one third of the tongue, and anaesthesia of the posterior one third of the tongue, soft palate, pharynx, larynx and uvula, due to glossopharyngeal and vagus nerve involvement.
- Ipsilateral atrophy and weakness of sternocleidomastoid and trapezius muscles due to accessory nerve involvement (atrophy may be more evident than weakness, hence the importance of palpating the muscle bellies).

Recognised causes of the jugular foramen syndrome include:

- Skull base trauma/fracture.
- Glomus jugulare tumour.
- Inflammatory/infective collection at the skull base.
- Ischaemia.

The differential diagnosis includes retropharyngeal or retroparotid space occupying lesions, which may additionally involve the hypoglossal nerve (XII; Collet-Sicard syndrome) and the sympathetic chain with or without the facial nerve (VII; Villaret's syndrome).

Cross References
Dysphagia; Dysphonia; Gag reflex

Junctional Scotoma, Junctional Scotoma of Traquair
Despite the similarity of these terms, they are used to refer to different types of scotoma:

- *Junctional scotoma*:
    Unilateral central scotoma with contralateral superior temporal defect, seen with lesions at the anterior angle of the chiasm. Such lesions have been said to damage the ipsilateral optic nerve plus the crossing loop of fibres (Wilbrand's knee) originating from the inferonasal portion of the contralateral eye, although it may be noted that some authors have questioned whether such a loop in fact exists.

- *Junctional scotoma of Traquair*:
    A monocular temporal scotoma, sometimes even hemianopia, seen with optic nerve involvement sufficiently close to the chiasm to involve only ipsilateral crossing nasal axons, which subserve the temporal visual field, but sparing nasal axons crossing from the contralateral eye.

Reference
Larner AJ. A developing visual field defect. *Postgrad Med J*. 2002; **78**: 106, 112–113.
Cross References
Scotoma; Visual field defects

K

Kayser-Fleischer Rings

Kayser-Fleischer rings are deposits of copper, seen as a brownish discoloration, in Descemet's membrane. Although often visible to the naked eye (difficult in people with a brown iris), they are best seen with slit-lamp examination. Since they are a highly reliable sign of intracerebral copper deposition in Wilson's disease (hepatolenticular degeneration), any patient suspected of this diagnosis (*i.e.* with parkinsonism or dystonia presenting before age 40, or possibly 50, years) should have a slit-lamp examination (as well as blood copper and caeruloplasmin, and urinary copper, measurements). Very occasionally cases of neurological Wilson's disease without Kayser-Fleischer rings have been reported, likewise presence of rings has been reported in patients with other hepatic conditions.

References
Schrag A, Schott JM. Images in clinical medicine: Kayser-Fleischer rings in Wilson's disease. *N Engl J Med*. 2012; **366**: e18.
Suvarna JC. Kayser-Fleischer ring. *J Postgrad Med*. 2008; **54**: 238–40.

Cross References
Dystonia; Parkinsonism

Kernig's Sign

Kernig's sign is pain in the lower back (and also sometimes in the neck) and resistance to movement during passive extension of the knee on the flexed thigh in a recumbent patient. It is indicative of meningeal mechanosensitivity due to inflammation, either infective (meningitis) or chemical (subarachnoid haemorrhage), in which case it may coexist with nuchal rigidity and Brudzinski's (neck) sign. If unilateral it may indicate irritation of the lumbosacral nerve roots from a ruptured intervertebral disc (in which case Lasègue's sign may also be present).

Kernig's sign is reported to have low sensitivity (0.05) and does not accurately discriminate between adult patients with and without meningitis, although the sensitivity is better in children (0.53; specificity 0.85).

References
Curtis S, Stobart K, Vandermeer B, Simel DL, Klassen T. Clinical features suggestive of meningitis in children. A systematic review of prospective data. *Pediatrics*. 2010; **126**: 952–60.
Thomas KE, Hasbun R, Jekel J, Quagliarello VJ. The diagnostic accuracy of Kernig's sign, Brudzinski's sign, and nuchal rigidity in adults with suspected meningitis. *Clin Infect Dis*. 2002; **35**: 46–52.
Ward MA, Greenwood TM, Kumar DR, Mazza JJ, Yale SH. Josef Brudzinski and Vladimir Mikhailovich Kernig: signs for diagnosing meningitis. *Clin Med Res*. 2010; **8**: 13–7.

Cross References
Brudzinski's (neck) sign; Lasègue's sign; Nuchal rigidity

Kernohan's Notch Syndrome

Raised intracranial pressure as a result of an expanding supratentorial lesion (*e.g.* tumour, subdural haematoma) may cause herniation of brain tissue through the tentorium into the subtentorial space, putting pressure on the midbrain. If the midbrain is shifted against the contralateral margin (free edge) of the tentorium, the cerebral peduncle on that side may be compressed, resulting in a hemiparesis which is ipsilateral to the supratentorial lesion (and hence may be considered "false-localising"), a phenomenon first described by

© Springer International Publishing Switzerland 2016
A.J. Larner, *A Dictionary of Neurological Signs*,
DOI 10.1007/978-3-319-29821-4_11

Kernohan and Woltman in 1929. There may also be an oculomotor (III) nerve palsy ipsilateral to the lesion, which may be partial (unilateral pupil dilatation).
References
Camacho Velasquez JL, Rivero Sanz E, Santos Lasaosa S, Lopez del Val J. Kernohan's notch. *Pract Neurol.* 2015; **15**: 221.
Kernohan JW, Woltman HW. Incisura of the crus due to contralateral brain tumor. *Arch Neurol Psychiatry.* 1929; **21**: 274–87.
Cross References
"False-localising signs"; Hemiparesis; Hutchinson's pupil

Kinesis Paradoxica
Kinesis paradoxica or paradoxical kinesis is the brief but remarkably rapid and effective movement sometimes observed temporarily in patients with Parkinson's disease or postencephalitic parkinsonism, despite the poverty and slowness of spontaneous movement (akinesia, hypokinesia; bradykinesia) seen in these conditions. First described by Souques in 1921, *kinesis paradoxica* often occurs in response to alarm, excitement or emotion (*e.g.* in response to a genuinely funny joke), in other words highly alerting situations.
References
Bonanni L, Thomas A, Onofrj M. Paradoxical kinesis in parkinsonian patients surviving earthquake. *Mov Disord.* 2010; **25**: 1302–4.
Souques AA. Rapport sur les syndromes parkinsoniens. *Rev Neurol (Paris).* 1921; **28**: 534–73.
Cross References
Akinesia; Bradykinesia; Hypokinesia; Parkinsonism

Kissing
- see OSCULATION

Klazomania
Klazomania was the term applied to the motor and vocal tics ("compulsive or compulsory shouting") seen as a sequel to encephalitis lethargica (von Economo's disease), along with parkinsonism and oculogyric crises. This observation helped to promote the idea that tics were due to neurological disease rather than being psychogenic, for example in Tourette syndrome.
References
Hategan A, Bourgeois JA. Compulsive shouting (klazomania) responsive to electroconvulsive therapy. *Psychosomatics.* 2013; **54**: 402–3.
Wohlfart G, Ingvar DH, Hellberg AM. Compulsory shouting (Benedek's "klazomania") associated with oculogyric spasm in chronic epidemic encephalitis. *Acta Psychiatr Scand.* 1961; **36**: 369–77.
Cross References
Coprolalia; Echolalia; Parakinesia, Parakinesis; Tic

Kleptomania
Kleptomania, a morbid impulse to steal, has been related to the obsessive-compulsive spectrum of behaviours in patients with frontal lobe dysfunction, substance abuse, and sometimes as an impulse control disorder in Parkinson's disease.
Reference
Bonfanti AB, Gatto EM. Kleptomania, an unusual impulsive control disorder in Parkinson's disease? *Parkinsonism Relat Disord.* 2010; **16**: 358–9.
Cross Reference
Frontal lobe syndromes

Klüver-Bucy Syndrome

The Klüver-Bucy syndrome consists of a variety of neurobehavioural changes, originally observed following bilateral temporal lobectomy (especially anterior tip) in monkeys, but subsequently described in man. The characteristic features, some or all of which may be present, are:

- Visual agnosia (*e.g.* misrecognition of others).
- Hyperorality.
- Hyperphagia, binge eating.
- Hypermetamorphosis.
- Hypersexuality.
- Emotional changes: apathy; loss of fear, rage reactions.

Recognised clinical causes of the Klüver-Bucy syndrome include:

- Sequel of bilateral temporal lobectomy.
- Post-ictal phenomenon in a patient with a previous unilateral temporal lobectomy.
- Sequel to minor head trauma; subdural haematoma.
- Tumour.
- Meningoencephalitis.
- Frontotemporal dementia (Pick's disease).
- Alzheimer's disease: especially hyperorality and hyperphagia, but it is rare to have all the features.

References
Anson JA, Kuhlman DT. Post-ictal Klüver-Bucy syndrome after temporal lobectomy. *J Neurol Neurosurg Psychiatry*. 1993; **56**: 311–3.
Klüver H, Bucy P. Preliminary analysis of functions of the temporal lobes in monkeys. *Arch Neurol Psychiatry*. 1939; **42**: 979–1000.
Cross References
Apathy; Hypermetamorphosis; Hyperorality; Hyperphagia; Hypersexuality; Visual agnosia

Knee Bobbing, Knee Tremor

A characteristic tremor of the patellae, sometimes known as knee bobbing, juddering, or quivering, may be seen in primary orthostatic tremor (POT; "shaky legs syndrome", "White rabbit syndrome"). It is due to rapid rhythmic contractions of the leg muscles on standing, which dampen or subside on walking, leaning against a wall, or being lifted off the ground, with disappearance of the knee tremor; hence this is a task-specific tremor. Auscultation with the diaphragm of a stethoscope over the lower limb muscles reveals a regular thumping sound, likened to the sound of a distant helicopter. EMG studies show pathognomonic synchronous activity in the leg muscles with a frequency of 14–18 Hz, thought to be generated by a central oscillator (peripheral loading does not alter tremor frequency).

A number of drugs have anecdotally been reported to be helpful in POT, including phenobarbitone, primidone, clonazepam, pramipexole and levodopa, although the only blinded placebo-controlled study suggesting efficacy is with gabapentin. Unlike the situation in essential tremor, propranolol is not helpful.

Knee bobbing has also been described in Charcot-Marie-Tooth disease, as repetitive knee flexion/extension that looks like bobbing but with the feet remaining fixed. A flexed knee posture is characteristic.

References
Brown P. New clinical sign for orthostatic tremor. *Lancet*. 1995; **346**: 306–7.
Heilman KM. Orthostatic tremor. *Arch Neurol*. 1984; **41**: 880–1.
Rossor AM, Murphy S, Reilly MM. Knee bobbing in Charcot-Marie-Tooth disease. *Pract Neurol*. 2012; **12**: 182–3.
Cross Reference
Tremor

Knee Jerk
The knee jerk, also sometimes known as the knee phenomenon, patellar reflex, or Westphal phenomenon, was probably the first of the (so-called) tendon reflexes to be introduced into clinical practice, largely through the teachings of Gowers. A blow to the quadriceps (patellar) tendon with the knee held slightly flexed leads to a brief extension movement at the joint.
References
Gowers WR. A study of the so-called tendon reflex phenomena. *Lancet*. 1879; **113**: 156–7.
Tyler KL, McHenry LC Jr. Fragments of neurological history. The knee jerk and other tendon reflexes. *Neurology*. 1983; **33**: 609–10.
Cross Reference
Reflexes

Körber-Salus-Elschnig Syndrome
This term describes convergence-retraction nystagmus, in which adducting saccades (medial rectus contraction) occur spontaneously or on attempted upgaze, often accompanied by retraction of the eyes into the orbits. This is associated with mesencephalic lesions of the pretectal region (*e.g.* pinealoma). The term may be used interchangeably with Parinaud's syndrome or pretectal syndrome.
Cross References
Nystagmus; Parinaud's syndrome

Kyphoscoliosis
Kyphoscoliosis is twisting of the spinal column in both the anteroposterior (kyphosis) and lateral (scoliosis) planes. Although such deformity is often primary or idiopathic, thus falling within the orthopaedic field of expertise, it may also be a consequence of neurological disease which causes weakness of paraspinal muscles. Recognised neurological associations of kyphoscoliosis and scoliosis include:

- Chiari I malformation, syringomyelia.
- Myelopathy (cause or effect? Skeletal disease such as achondroplasia is more likely to be associated with myelopathy than idiopathic scoliosis).
- Cerebral palsy.
- Friedreich's ataxia.
- Neurofibromatosis.
- Hereditary motor and sensory neuropathies.
- Spinal muscular atrophies.
- Myopathies, *e.g.* Duchenne muscular dystrophy.

Stiff person syndrome may produce a characteristic hyperlordotic spine. Some degree of scoliosis occurs in virtually all patients who suffer from paralytic poliomyelitis before the pubertal growth spurt.
Cross References
Camptocormia; Stiffness

L

Lagophthalmos

Lagophthalmos is an inability to close the eyelid in a peripheral facial (VII) nerve palsy, leaving the palpebral fissure partially open. Exposure of the corneal surface increases the risk of keratitis, ulceration, and potentially visual loss.

A similar phenomenon may be observed with aberrant regeneration of the oculomotor (III) nerve, thought to be due to co-contraction of the levator palpebrae superioris and superior rectus muscles during Bell's phenomenon.

Reference
Vasquez LM, Medel R. Lagophthalmos after facial palsy: current therapeutic options. *Ophthal Res.* 2014; **52**: 165–9.

Cross References
Bell's palsy; Bell's phenomenon, Bell's sign; Facial paresis, Facial weakness

Lambert's Sign

Lambert's sign is the gradual increase in force over a few seconds when a patient with Lambert-Eaton myasthenic syndrome is asked to squeeze the examiner's hand as hard as possible, reflecting increased power with sustained exercise (post-tetanic potentiation). This may also be known as augmentation.

Cross References
Augmentation; Facilitation

Lasègue's Sign

Lasègue's sign is pain along the course of the sciatic nerve induced by exerting traction on the nerve, which is achieved by flexing the thigh at the hip while the leg is extended at the knee ("straight leg raising"). This is similar to the manoeuvre used in Kernig's sign (gradual extension of knee with thigh flexed at the hip). Both indicate irritation of the lower lumbosacral nerve roots and/or meninges. The test is said to have good sensitivity but poor specificity for herniated discs (0.91 and 0.26 in one meta-analysis). The test is non-specific with respect to aetiology, as it may be positive not only with disc protrusion but also with intraspinal tumour or inflammatory radiculopathy.

Various modifications of Lasègue's sign have been described. Pain may be aggravated or elicited sooner using Bragard's test, which is dorsiflexing the foot while raising the leg thus increasing sciatic nerve stretch, or Neri's test, flexing the neck to bring the head on to the chest, indicating dural irritation. Crossed straight leg raising, when the complaint of pain on the affected side occurs when raising the contralateral leg, is said to be less sensitive but highly specific. The femoral nerve stretch test, or "reverse straight leg raising", may detect L3 root or femoral nerve irritation by exerting traction on the femoral nerve.

References
Cook C, Cleland J, Huijbregts P. Creation and critique of studies of diagnostic accuracy: use of the STARD and QUADAS methodological quality assessment tools. *J Man Manip Ther.* 2007; **15**: 93–102 [at 96].

Dalfardi B, Mahmoudi Nezhad GS. Ernest-Charles Lasègue (1816–1883). *J Neurol.* 2014; **261**: 2247–8.

Deville WL, van der Windt DA, Dzaferagic A, Bezemer PD, Bouter LM. The test of Lasègue: systematic review of the accuracy in diagnosing herniated discs. *Spine.* 2000; **25**: 1140–7.

Cross References
Femoral nerve stretch test; Kernig's sign

© Springer International Publishing Switzerland 2016
A.J. Larner, *A Dictionary of Neurological Signs*,
DOI 10.1007/978-3-319-29821-4_12

Lateral Medullary Syndrome

The lateral medullary syndrome (or Wallenberg's syndrome, after the neurologist who described it in 1895) results from damage (usually infarction) of the posterolateral medulla with or without involvement of the inferior cerebellum, producing the following clinical features:

- Nausea, vomiting, vertigo, oscillopsia (involvement of vestibular nuclei).
- Contralateral hypoalgesia, thermoanaesthesia (spinothalamic tract).
- Ipsilateral facial hypoalgesia, thermoanaesthesia, + facial pain (trigeminal spinal nucleus and tract).
- Horner's syndrome (descending sympathetic tract), ± ipsilateral hypohidrosis of the body.
- Ipsilateral ataxia of limbs (olivocerebellar/spinocerebellar fibres, inferior cerebellum).
- Dysphagia, dysphonia, impaired gag reflex.
- ± eye movement disorders, including nystagmus, abnormalities of ocular alignment (skew deviation, ocular tilt reaction, environmental tilt), smooth pursuit and gaze holding, and saccades (lateropulsion, ipsipulsion).
- ± hiccups (singultus); loss of sneezing.

Infarction due to vertebral artery occlusion (occasionally posterior inferior cerebellar artery) or dissection is the most common cause of lateral medullary syndrome, although tumour, demyelination, and trauma are also recognised causes.

References

Fisher CM, Karnes W, Kubik C. Lateral medullary infarction: the pattern of vascular occlusion. *J Neuropathol Exp Neurol.* 1961; **20**: 103–13.
Sacco RL, Freddo L, Bello JA, Odel JG, Onesti ST, Mohr JP. Wallenberg's lateral medullary syndrome. Clinical-magnetic resonance imaging correlations. *Arch Neurol.* 1993; **50**: 609–14.

Cross References

Anaesthesia; Dysphagia; Dysphonia; Environmental tilt; Gag reflex; Hemiataxia; Hiccups; Horner's syndrome; Hypoalgesia; Hypohidrosis; Lateropulsion; Medial medullary syndrome; Nystagmus; Ocular tilt reaction; Oscillopsia; Saccades; Skew deviation; Sneezing; Vertigo

Lateral Rectus Palsy

- see ABDUCENS (VI) NERVE PALSY

Laterocollis

Laterocollis is a lateral head tilt; this may be seen in 10–15% of patients with torticollis.

Cross Reference

Torticollis

Lateropulsion

Lateropulsion or ipsipulsion is literally pulling to one side. The term may be used to describe ipsilateral axial lateropulsion after cerebellar infarcts preventing patients from standing upright, causing them to lean to towards the opposite side. Lateral medullary syndrome may be associated with lateropulsion of the eye toward the involved medulla, and there may also be lateropulsion of voluntary saccadic eye movements (hypermetric to the side of the lesion, hypometric towards the opposite side).

Laughter

- see AUTOMATISM; PATHOLOGICAL CRYING, PATHOLOGICAL LAUGHTER

Lazarus Sign

Various spontaneous and reflex movements are described in brain death, the most dramatic of which has been labelled the Lazarus sign, after Lazarus, raised from the dead by Christ (John 11:1–44). This spinal reflex manifests as flexion of the arms at the elbow, adduction of the shoulders, lifting of the arms, dystonic posturing of the hands and crossing of the hands.

Reference
Bueri JA, Saposnik G, Mauriño J, Saizar R, Garretto NS. Lazarus' sign in brain death. *Mov Disord*. 2000; **15**: 583–6.
Cross Reference
Spinal mass reflex

Leadpipe Rigidity
- see RIGIDITY

Leucocoria
Leucocoria is a white pupillary reflex, in contrast to the normal red reflex. Causes include retinoblastoma, retinal detachment, toxocara infection, congenital cataract, and benign retinal hypopigmentation.

Levator Inhibition
- see EYELID APRAXIA

Levitation
Spontaneous levitation may be displayed by an alien limb, more usually an arm than a leg, indicative of parietal lobe pathology. It is most often seen in corticobasal (ganglionic) degeneration, but a few cases with pathologically confirmed progressive supranuclear palsy have been reported. This has sometimes been called the posterior variant of alien limb.
References
Barclay CL, Bergeron C, Lang AE. Arm levitation in progressive supranuclear palsy. *Neurology*. 1999; **52**: 879–82.
Brunt ER, van Weerden TW, Pruim J, Lakke JW. Unique myoclonic pattern in corticobasal degeneration. *Mov Disord*. 1995; **10**: 132–42.
Cross Reference
Alien hand, Alien limb

Lhermitte's Sign
Lhermitte's sign, or the "barber's chair syndrome", is a painless but unpleasant tingling or electric shock-like sensation in the back and spreading instantaneously down the arms and legs following neck flexion (active or passive). It is associated with pathology within the cervical spinal cord. Although most commonly encountered (and originally described in) multiple sclerosis, it is not pathognomonic of demyelination, and has been described with other local pathologies such as:

- subacute combined degeneration of the cord (vitamin B_{12} deficiency); nitrous oxide (N_2O) exposure.
- traumatic or compressive cervical myelopathy (*e.g.* cervical spondylotic myelopathy).
- epidural/subdural/intraparenchymal tumour.
- radiation myelitis.
- pyridoxine toxicity.
- inflammation, *e.g.* systemic lupus erythematosus, Behçet's disease.
- cervical herpes zoster myelitis.
- cavernous angioma of the cervical cord.

Pathophysiologically, this movement-induced symptom may reflect the exquisite mechanosensitivity of axons which are demyelinated, or damaged in some other way.
A "motor equivalent" of Lhermitte's sign, McArdle's sign, has been described, as has "reverse Lhermitte's sign", a label applied either to the aforementioned symptoms occurring on neck extension, or in which neck flexion induces electrical shock-like sensation travelling from the feet upward.

References
Lhermitte J, Bollack J, Nicolas M. Les douleurs à type de décharge electrique consécutives à la flexion céphalique dans la sclérose en plaques: un case de forme sensitive de la sclérose multiple. *Rev Neurol (Paris)*. 1924; **39**: 56–62.
Pearce JMS. Lhermitte's sign. In: Fragments of neurological history. London: Imperial College Press; 2003. p. 367–9.
Smith KJ. Conduction properties of central demyelinated axons: the generation of symptoms in demyelinating disease. In: Bostock H, Kirkwood PA, Pullen AH, editors. The neurobiology of disease: contributions from neuroscience to clinical neurology. Cambridge: Cambridge University Press; 1996. p. 95–117.
Cross References
McArdle's sign; Myelopathy

Lid Lag
Lid lag is present if a band of sclera is visible between the upper eyelid and the corneal limbus on attempted downgaze (*cf.* lid retraction), seen for example in thyroid eye disease (von Graefe's sign), progressive supranuclear palsy (Steele-Richardson-Olszewski syndrome), and Guillain-Barré syndrome.
Cross References
Lid retraction; Von Graefe's sign

Lid Retraction
Lid (eyelid) retraction is present if a band of sclera is visible between the upper eyelid and the corneal limbus in the primary position (*cf.* lid lag). This should be distinguished from contra-lateral ptosis. Recognised causes of lid retraction include:

- Overactivity of levator palpebrae superioris:
  Dorsal mesencephalic lesion (Collier's sign).
  Opposite to unilateral ptosis, *e.g.* in myasthenia gravis; retracted lid may fall when ptotic lid raised (enhanced ptosis); frontalis overactivity usually evident.
  Paradoxical lid retraction with jaw movement (jaw winking, Marcus Gunn phenomenon).
- Overactivity of Müller's muscle:
  irritative oculosympathetic lesions (Claude-Bernard syndrome).
- Contracture of the levator muscle:
  Hyperthyroidism, Graves' ophthalmopathy (Dalrymple's sign): may be associated lid lag.
  Myotonic syndromes.
  Aberrant oculomotor (III) nerve regeneration (pseudo-von Graefe's sign).
- Central lesion:
  progressive supranuclear palsy.
  dementia with Lewy bodies.
  Parkinson's disease.
- Cicatricial retraction of the lid, *e.g.* following trauma.
- Hepatic disease (Summerskill's sign).
- Guillain-Barré syndrome.

Lower lid retraction may be congenital, or a sign of proptosis. Ectropion may also be seen with lower lid tumour or chalazion, trauma with scarring, and ageing.
Reference
Onofrj M, Monaco D, Bonanni L, et al. Eyelid retraction in dementia with Lewy bodies and Parkinson's disease. *J Neurol*. 2011; **258**: 1542–4.

Cross References
Collier's sign; Contracture; Dalrymple's sign; Jaw winking; Lid lag; Proptosis; Pseudo-von Graefe's sign; Ptosis; Stellwag's sign; Sunset sign

Light-Near Pupillary Dissociation
Light-near pupillary dissociation refers to the loss of pupillary light reflexes, whilst the convergence-accommodation reaction is preserved (see Pupillary Reflexes). This dissociation may be seen in a variety of clinical circumstances:

- Argyll Robertson pupil: small irregular pupils with reduced reaction to light, typically seen in neurosyphilis; the absence of miosis and/or pupillary irregularity has been referred to as pseudo-Argyll Robertson pupil, which may occur in neurosarcoidosis, diabetes mellitus, and aberrant regeneration of the oculomotor (III) nerve.
- Holmes-Adie pupil: dilated pupil showing strong but slow reaction to accommodation but minimal reaction to light (tonic > phasic).
- Parinaud's syndrome (dorsal rostral midbrain syndrome): due to a lesion at the level of the posterior commissure, and characterized by vertical gaze palsy, lid retraction (Collier's sign) or ptosis, and large regular pupils responding to accommodation but not light.

Reference
Kawasaki A. Approach to the patient with abnormal pupils. In: Biller J, editor. Practical neurology. 2nd ed. Philadelphia: Lippincott Williams & Wilkins; 2002. p. 135–46.
Cross References
Argyll Robertson pupil; Collier's sign; Holmes-Adie pupil, Holmes-Adie syndrome; Lid retraction; Parinaud's syndrome; Pseudo-Argyll Robertson pupil; Pupillary reflexes

Light Reflex
- see PUPILLARY REFLEXES

Locked-in Syndrome
The locked-in syndrome results from de-efferentation, such that a patient is awake, self-ventilating and alert, but unable to speak or move; vertical eye movements and blinking are usually preserved, affording a channel for simple (yes/no) communication.

The most common cause of the locked-in syndrome is basilar artery thrombosis causing ventral pontine infarction (both pathological laughter and pathological crying have on occasion been reported to herald this event). Other pathologies include pontine haemorrhage and central pontine myelinolysis. Bilateral ventral midbrain and internal capsule infarcts can produce a similar picture. Generally this is irreversible, although recovery has on occasion been recorded.

The locked-in syndrome may be mistaken for abulia, akinetic mutism, coma, and catatonia.
References
Bauby J-D. The diving-bell and the butterfly. London: Fourth Estate; 1997.
Laureys S, Pellas F, van Eeckhout P, et al. The locked-in syndrome: what is it like to be conscious but paralyzed and voiceless? *Prog Brain Res*. 2005; **150**: 495–511.
Smith E, Delargy M. Locked-in syndrome. *BMJ*. 2005; **330**: 406–9.
Cross References
Abulia; Akinetic mutism; Blinking; Catatonia; Coma; Pathological crying, Pathological laughter; Vegetative states

Lockjaw
- see TRISMUS

Logoclonia

Logoclonia is the tendency for a patient to repeat the final syllable of a word when speaking; hence it is one of the reiterative speech disorders (*cf.* echolalia, palilalia). Liepmann apparently coined this term in 1905 to indicate "continuous perseveration". It may be described as the festinating repetition of individual phonemes.

Logoclonia is an indicator of bilateral brain injury, usually involving subcortical structures, and may be seen in the late stages of dementia of Alzheimer type (but not in semantic dementia).

Reference

Kertesz A. Language in Alzheimer's disease. In: Morris R, Becker JT, editors. Cognitive neuropsychology of Alzheimer's disease. 2nd ed. Oxford: Oxford University Press; 2004. p. 197–218 [at 202].

Cross References

Echolalia; Festination, Festinant gait; Palilalia; Perseveration

Logopenia

Logopenia denotes a language disorder characterised by word finding pauses, but with relatively preserved phrase length and syntactically complete language, but with impaired repetition of phrases and sentences. A logopenic variant of primary progressive aphasia has been delineated in recent years, with Alzheimer-type pathology as the most common neuropathological substrate, hence this is one of the acknowledged variant forms of Alzheimer's disease.

References

Dubois B, Feldman HH, Jacova C et al. Advancing research diagnostic criteria for Alzheimer's disease: the IWG-2 criteria. *Lancet Neurol.* 2014; **13**: 614–29 [Erratum *Lancet Neurol.* 2014; **13**: 757].
Gorno-Tempini ML, Hillis AE, Weintraub S, et al. Classification of primary progressive aphasia and its variants. *Neurology.* 2011; **76**: 1006–14.

Cross Reference

Aphasia

Logorrhoea

Logorrhoea is literally a flow of speech, or pressure of speech, denoting an excessive verbal output, an abnormal number of words produced during each utterance. Content is often irrelevant, disconnected and difficult to interpret. The term may be used to describe the output in the Wernicke/posterior/sensory type of aphasia, or an output which superficially resembles Wernicke aphasia but in which syntax and morphology are intact, rhythm and articulation are usually normal, and paraphasias and neologisms are few. Moreover comprehension is better than anticipated in the Wernicke type of aphasia. Patients may be unaware of their impaired output (anosognosia) due to a failure of self-monitoring.

Logorrhoea may be observed in subcortical (thalamic) aphasia, usually following recovery from lesions (usually haemorrhage) to the anterolateral nuclei. Similar speech output may be observed in psychiatric disorders such as mania and schizophrenia (schizophasia).

Reference

Damasio AR. Aphasia. *N Engl J Med.* 1992; **326**: 531–9.

Cross References

Aphasia; Delirium; Echolalia; Jargon aphasia; Schizophasia; Wernicke's aphasia

Lombard Effect

The Lombard effect is the reflex increase in spoken sound volume in a noisy environment, named after Etienne Lombard, a French ENT surgeon who first described the phenomenon in the early 1900s. Something similar may be noted when attempting conversation with those wearing headphones.

Reference
Zollinger SA, Brumm H. The Lombard effect. *Curr Biol.* 2011; **21**: R614–5.

Long Tract Signs
- see UPPER MOTOR NEURONE (UMN) SYNDROME

"Looking Glass Syndrome"
- see MIRROR AGNOSIA

Lower Motor Neurone (LMN) Syndrome
A lower motor neurone (LMN) syndrome constitutes a constellation of motor signs resulting from damage to lower motor neurone pathways, *i.e.* from anterior horn cell distally, encompassing the motor roots, nerve plexuses, peripheral nerves, and neuromuscular junction. Following the standard order of neurological examination of the motor system, the signs include:

- *Appearance*:
  muscle wasting; fasciculations (or "fibrillations") may be observed or induced, particularly if the pathology is at the level of the anterior horn cell.
- *Tone*:
  reduced tone (flaccidity, hypotonus), although this may simply reflect weakness.
- *Power*:
  weakness, often marked; depending on the precise pathological process, weakness often affects both flexor and extensor muscles equally (although this is not always the case).
- *Co-ordination*:
  depending on the degree of weakness, it may not be possible to comment on the integrity or otherwise of co-ordination in LMN syndromes; in a pure LMN syndrome co-ordination will be normal.
- *Reflexes*:
  depressed (hyporeflexia) or absent (areflexia); plantar responses are flexor.

It is often possible to draw a clinical distinction between motor symptoms resulting from lower or upper motor neurone pathology and hence to formulate a differential diagnosis and direct investigations accordingly. Sensory features may also be present in LMN syndromes if the pathology affects sensory as well as motor roots, or both motor and sensory fibres in peripheral nerves.

Cross References
Areflexia; Fasciculation; Fibrillation; Flaccidity; Hyporeflexia; Hypotonia, Hypotonus; Neuropathy; Reflexes; Upper motor neurone (UMN) syndrome; Weakness

Luria Test
- see FIST-EDGE-PALM TEST

M

Macrographia

Macrographia is abnormally large handwriting. It may be seen in cerebellar disease, possibly as a reflection of the kinetic tremor and/or the impaired checking response seen therein (*cf.* micrographia), and in essential tremor.

Reference

Martinez-Hernandez HR, Louis ED. Macrographia in essential tremor: a study of patients with and without rest tremor. *Mov Disord.* 2014; **29**: 960–1.

Cross References

Micrographia; Tremor

Macropsia

Macropsia, or "Brobdingnagian sight" (after Swift's *Gulliver's Travels*), is an illusory phenomenon in which the size of a normally recognized object is overestimated.

Cross Reference

Metamorphopsia

Macrosomatognosia

- see "ALICE IN WONDERLAND" SYNDROME

Macro-Square-Wave Jerks

- see SQUARE-WAVE JERKS

Macula Sparing, Macula Splitting

Macula sparing is a feature of an homonymous hemianopia in which central vision is intact, due to damage confined to the occipital cortex without involving the occipital pole. This may occur because anastomoses between the middle and posterior cerebral arteries maintain blood supply to that part of area 17 necessary for central vision after occlusion of the posterior cerebral artery.

Cortical blindness due to bilateral (sequential or simultaneous) posterior cerebral artery occlusion may leave a small central field around the fixation point intact, also known as macula sparing.

Macula splitting describes an homonymous hemianopia which cuts through the vertical meridian of the macula, as seen with lesions of the optic radiation.

Hence, macula sparing and macula spiltting have localising value in the assessment of a homonymous hemianopia.

Cross References

Cortical blindness; Hemianopia; Visual field defects

Maculopathy

Maculopathy describes any process affecting the macula, with changes observable on ophthalmoscopy. These processes may produce visual field defects such as a central or ring scotoma, or visual failure. Common causes include:

- Diabetes mellitus: oedema and hard exudates at the macula are a common cause of visual impairment, especially in non-insulin dependent diabetes mellitus.
- Hypertension: abnormal vascular permeability around the fovea may produce a macular star.

© Springer International Publishing Switzerland 2016

A.J. Larner, *A Dictionary of Neurological Signs*,

DOI 10.1007/978-3-319-29821-4_13

- Drug-induced: *e.g.* "bull's-eye" maculopathy of chloroquine.
- "Cherry red spot at the macula": this appearance may occur in sialidosis ("cherry red spot-myoclonus syndrome") and gangliosidoses (*e.g.* Tay-Sachs disease).

Cross References
Cherry red spot at the macula; Retinopathy; Scotoma; Visual field defects

Magnetic Movements
Movements may be described as magnetic in varying contexts:

- following or tracking movements made by an alien hand in corticobasal degeneration; reaching out to touch or grasp the examiner's hand or clothing, as in forced groping; also known as compusive tactile exploration.
- in a hesitant gait (ignition failure), with seeming inability to lift the feet ("stuck to the floor") in gait apraxia.

Reference
Denny-Brown D. The nature of apraxia. *J Nerv Ment Dis*. 1958; **126**: 9–32.
Cross References
Alien hand, Alien limb; Forced groping; Gait apraxia; Grasp reflex

Main D'Accoucheur
Main d'accoucheur, or carpopedal spasm, is a posture of the hand with wrist flexion in which the muscles are rigid and painful. *Main d'accoucheur* is so called because of its resemblance to the posture of the hand adopted for the manual delivery of a baby ("obstetrical hand").

This tetanic posture may develop in acute hypocalcaemia (induced by hyperventilation, for instance) or hypomagnesaemia, and reflects muscle hyperexcitability. Development of *main d'accoucheur* within 4 min of inflation of a sphygmomanometer cuff above arterial pressure (Trousseau's sign) indicates latent tetany. Mechanosensitivity of nerves may also be present elsewhere (*e.g.* Chvostek's sign).
Reference
Athappan G, Ariyamuthu VK. Images in clinical medicine. Chvostek's sign and carpopedal spasm. *N Engl J Med*. 2009; **360**: e24.
Cross References
Chvostek's sign; Trousseau's sign

Main En Griffe
- see CLAW HAND

Main Étranger
- see ALIEN HAND, ALIEN LIMB

Main Succulente
Main succulente refers to a swollen hand with thickened subcutaneous tissues, hyperkeratosis and cyanosis, a constellation of trophic changes which may be observed in an analgesic hand, *e.g.* in syringomyelia.
Cross Reference
Charcot joint

Malapropisms
Malapropisms describe a misuse or inappropriate use of language, usually with unanticipated comic effect, named after the character Mrs Malaprop (derived from the French *mal à propos*, meaning inappropriate) in Richard Brinsley Sheridan's play *The Rivals* (1775).

Malapropisms have been reported as a feature of behavioural variant frontotemporal dementia.

Reference
Mendez MF. Malapropisms, or "the Archie Bunker syndrome", and frontotemporal dementia. *J Neuropsychiatry Clin Neurosci.* 2011; **23**: E3.

"Man-in-the-Barrel"
"Man-in-the-barrel" describes a clinical syndrome of brachial diplegia with preservation of brainstem function and of muscle strength in the legs; this clinical phenotype may result from central or peripheral nervous system pathology.

This most usually occurs as a result of bilateral borderzone infarcts in the territories between the anterior and middle cerebral arteries ("watershed infarction"). This may be as a consequence of cerebral hypoperfusion (*e.g.* during cardiac arrest, cardiac surgery), in which case the prognosis is poor. The clinical picture has also been reported with cerebral metastases. Acute central cervical cord lesions may also produce a "man-in-the-barrel" syndrome, for example after severe hyperextension injury, or after unilateral vertebral artery dissection causing anterior cervical spinal cord infarction. This may follow a transient quadriplegia, and considerable recovery is possible.

A neurogenic man-in-the-barrel syndrome has been reported ("flail arm syndrome"), which is a variant of motor neurone disease. Likewise, bilateral neuralgic amyotrophy can produce an acute man-in-the-barrel phenotype.

References
Moore AP, Humphrey PR. Man-in-the-barrel syndrome caused by cerebral metastases. *Neurology.* 1989; **39**: 1134–5.
Sage JI, van Uitert RL. Man-in-the-barrel syndrome. *Neurology.* 1986; **36**: 1102–3.
Yague S, Moraleda M, Girones D. Peripheral "man-in-the-barrel" syndrome: two cases of acute bilateral neuralgic amyotrophy. *J Neurol.* 2009; **256**(Suppl 2):S117 (abstract P332).

Cross References
Flail limb; Quadriparesis, Quadriplegia

Marche À Petit Pas
Marche à petit pas is a disorder of gait characterized by impairments of balance, gait ignition, and locomotion. There is shortened stride length (literally *marche à petit pas*) and a variably wide base.

This gait disorder is often associated with dementia, frontal release signs, and urinary incontinence, and sometimes with apraxia, parkinsonism, and pyramidal signs. This constellation of clinical signs reflects underlying pathology in the frontal lobe and subjacent white matter, most usually of vascular origin, and is often associated with a subcortical vascular dementia. Modern clinical classifications of gait disorders have subsumed *marche à petit pas* into the category of frontal gait disorder.

Reference
Nutt JG, Marsden CD, Thompson PD. Human walking and higher-level gait disorders, particularly in the elderly. *Neurology.* 1993; **43**: 268–79.

Cross References
Apraxia; Dementia; Frontal release signs; Parkinsonism; Urinary incontinence

Marcus Gunn Phenomenon
- see JAW WINKING

Marcus Gunn Pupil, Marcus Gunn Sign
The Marcus Gunn pupil or sign, first described in 1902 by the ophthalmologist Robert Marcus Gunn (1850–1909), is the adaptation of the pupillary light reflex to persistent light stimulation, that is, a dilatation of the pupil is observed with continuing stimulation with

incident light ("dynamic anisocoria"). This is indicative of an afferent pathway defect, such as retrobulbar neuritis.

The swinging flashlight sign or test may be used to demonstrate this by comparing direct and consensual pupillary light reflexes in one eye. Normally the responses are equal but in the presence of an afferent conduction defect an inequality is manifest as pupillary dilatation.

References
Ha A, Jankovic J. Sorting out the Marcus Gunn phenomena. *World Neurol*. 2010; **25**(6):3.
Mahmoudi Nezhad GS, Jalalpour MH, Dalfardi B. Robert Marcus Gunn (1850–1909). *J Neurol*. 2015; **262**: 2599–600.

Cross References
Pupillary reflexes; Relative afferent pupillary defect (RAPD); Swinging flashlight sign

Mask-Like Facies
The poverty of spontaneous facial expression, hypomimia, seen in extrapyramidal disorders such as idiopathic Parkinson's disease is sometimes described as mask-like.

Cross References
Hypomimia; Parkinsonism

Masseter Hypertrophy
Masseter hypertrophy, either unilateral or bilateral, may be a benign variant. It may occur in individuals prone to bruxism. A familial syndrome of masseter hypertrophy has been described.

Reference
Matinelli P, Fabbri R, Gabellini AS. Familial hypertrophy of the masseter muscles. *J Neurol*. 1987; **234**: 251–3.

Cross Reference
Bruxism

Masseter Reflex
- see JAW JERK

Masticatory Claudication
- see JAW CLAUDICATION

McArdle's Sign
McArdle's sign is the combination of reduced lower limb strength, increased lower limb stiffness and impaired mobility following neck flexion. The difference may best be appreciated by comparing leg strength (*e.g.* hip flexion) with the neck fully extended and fully flexed.

The sign was initially described in multiple sclerosis but may occur in other myelopathies affecting the cord at any point between the foramen magnum and the lower thoracic region. The mechanism is presumed to be stretch-induced conduction block, due to demyelinated plaques or other pathologies, in the axons in the corticospinal tracts. McArdle's sign may be envisaged as the motor equivalent of Lhermitte's sign.

References
McArdle MJ. McArdle's sign in multiple sclerosis. *J Neurol Neurosurg Psychiatry*. 1988; **51**: 1110.
O'Neill JH, Mills KR, Murray NMF. McArdle's sign in multiple sclerosis. *J Neurol Neurosurg Psychiatry*. 1987; **50**: 1691–3.

Cross References
Lhermitte's sign; Myelopathy

Medial Medullary Syndrome
The medial medullary syndrome, or Dejerine's anterior bulbar syndrome, results from damage to the medial medulla, most usually infarction as a consequence of anterior spinal artery or vertebral artery occlusion. The clinical picture is of:

- Ipsilateral tongue paresis and atrophy, fasciculations (due to hypoglossal nerve involvement).
- Contralateral hemiplegia with sparing of the face (pyramid).
- Contralateral loss of position and vibration sense (medial lemniscus) with pain and temperature sensation spared.
- ± upbeat nystagmus (possibly due to involvement of the nucleus intercalatus of Staderini).

References
Hirose G, Ogasawara T, Shirakawa T, et al. Primary position upbeat nystagmus due to unilateral medial medullary infarction. *Ann Neurol*. 1998; **43**: 403–6.
Sawada H, Seriu N, Udaka F, Kameyama M. Magnetic resonance imaging of medial medullary infarction. *Stroke*. 1990; **21**: 963–6.
Cross References
Fasciculation; Hemiplegia; Lateral medullary syndrome; Nystagmus

Menace Reflex
The menace reflex, a blink reflex to visual threat (also known as the threat reflex, or visuopalpebral reflex), may be used at the bedside to test visual processing in patients unable to comply with standard confrontation visual field testing. Failure to respond to a stimulus moving into the temporal field of vision may indicate a hemianopic field defect. The stimulus should be unexpected or unanticipated since the reflex can be voluntarily suppressed, hence it is recommended that the examiner stand behind the patient. Care should be taken to avoid generating air currents with the hand movement as this may stimulate the corneal reflex which may simulate the menace reflex.

It is probable that the menace reflex requires cortical processing: it is lost in persistent vegetative states and is not present in anencephalics. Loss of this reflex may occur in Balint's syndrome, ascribed to inability to recognise the nearness of the threatening object. Experimental and clinical studies have shown that occipital lobe lesions can abolish the menace reflex, as can lesions in parietal and even frontal lobes. Hence the presence of the menace reflex may be used to exclude hemianopia but its absence is not necessarily of localising value.
Reference
Van Ballegoij WJC, Koehler PJ, Ter Meulen BC. The menace reflex. *Pract Neurol*. 2015; **15**: 233–5.
Cross References
Blink reflex; Corneal reflex; Hemianopia; Visual field defects

Meningism
Meningism (meningismus, nuchal rigidity) is a stiffness or discomfort on passive movement (especially flexion) of the neck in the presence of meningeal irritation (*e.g.* infective meningitis, subarachnoid haemorrhage). A number of other, eponymous, signs of meningeal irritation have been described, of which the best known are those of Kernig and Brudzinski.

Meningism is not synonymous with meningitis, since it may occur in acute systemic pyrexial illnesses (pneumonia, bronchitis), especially in children. Moreover, meningism may be absent despite the presence of meningitis in the elderly and those receiving immunosuppressive medication.
Cross References
Brudzinski's (neck) sign; Kernig's sign; Nuchal rigidity

Metamorphopsia

Metamorphopsia is an illusory visual phenomenon characterized by objects appearing distorted or misshapen in form. As with neglect, these phenomena may be classified as object- or person-centred:

- *Object-centred*: affecting size and spatial relationships.
    - Macropsia: objects appear larger than normal.
    - Micropsia: objects appear smaller than normal.
    - Peliopsia: objects appear closer to the observer than they actually are.
    - Porropsia: objects appear farther away from the observer than actually.
    - Zoom effect: sequential increase and decrease in object size.
- *Person centred*:
    - Micro- and macrosomatognosia: body image appears smaller or larger than normal ("Alice in Wonderland" syndrome).

Metamorphopsias are often transient and episodic, occurring for example during migraine attacks, epileptic seizures, with psychotropic drug use, and following petechial intraparenchymal haemorrhages. Rarely, they are long-lasting or permanent, for example following brain infarction (most commonly involving the occipito-parietal or temporo-parietal cortex: lesions on the right are more likely than those on the left to give metamorphopsia) or tumours. Metamorphopsia may be associated with visual hallucinations.

Retinal disease causing displacement of photoreceptors may produce metamorphopsia: micropsia due to receptor separation in retinal oedema, macropsia due to receptor approximation in retinal scarring.

Occasional cases of metamorphopsia have been reported with lesions of the optic chiasm, optic radiation, and retrosplenial region. Indeed, it seems that metamorphopsia may occur with pathology at any point along the visual pathway from retina to cortex.

Differing patterns of metamorphoposia may assist with clinico-anatomical correlation:

- retinal lesions: ipsilateral monocular.
- chiasmal lesions: bitemporal.
- occipitoparietal lesions: contralateral homonymous.

The Amsler Chart Manual (test charts to determine the quality of central vision, by Prof. Dr. Marc Amsler of Zurich) includes charts to demonstrate metamorphopsia (numbers 5 and 6).

Reference
Simunovic MP. Metamorphopsia and its quantification. *Retina*. 2015; **35**: 1285–91.

Cross References
"Alice in Wonderland" syndrome; Hallucination; Hemiprosopometamorphopsia; Illusion; Macropsia; Micropsia; Peliopsia; Porropsia; Teliopsia; Zoom effect

Micrographia

Micrographia is small handwriting. It is most often recognised in association with the extrapyramidal features of idiopathic Parkinson's disease (indeed it may be the presenting sign), but may occasionally occur with other parkinsonian syndromes (*e.g.* progressive supranuclear palsy [PSP]) or in isolation with focal lesions of the midbrain or basal ganglia.

In Parkinson's disease (PD), handwriting may initially be of normal size but then become progressively smaller, slower, and more illegible as writing proceeds, an example of parkinsonian fatigue, a gradual decline in the amplitude and speed of initiation of voluntary movements. Such "slow" micrographia may be distinguished from "fast" micrographia in which letters are small throughout although written at normal speed without fatigue, which may be seen in PSP or other pallidal pathologies. A distinction has also been made between consistent or progressive reduction in the size of handwriting in Parkinson's disease.

Whereas a poor correlation between micrographia and the side, severity or duration of classical parkinsonian features was once reported, more recent studies have found disease severity and impaired cognition to be important clinical correlates, with a relationship to bradykinesia and hypophonia, suggesting overlapping pathophysiology. This again contrasts with previous reports of variable response of micrographia to levodopa preparations. A functional MRI study of micrographia in PD has suggested that so-called consistent micrographia is associated with decreased activity and connectivity in the basal ganglia motor circuit and responds to levodopa, whereas progressive micrographia involves not only the basal ganglia but also the rostral supplementary and cingulate motor areas and cerebellum and is unresponsive to levodopa.

Reports of isolated micrographia with cortical lesions demonstrated by neuroimaging, suggest that the anatomical basis of micrographia may in some cases be at the level of the cortex (dominant parietal lobe) rather than the basal ganglia. Micrographia has also been described following large right anterior cerebral artery infarcts and lacunar infarcts involving the putamen and genu of the internal capsule. Isolated micrographia has been reported with lenticular haematoma.

References

McLennan JE, Nakano K, Tyler HR, Schwab RS. Micrographia in Parkinson's disease. *J Neurol Sci.* 1972; **15**: 141–52.

Scolding NJ, Lees AJ. Micrographia associated with a parietal lobe lesion in multiple sclerosis. *J Neurol Neurosurg Psychiatry*. 1994; **57**: 739–41.

Wagle Shukla A, Ounpraseuth S, Okun MS, Gray V, Schwankhaus J, Metzer WS. Micrographia and related deficits in Parkinson's disease: a cross-sectional study. *BMJ Open*. 2012; **2**(3). pii: e000628.

Wu T, Zhang J, Hallett M, Feng T, Hou Y, Chan P. Neural correlates underlying micrographia in Parkinson's disease. *Brain*. 2016; **139**: 144–60.

Cross References

Fast micrographia; Fatigue; Parkinsonism

Micropsia

Micropsia, or "Lilliput sight" (after Swift's *Gulliver's Travels*, 1726), is an illusory phenomenon in which the size of a normally recognized object is underestimated. It is the most common form of metamorphopsia, and is most often associated with lesions of the right temporo-parietal cortex, although macular oedema and optic chiasm lesions may also cause micropsia. Transient micropsia may occur in migraine. Hemimicropsia, micropsia confined to one visual hemifield, has been recorded. The entirely subjective nature of the disorder may account for the relative rarity of reports. "Lilliputian hallucinations" have been claimed to be distinctive in belladonna poisoning.

References

Allison RS. The senile brain. A clinical study. London: Edward Arnold; 1962. p. 228.

Ceriani F, Gentileschi V, Muggia S, Spinnler H. Seeing objects smaller than they are: micropsia following right temporo-parietal infarction. *Cortex*. 1998; **34**: 131–8.

Cohen L, Gray F, Meyrignac C, et al. Selective deficit of visual size perception: two cases of hemimicropsia. *J Neurol Neurosurg Psychiatry*. 1994; **57**: 73–8.

Cross Reference

Metamorphopsia

Microsomatognosia

- see "ALICE IN WONDERLAND" SYNDROME

Milkmaid's Grip

Milkmaid's grip is the descriptive term applied to the inability to maintain a firm grip (*e.g.* of the examiner's fingers), detected as an alternating squeezing and releasing (as required for successful milking by hand). Seen in Huntington's disease, this may reflect a combination of chorea and motor impersistence.

Cross References
Chorea, Choreoathetosis; Impersistence; Trombone tongue

Minimally Conscious State

The minimally conscious state is characterized by wakefulness with minimal awareness. It is a state of severely altered consciousness in which minimal but clearly discernible behavioural evidence of self- or environmental awareness is demonstrated. It is characterized by inconsistent but reproducible responses above the level of spontaneous or reflexive behavior, which indicate some degree of interaction of the patient with their surroundings.

References
Giacino JT, Kalmar K. Diagnostic and prognostic guidelines for the vegetative and minimally conscious states. *Neuropsychol Rehabil*. 2005; **15**: 166–74.
Royal College of Physicians. Prolonged disorders of consciousness: national clinical guidelines. London: Royal College of Physicians; 2013. p. 3, 12.

Cross References
Coma; Vegetative states

Miosis

Miosis is abnormal reduction in pupillary size, which may be unilateral or bilateral. Recognised causes include:

- Oculosympathetic paresis of whatever cause, *e.g.* Horner's syndrome (unilateral), pontine haemorrhage (bilateral), early stages of central cephalic herniation (bilateral).
- Drug-induced: *e.g.* opiates (bilateral).
- Pupils tend to be small and reactive in metabolic-toxic encephalopathies (bilateral).
- "Senile miosis" (bilateral): age-related.

If only one pupil appears small (anisocoria), it is important to distinguish miosis from contralateral mydriasis, when a different differential will apply.

Reference
Kawasaki A. Approach to the patient with abnormal pupils. In: Biller J, editor. Practical neurology, 2nd ed. Philadelphia: Lippincott Williams & Wilkins; 2002. p. 135–46.

Cross References
Age-related signs; Anisocoria; Argyll Robertson pupil; Horner's syndrome; Mydriasis

Mirror Agnosia, Mirror Apraxia, Mirror Ataxia

Mirror agnosia is a deficit in which patients are unable to use mirror knowledge when interacting with mirrors (a definition which might also encompass mirror sign and mirrored self-misidentification). Also sometimes known as the "looking glass syndrome", or "Ramachandran's sign" after the first description, patients are unable to point to the real object when it is seen in a mirror. They may attempt to reach "into" the mirror even when the actual location of the target has been shown, suggesting an inability to distinguish between the real and virtual images. This reaching for the virtual object has been termed mirror apraxia. Reaching for the real object but with increased errors in direction of reaching has been termed mirror ataxia, suggesting that visual information is not adequately transformed into a body-centred frame of reference.

Parietal lobe lesions with associated hemispatial neglect may underlie these signs, with dissociation of retinotopic (allocentric) space and body schema (egocentric space). A lesion study suggested different areas of parietal lobe might underpin mirror agnosia (posterior angular gyrus and superior temporal gyrus) and mirror ataxia (postcentral sulcus).

References

Binkofski F, Buccino G, Dohle C, Seitz RJ, Freund H-J. Mirror agnosia and mirror ataxia constitute different parietal lobe disorders. *Ann Neurol*. 1999; **46**: 51–61.
Binkofski F, Butler AJ, Buccino G, et al. Mirror apraxia is affecting the peripersonal mirror space. A combined lesion and cerebral activation study. *Exp Brain Res*. 2003; **153**: 210–19.
Ramachandran VS, Altschuler EL, Hillyer S. Mirror agnosia. *Proc Royal Soc London, Ser B*. 1997; **264**: 645–7.

Cross References

Agnosia; "Mirror sign"; Neglect

Mirror Dystonia
- see WRITER'S CRAMP

Mirror Hallucination
- see AUTOSCOPY

Mirror Movements

Mirror movements are involuntary movements of one side of the body that accompany and "mirror" (reflect) intentional movements on the opposite side of the body (also known as imitation synkinesis). They are usually symmetrical and most often seen when using distal muscles of the upper limb. Mirror movements are frequently present in young children but the prevalence decreases with age. Persistence of mirror movements into adult life ("congenital mirror movements") is pathological, as is acquisition in adult life. These movements are uncommon after acquired brain lesions with no relationship to specific anatomical areas.

Congenital mirror movements are associated with skeletal developmental abnormalities, especially of the atlanto-occipital region, such as Klippel-Feil syndrome. They are also seen in 85% of patients with X-linked Kallmann syndrome (hypogonadotrophic hypogonadism and anosmia).

Acquired mirror movements have been described following thalamic lesions, and in association with spastic paraparesis, extrapyramidal disorders (Parkinson's disease, multiple system atrophy), Friedreich's ataxia, phenylketonuria, and affecting hemiparetic limbs following stroke in young children.

There is some neurophysiological evidence from patients with X-linked Kallmann syndrome for the existence of an ipsilateral corticospinal pathway, consistent with other evidence that the congenital condition is primarily a disorder of axonal guidance during development. Concurrent activity within ipsilateral and contralateral corticospinal pathways may explain mirroring of movements. Alternatively, a failure of transcallosal inhibition, acquired at the time of myelination of these pathways, may contribute to the genesis of mirror movements. Loss of joint position sense following thalamic lesions may be of relevance. A deficit of sustained attention has also been postulated as the cause of mirror movements.

References

Espay AJ, Li JY, Johnston L, Lang AE. Mirror movements in parkinsonism: evaluation of a new clinical sign. *J Neurol Neurosurg Psychiatry*. 2005; **76**: 1355–8.
Farmer SF, Harrison LM, Mayston MJ, Parekh A, James LM, Stephens JA. Abnormal cortex-muscle interactions in subjects with X-linked Kallmann's syndrome and mirror movements. *Brain*. 2004; **127**: 385–97.
Galléa C, Popa T, Billot S, Méneret A, Depienne C, Roze E. Congenital mirror movements: a clue to understanding bimanual motor control. *J Neurol*. 2011; **258**: 1911–9.

Cross References

Anosmia; Attention; Mirror writing; Proprioception; Synkinesia, Synkinesis

M

"Mirror Pain"
- see ALLOAESTHESIA

"Mirror Sign"
"Mirror sign" refers to the failure to recognise ones' own reflection in a mirror. In addition to this failure, patients may sometimes develop a delusional belief that their reflection is in fact that of a stranger, a phenomenon which has been termed "mirrored self-misidentification". This might contribute to the "phantom boarder sign", the belief that there is someone else living in the house. Hence these phenomena may be classified with the delusional misidentification syndromes. Some authors believe "the phenomenon of the mirror" to be an extreme example of prosopagnosia, but other studies have not found an association.

Mirror sign occurs in the context of cognitive decline, for example in Alzheimer's disease (AD) or dementia with Lewy bodies. The right dorsolateral prefrontal cortex may be important for self-recognition.

Failure to recognise oneself in a mirror may also be a dissociative symptom, a symptom of depersonalisation.

Reference
Larner AJ. Neurological signs: mirror phenomena. *Adv Clin Neurosci Rehabil*. 2015; **15**(4): 14.
Cross References
Confabulation; Depersonalisation; Misidentification syndromes; "Picture sign"; Prosopagnosia

Mirror Writing
As the name implies, mirror writing is a mirror image of normal writing, hence running from right to left, with characters back to front. This may occur spontaneously, apparently more often in left-handers, or in right-handers attempting to write with the left hand following left-sided brain injury (*e.g.* stroke).

Leonardo da Vinci (1452–1519) is the most celebrated mirror writer: it is possible his left-handedness, and hence mirror writing, followed an injury to his right hand. The author Lewis Carroll occasionally wrote mirror letters but these differ from his normal script, unlike the situation with Leonardo whose two scripts are faithful mirror images. Carroll's letters may thus reflect not an inherent capacity but a contrivance, designed to amuse children who corresponded with him. The device was also used by the author Arthur Ransome in his 1939 novel *Secret Water*. Jane Austen wrote one letter (1817) to a young niece in which script runs from right to left but with word order reversed within words (*i.e.* not mirror writing).

Various neural mechanisms are proposed to explain mirror writing, including bilateral cerebral representation of language, motor programmes or visual memory traces or engrams. The mechanisms may differ between a true mirror writer like Leonardo and someone performing the task for amusement like Carroll.

Double mirror writing (*écriture en double miroir*) is inverted top to bottom (*i.e.* script goes up the page, upside down) in addition to being mirror reversed.

The ability to read mirror reversed text as quickly as normally oriented text has been reported in some autistic individuals.

References
Critchley M. Mirror-writing. London: Kegan Paul, Trench and Trubner; 1928.
Larner AJ. The neurology of "Alice". *Adv Clin Neurosci Rehabil*. 2005; **4**(6):35–6.
Le Faye D, editor. Jane Austen's letters. 4th ed. Oxford: Oxford University Press; 2011. p. 338–9 [Letter 148].
McManus C. Right hand, left hand. The origins of asymmetry in brains, bodies, atoms and culture. London: Phoenix; 2003. p. 348–50.
Schott GD. Mirror writing: neurological reflections on an unusual phenomenon. *J Neurol Neurosurg Psychiatry*. 2007; **78**: 5–13.

Misidentification Syndromes
These are defined as delusional conditions in which patients incorrectly identify and redupli-
cate people, places, objects, or events. Examples include:

- Capgras syndrome; may be related to reduplicative paramnesia.
- Fregoli syndrome.
- Intermetamorphosis.
- Phantom boarder sign.
- Mirror sign.

Reference
Cipriani G, Vedovello M, Ulivi M, Lucetti C, Di Fiorino A, Nuti A. Delusional misidentifica-
tion syndromes and dementia: a border zone between neurology and psychiatry. *Am J
Alzheimer's Dis Other Demen.* 2013; **28**: 671–8.
Cross References
Delusion; Intermetamorphosis; "Mirror sign"; Reduplicative paramnesia

Misophonia
Misophonia, or selective sound sensitivity syndrome, is characterised clinically by sensitivity
to everyday sounds such as chewing, breathing, or keyboard typing, evoking feelings of anger,
panic or anxiety and an urge to escape from the situation producing these sounds. It may be
a disorder of emotion processing of sounds.
References
Cavanna AE. What is misophonia and how can we treat it? *Exp Rev Neurother.* 2014; **14**:
357–9.
Kumar S, Hancock O, Cope T, Sedley W, Winston J, Griffiths TD. Misophonia: a disorder of
emotion processing of sounds. *J Neurol Neurosurg Psychiatry.* 2014; **85**: e3. doi:10.1136/
jnnp-2014-308883.38.

Misoplegia
Misoplegia is a disorder of body schema in which there is active hatred of a paralysed limb, with
or without personification of the limb, and attempts to injure the paralysed limb. It occurs with
right parietal lobe injury (hence left sided limbs are most often involved) and may occur in conjunction with anosognosia, left hemispatial neglect, and (so called) constructional apraxia.
References
Critchley M. Misoplegia, a hatred of hemiplegia. *Mt Sinai J Med.* 1974; **41**: 82–7 [reprinted
in Critchley M. The divine banquet of the brain and other essays. New York: Raven Press;
1979. p. 115–20].
Loetscher T, Regard M, Brugger P. Misoplegia: a review of the literature and a case without
hemiplegia. *J Neurol Neurosurg Psychiatry.* 2006; **77**: 1099–100.
Moss AD, Turnbull OH. Hatred of hemiparetic limbs (misoplegia) in a 10 year old child.
J Neurol Neurosurg Psychiatry. 1996; **61**: 210–11.
Cross References
Anosognosia; Apraxia; Hemiparesis; Hemiplegia; Neglect

Mitbewegungen
- see SYNKINESIA, SYNKINESIS

Mitgehen
An abnormality of induced movement, in which limb movement occurs in response to appli-
cation of the slightest pressure despite the patient having been told to resist (German: to go
too); a manifestation of negativism.
Cross Reference
Negativism

Mitmachen

A motor disorder in which the patient acquiesces to every passive movement of the body made by the examiner, but as soon as the examiner releases the body part, the patient returns it to the resting position.

Monoballismus

Monoballismus is ballism affecting a single limb.

Cross References

Ballism, Ballismus; Hemiballismus

"Monochromatopsia"

The author has seen a patient with a diagnosis of frontotemporal dementia who persistently and consistently complained that everything he saw was red, even though he was aware that they were not red, for example that his wife's hair was grey. His speech was fluent without paraphasia although impoverished in content, with recurrent themes repeated almost verbatim. He had mild orofacial dyspraxia. There was no alexia. Confronted with objects of different colours, he was unable to point to them by colour since all appeared red to him. The features seem to be distinct from erythropsia (in that they were persistent) or phantom chromatopsia (visual acuity was normal). The author proposes that this phenomenon might be termed "monochromatopsia".

Cross References

Erythropsia; Phantom chromatopsia; Xanthopsia

Monomelia

- see MONOPARESIS, MONOPLEGIA

Mononeuritis Multiplex, Mononeuropathy Multiplex

- see NEUROPATHY

Mononeuropathy

- see NEUROPATHY

Monoparesis, Monoplegia

Monoparesis is weakness, monoplegia complete weakness ("paralysis"), of a single limb. Monoparesis of the arm or of the leg ("hemiparaplegia") of upper motor neurone type is usually cortical in origin, although may unusually arise from a cord lesion (leg more frequently than arm). Hoover's sign and Babinski's trunk-thigh test may be helpful in deciding whether monoparetic/monoplegic leg weakness is of non-organic origin, and the "arm drop" or "face-hand test" in arm weakness.

Peripheral disorders can sometimes present exclusively with single limb weakness, such as monomelic motor neurone disease (Hirayama disease), multifocal motor neuropathy with conduction block, and Guillain-Barré syndrome.

Cross References

"Arm drop"; Babinski's trunk-thigh test; Hemiparesis; Hoover's sign; Paraplegia

Monophasia

- see RECURRENT UTTERANCES

Monotonia

Monotonia is a restricted range of speech inflection, occurring with hypophonia as part of the hypokinetic dysarthria observed in parkinsonism.

Cross References

Dysarthria; Hypophonia; Parkinsonism

Moria

Moria is literally folly, (as in Desiderius Erasmus' *Moriae Encomium* of 1509, literally "praise of folly"). In clinical usage, the meaning overlaps with that of emotional lability but has also be used in the context of pathological laughter. It may be seen in frontotemporal dementia.

Reference

Mendez MF. Moria and Witzelsucht from frontotemporal dementia. *J Neuropsychiatry Clin Neurosci*. 2005; **17**: 429–30.

Cross References

Emotionalism, Emotional lability; Pathological crying, Pathological laughter; *Witzelsucht*

Motor Neglect

Motor neglect describes impairment in the ability to initiate movement which cannot be attributed to muscular weakness, a more severe impairment than directional hypokinesia. Task performance may be awkward, and accomplished with effort. Damage to fibre tracts connecting the posterior limb of the internal capsule, supplementary motor area and posterior aspect of the thalamus may underpin motor neglect

Reference

Likitjaroen Y, Suwanwela NC, Mitchell AJ, Lerdlum S, Phanthumchinda K, Teipel SJ. Isolated motor neglect following infarction of the posterior limb of the right internal capsule: a case study with diffusion tensor imaging-based tractography. *J Neurol*. 2012; **259**: 100–5.

Cross References

Directional hypokinesia; Eastchester clapping sign; Neglect

Motor Tinel Sign

- see TINEL'S SIGN

Moving Ear

Moving ear is a focal dyskinesia. This may be a focal myoclonus involving temporal muscles, amenable to treatment with botulinum toxin injections.

References

Chaudhuri KR, Leigh PN, Gibb WR, Pye IF. The moving ear syndrome: a focal dyskinesia. *J Neurol Neurosurg Psychiatry*. 1996; **60**: 106.

Godeiro-Junior C, Felicio AC, Felix EP, et al. Moving ear syndrome: the role of botulinum toxin. *Mov Disord*. 2008; **23**: 122–4.

Cross References

Dyskinesia; Myoclonus

Multiplication of Images

- see POLYOPIA

Muscle Atrophy

- see AMYOTROPHY; ATROPHY

Muscle Hypertrophy

Muscle hypertrophy is muscle enlargement due to an increase in the size of its myofibrils. Muscle hypertrophy may be generalised or focal; and occur in response to repetitive voluntary contraction (physiological) or repetitive abnormal electrical activity (pathological, *e.g.* myotonia in Thomsen's disease; primary orthostatic tremor). Muscle enlargement may also result from replacement of myofibrils by other tissues such as fat or amyloid, a situation better described as pseudhypertrophy.

Cross References

Calf hypertrophy; Masseter hypertrophy; Myotonia

Mutism

Mutism is absence of speech output. This may be psychogenic, as in schizophrenia or affective disorders, with or without catatonia; or a consequence of neurological disease, for example:

- Akinetic mutism.
- Dementia syndromes, especially frontal lobe dementia, late stages of primary non-fluent aphasia.
- Encephalopathy (toxic/drug-induced/metabolic).
- Damage to Broca's area, supplementary motor area; severe pseudobulbar palsy, bilateral thalamic damage.
- Cerebellar mutism: rare, following midline cerebellar surgery in children. Thought to be due to dentatothalamocortical tract damage, bilateral oedema in cerebellar peduncles (rather than surgical trauma or infaction).
- Bilateral vocal cord paralysis (although this may be better termed aphonia).
- Autism

In neurological disorders there may be difficulty initiating movements, completing motor sequences, or inhibition of appropriate responses.

References
Altshuler LL, Cummings JL, Mills MJ. Mutism: review, differential diagnosis and report of 22 cases. *Am J Psychiatry*. 1986; **143**: 1409–14 (Erratum: *Am J Psychiatry*. 1987; **144**: 542).
Wang MC, Winston KR, Breeze RE. Cerebellar mutism associated with a midbrain cavernous malformation. Case report and review of the literature. *J Neurosurg*. 2002; **96**: 607–10.
Cross References
Aphasia; Aphonia

"Myasthenic Snarl"

Patients with weakness of facial musculature as a consequence of myasthenia gravis may have a "transverse smile", with lack of elevation of the corners of the mouth, and hence may appear to snarl when asked to smile or laugh. This may give the impression that they seem peculiarly unamused by an examiner's attempted witticisms. These phenomena may be seen with other causes of facial weakness, such as facioscapulohumeral (FSH) dystrophy.

References
Gowers WR. Remarks on myasthenia and ophthalmoplegia. *BMJ*. 1902; **1**: 1253–6.
Howard JF. The myasthenic facies and snarl. *J Clin Neuromuscul Dis*. 2000; **1**: 214–5.

Mydriasis

Mydriasis is an abnormal dilatation of the pupil, either unilateral or bilateral. Causes include:

- Oculoparasympathetic paresis, from lesions at the Edinger-Westphal nucleus or anywhere along the course of the oculomotor (III) nerve (usually unilateral).
- Tonic enlargement of the pupil (Holmes-Adie pupil, usually unilateral).
- Sympathomimetic drugs, *e.g.* adrenaline (usually bilateral).
- Later stages of central cephalic herniation.
- A syndrome of benign episodic unilateral mydriasis has been described, sometimes related to migraine.

If only one pupil appears large (anisocoria), it is important to distinguish mydriasis from contralateral miosis, when a different differential will apply (*e.g.* Horner's syndrome).

References
Jacobson DM. Benign episodic unilateral mydriasis: clinical characteristics. *Ophthalmology*. 1995; **102**: 1623–7.

Kawasaki A. Approach to the patient with abnormal pupils. In: Biller J, editor. Practical neurology. 2nd ed. Philadelphia: Lippincott Williams & Wilkins; 2002. p. 135–46.
Sarkies NJ, Sanders MD, Gautier-Smith PC. Episodic unilateral mydriasis and migraine. *Am J Ophthalmol.* 1985; **99**: 217–8.

Cross References
Anisocoria; Holmes-Adie pupil, Holmes-Adie syndrome; Horner's syndrome; Hutchinson's pupil; Miosis; Oculomotor (III) nerve palsy

Myelopathy
Myelopathy is a disorder of the spinal cord. Such disorders may be further characterized according to whether the responsible lesion lies within (intramedullary) or outside (extramedullary) the spinal cord: intrinsic or intramedullary lesions are always intradural; extrinsic or extramedullary lesions may be intradural or extradural. It may be possible to differentiate intramedullary from extramedullary lesions on clinical grounds, although this distinction is never absolute because of clinical overlap.

- *Clinical features of extrinsic/extramedullary myelopathy*:
  Motor: sequential spastic paraparesis below the level of the lesion; upper motor neurone (UMN) signs occur early; lower motor neurone (LMN) signs are unusual and have a segmental (radicular) distribution if present.
  Sensory: symptoms of pain may be radicular (*e.g.* secondary to a neurofibroma) or verterbal (*e.g.* secondary to neoplastic or inflammatory processes); sensory signs are not usually marked until the later stages, and all modalities are often involved. A Brown-Séquard syndrome may be more common in extrinsic than intrinsic myelopathies.
  Sphincters: may have bladder urgency, impotence.

  Pathologies commonly causing extrinsic myelopathy include:
  prolapsed disc, osteophyte bar.
  tumour (primary, secondary).
  arteriovenous malformation/haematoma.
  abscess.

- *Clinical features of intrinsic/intramedullary myelopathy*:
  Motor: LMN signs may be prominent and diffuse; UMN signs tend to occur late (spastic paraparesis below level of lesion). A combination of UMN and LMN signs is much more likely to reflect intrinsic than extrinsic pathology.
  Sensory: symptoms of central (funicular) pain may occur; dissociated sensory loss (spinothalamic > dorsal column involvement, or *vice versa*), suspended sensory loss, and sacral sparing are characteristic of intramedullary lesions; a Brown-Séquard syndrome may occur. Vibratory sensibility is more often affected than proprioception.
  Sphincters: bladder involvement common, often early and slow to recover.

  These features are dependent on the extent to which the cord is involved: some pathologies have a predilection for posterior columns, central cord, *etc.*
  Pathologies commonly causing intrinsic myelopathy include:
  multiple sclerosis or other inflammatory process causing transverse myelitis (complete or partial), *e.g.* viral infection, HTLV-1 infection, tabes dorsalis.
  longitudinal myelitis (abnormal MRI signal over several contiguous spinal segments), unlike the pattern typical of MS, may be seen in neuromyelitis optica; infective (viral), post-infectious, and post-vaccination myelitides; and collagen vascular diseases.

tumour (primary, secondary).

syringomyelia.

infarction, *e.g.* anterior spinal artery syndrome.

metabolic causes: vitamin B_{12} deficiency producing subacute combined degeneration of the cord.

Imaging of the cord, ideally with MRI, may be helpful in defining the cause of myelopathy.

References

Jacob A, Larner AJ. Diseases of the spinal cord. In: Cox TM, et al. editors. Oxford textbook of medicine. 6th ed. Oxford: Oxford University Press; 2016: in press.

Wong SH, Boggild M, Enevoldson TP, Fletcher NA. Myelopathy but normal MRI: where next? *Pract Neurol.* 2008; **8**: 90–102.

Cross References

Brown-Séquard syndrome; Lower motor neurone (LMN) syndrome; Paraparesis; Proprioception; Sacral sparing; Suspended sensory loss; Upper motor neurone (UMN) syndrome; Vibration

Myerson's Sign

- see GLABELLAR TAP REFLEX

Myoclonus

Myoclonus describes an involuntary, "shock-like", muscle jerking, arrhythmic more often than regular, of central nervous system (CNS) origin. This may be focal, multifocal, or generalised. Multiple irregular asynchronous myoclonic jerks may be termed polymyoclonus. Myoclonus may be characterized in several ways:

- Clinical classification (by observation, examination):

    Spontaneous.

    Action or intention: following voluntary action; may be elicited by asking patient to reach out to touch the examiner's hand.

    Reflex, stimulus-sensitive: jerks produced by somaesthetic stimulation of a limb, or in response to loud noises.

- Anatomical/pathophysiological classification (by neurophysiological recordings):

    Cortical.

    Subcortical/reticular.

    Propriospinal/segmental.

- Aetiological classification:

    Physiological, *e.g.* "sleep starts" (hypnic jerks).

    Essential: in the absence of any other abnormality of the CNS.

    Epileptic: as a manifestation of idiopathic epilepsy.

    Symptomatic: of other neurological diseases, of which there are many, including:

        Anoxic brain injury (Lance-Adams syndrome).

        Cerebrovascular lesions.

        Neoplasia.

        Encephalopathies: especially of metabolic origin (hepatic, renal), but also toxic, viral, paraneoplastic, mitochondrial.

        Degenerations: basal ganglia, spinocerebellar.

        Malabsorption syndromes: coeliac disease, Whipple's disease.

        Storage disorders, *e.g.* Lafora body disease, Tay-Sachs disease, sialidosis.

        Dementias: Alzheimer's disease (usually late), prion disease (usually early in sporadic Creutzfeldt-Jakob disease); not seen in frontotemporal lobar degenerations.

Inherited disorders: myoclonus-dystonia syndrome (DYT11).

The clinical differential diagnosis of myoclonus includes chorea, tic, tremor (especially with rhythmic myoclonus), and certain peripheral nerve disorders (fasciculation, myokymia). Periodic limb movement disorder or periodic leg movements of sleep, frequently found in association with restless legs syndrome, is sometimes called "nocturnal myoclonus". Brief lapses of muscle contraction with loss of posture are in some ways the converse of myoclonus and have in the past been labelled "negative myoclonus", although the term asterixis is now preferred.

Drugs useful in the symptomatic treatment of myoclonus include clonazepam, sodium valproate, primidone, and piracetam. These may need to be given in combination to suppress severe action myoclonus.

References
Dijk JM, Tijssen MA. Management of patients with myoclonus: available therapies and the need for an evidence-based approach. *Lancet Neurol.* 2010; **9**: 1028–36.
Marsden CD, Hallett M, Fahn S. The nosology and pathophysiology of myoclonus. In: Marsden CD, Fahn S, editors. Movement disorders. London: Butterworth; 1982. p. 196–248.
Werhahn KJ. Myoclonus. In: Schmitz B, Tettenborn B, Schomer DL, editors. The paroxysmal disorders. Cambridge: Cambridge University Press; 2010. p. 145–57.

Cross References
Asterixis; Chorea, Choreoathetosis; Dystonia; Fasciculation; Hiccups; Jactitation; Myokymia; Palatal tremor; Tic; Tremor

Myoedema
Myoedema, or muscle mounding, provoked by mechanical stimuli or stretching of muscle, is a feature of rippling muscle disease, in which the muscle contractions are associated with electrical silence. It has also been reported as a neuromuscular feature of hypothyroidism.

Reference
Capistrano GG, Galdino GS. Teaching Video NeuroImages: myoedema in hypothyroidism. *Neurology.* 2015; **84**: e24.

Myokymia
Myokymia is an involuntary, spontaneous, wave-like, painless, undulation of a muscle surface (*cf.* fasciculation), sometimes likened to a "bag of worms", which often persists continuously for days or weeks. Neurophysiologically this corresponds to involuntary and disorganized continuous activation of motor units within the muscle. Multiplet discharges may be seen following stimulation of a nerve supplying a myokymic muscle. Myokymia may be related to other signs of peripheral nerve hyperexcitability such as neuromyotonia.

Myokymia may result from peripheral or central nervous system pathology: the former group includes peripheral neuropathies and radiculopathies; the latter multiple sclerosis and pontine lesions. Facial myokymia is a rare facial dyskinesia, possibly related to disinhibition of the facial (VII) nerve nucleus by focal pontine lesions (tumour, demyelination). It may be distinguished from hemifacial spasm by its persistent rather than paroxysmal nature.

A syndrome of superior oblique myokymia is described, often following superior oblique palsy, which produces a microtremor of the eye and causes symptoms of oscillopsia or transient diplopia.

Neurophysiological evidence of myokymia may be helpful in the assessment of a brachial plexopathy, since this is found in radiation-induced, but not neoplastic, lesions.

References
Lukas RV, Rezania K, Malec M, Salgia R. Teaching Video NeuroImages: myokymia and nerve hyperexcitability as components of Morvan syndrome due to malignant thymoma. *Neurology.* 2013; **80**: e55.

Meinck HM. Cramps, spasms, startles and related symptoms. In: Schmitz B, Tettenborn B, Schomer DL, editors. The paroxysmal disorders. Cambridge: Cambridge University Press; 2010. p. 130–44.

Thompson PD. Stiff people. In: Marsden CD, Fahn S, editors. Movement disorders 3. Boston: Butterworth; 1994. p. 373–405.

Cross References
Fasciculation; Hemifacial spasm; Myotonia; Neuromyotonia; Spasm; Stiffness

Myopathy

The term myopathy denotes a primary disorder of muscle causing wasting and/or weakness in the absence of sensory abnormalities. Clinically, myopathic processes need to be differentiated from neuropathies, particularly anterior horn cell diseases and motor neuropathies, and neuromuscular junction disorders.

Generally in primary muscle disease fasciculation is not seen, reflexes are lost late, and phenomena such as (peripheral) fatigue and facilitation do not occur.

Myopathies may be subdivided according to the clinical pattern of weakness, and/or their aetiology:

- *Proximal*: affecting predominantly shoulder abductors and hip flexors:

  Inflammatory: polymyositis, dermatomyositis.
  Progressive muscular dystrophies: Duchenne, Becker, limb-girdle, facioscapulo-humeral (FSH).
  Metabolic: acid-maltase deficiency (Pompe); thyroid dysfunction, Cushing's syndrome.
  Non-metastatic feature of malignant disease.
- *Distal*: an unusual pattern for myopathy, which needs to be differentiated from distal polyneuropathy:

  Myotonic dystrophy.
  Miyoshi dystrophy.
  Desmin myopathy.
- *Bulbar palsy.*
- *Facial paresis.*
- *Diaphragm weakness*:

  Acid-maltase deficiency.
  Acute polymyositis.
  Neuralgic amyotrophy.
- *Axial myopathy*:

  Camptocormia ("bent spine syndrome").
  Dropped head syndrome.

References
Barnes PRJ, Hilton-Jones D, Dalakas MC, Palace JA, Rose MR. Myopathy in clinical practice. London: Martin Dunitz; 2003.

Baumer D, Hammans S. An overview of muscle disease presenting in adulthood. *Br J Hosp Med.* 2015; **76**: 576–82.

Karpati G, Hilton-Jones D, Bushby K, Griggs RC, editors. Disorders of voluntary muscle. 8th ed. Cambridge: Cambridge Univesrity Press; 2010.

Cross References
Atrophy; Bulbar palsy; Camptocormia; Dropped head syndrome; Facial paresis, Facial weakness; Fatigue; Gowers' sign; Paradoxical breathing; Wasting; Weakness

Myorhythmia

Myorhythmia is an involuntary, repetitive, movement disorder characterized by rhythmic contraction (1–4 Hz) of muscles producing a coarse tremor, which may affect limbs, face, palate, head, jaw, neck, tongue, eyes or trunk. The movements are continuous and persist during sleep. They have been described in association with brainstem or thalamic vascular disease, trauma, alcohol-related nutritional deficiency, phenytoin intoxication, steroid-responsive encephalopathy (Hashimoto's encephalopathy), NMDA-receptor encephalitis, and Whipple's disease.

Although very rare, oculomasticatory myorhythmia is of diagnostic importance since it is pathognomonic for Whipple's disease of the nervous system. In this condition, there is also characteristic convergent-divergent pendular nystagmus with synchronous rhythmic movement of the mouth, tongue, jaw and sometimes proximal and distal skeletal muscles. The neurological manifestations of Whipple's disease are protean, and include dementia, ataxia, supranuclear ophthalmoplegia (with sparing of the pupils), epileptic seizures, myoclonus, nystagmus and psychosis. The condition is caused by the bacterium *Tropheryma whipplei*. Treatment is with antibiotics, usually a 2-week intravenous course of trimethoprim-sulphamethoxazole or ceftriazone followed by oral treatment for 1 year. Sodium valproate may be helpful for the involuntary movements which do not respond to antibiotics.

References
Anderson M. Neurology of Whipple's disease. *J Neurol Neurosurg Psychiatry*. 2000; **68**: 2–5.
Baizabal-Carvallo JF, Cardoso F, Jankovic J. Myorhythmia: phenomenology, etiology, and treatment. *Mov Disord*. 2015; **30**: 171–9.

Cross References
Ataxia; Dementia; Myoclonus; Nystagmus

Myotonia

Myotonia is a stiffness of muscles with inability to relax after voluntary contraction (action myotonia), or induced by electrical or mechanical (*e.g.* percussion myotonia) excitation. The phenomenon is often described by patients as "cramp" or stiffness. This is a reflection of primary muscle disease (*i.e.* myogenic; *cf.* neuromyotonia, neurogenic muscle stiffness, peripheral nerve hyperexcitability), which persists after peripheral nerve or neuromuscular junction blockade.

Neurophysiological assessment reveals myotonic discharges, with prolonged twitch relaxation phase, which may be provoked by movement, percussion, and electrical stimulation of muscle; discharges typically wax and wane.

Myotonia may be aggravated by hyperkalaemia, depolarizing neuromuscular blocking drugs (*e.g.* suxamethonium), and anticholinesterase drugs (neostigmine). Other factors that can induce myotonia include hypothermia, mechanical or electrical stimulation (including surgical incision and electrocautery), shivering, and use of inhalational anaesthetics.

A similar clinical phenomenon of slow muscle relaxation may be observed in other circumstances, for example hypothyroidism, but without the characteristic EMG findings of myotonia, hence this is labelled as pseudomyotonia. Paramyotonia is myotonia exacerbated by cold and exertion (paradoxical myotonia).

Recognised causes of myotonia include:

- myotonic dystrophy types 1 and 2.
- hyperkalaemic periodic paralysis.
- myotonia congenita (autosomal dominant Thomsen's disease, autosomal recessive Becker's myotonia).
- K^+-aggravated myotonia.
- Schwartz-Jampel syndrome (chondrodystrophic myotonia).

Mutations in genes encoding voltage-gated ion channels have been identified in some of the inherited myotonias, hence these are channelopathies: skeletal muscle voltage-gated Na^+ channel mutations have been found in K^+-aggravated myotonia, and also paramyotonia congenita and hyperkalaemic periodic paralysis. Chloride (Cl^-) channel mutations have been identified in myotonia congenita. These latter conditions respond best to mexilitene.

References

Quinn C, Salajegheh MK. Myotonic disorders and channelopathies. *Semi Neurol.* 2015; **35**: 360–8.

Turner C, Hilton-Jones D. The myotonic dystrophies: diagnosis and management. *J Neurol Neurosurg Psychiatry.* 2010; **81**: 358–67.

Cross References

Muscle hypertrophy; Neuromyotonia; Paramyotonia; Percussion myotonia; Pseudomyotonia; Stiffness; Warm-up phenomenon; Woltman's sign

N

Narcolepsy, Narcoleptic Syndrome
- see HYPERSOMNOLENCE

Nasopalpebral Reflex
- see GLABELLAR TAP REFLEX

Negative Myoclonus
- see ASTERIXIS

Negative Tremor
- see ASTERIXIS

Negativism

Negativism may be used to describe a motor sign consisting of the patient doing the opposite of what is asked and actively resisting efforts to persuade compliance. For example, movement of a limb in response to application of pressure despite the patient having been told to resist (*mitgehen*) may be one element of negativism. This may be observed in mental disorder, usually schizophrenia, and may also be a feature of catatonia. The similarity of some of these features to *gegenhalten* suggests the possibility of frontal lobe dysfunction as the underlying cause.

Negativism has also been used by Bleuler to describe an inner sensation in which the effort to start one action elicits a counter impulse which blocks or hinders the execution of the action, also known as conflict of intentions. This may reflect a callosal lesion.

References

Moore DP. Conflict of intentions or inner negativism? *J Neurol Neurosurg Psychiatry*. 2002; **72**: 681.

Nishikawa T, Okuda J, Mizuta I, et al. Conflict of intentions due to callosal disconnection. *J Neurol Neurosurg Psychiatry*. 2001; **71**: 462–71.

Cross References

Catatonia; *Gegenhalten*

Neglect

Neglect is a failure to orient toward, respond to, or report novel or meaningful stimuli. If failure to respond can be attributed to concurrent sensory or motor deficits (*e.g.* hemiparesis, hemianopia, visuospatial deficits) neglect is not present.

Neglect can involve stimuli in the extrapersonal environment (*e.g.* visual neglect) or personal space (*e.g.* personal neglect or asomatognosia). This dichotomy may also be characterised as egocentric (neglecting hemispace defined by the midplane of the body) and allocentric (neglecting one side of individual stimuli). Neglect of contralateral hemispace may also be called unilateral spatial neglect, hemi-inattention, or hemineglect. Lesser degrees of neglect may be manifest as extinction (double simultaneous stimulation). Motor neglect may be evident as hemiakinesia, hypokinesia, or motor impersistence. Alexia may sometimes be a consequence of neglect (neglect alexia). Alloaesthesia and allokinesia may also be features of neglect.

© Springer International Publishing Switzerland 2016
A.J. Larner, *A Dictionary of Neurological Signs*,
DOI 10.1007/978-3-319-29821-4_14

Neglect may be obvious (*e.g.* patient not dressing one side of the body), but is sometimes more subtle, in which case it may be tested for using various simple tests:

- Cancellation tests, *e.g.* stars (unstructured array), letters (structured array).
- Line bisection (part of the Behavioural Inattention Test), numbering a clock face.
- Figure copying, *e.g.* Rey-Osterrieth figure.
- Drawing from memory.

Neglect is more common after right rather than left brain damage, usually of vascular origin. The angular gyrus and parahippocampal gyrus may be central to the development of visual neglect. Marked degrees of neglect may seriously hamper attempts at neurorehabilitation.

References

Husain M. Hemispatial neglect. *Handbook Clin Neurol*. 2008; **88**: 359–72.

Li K, Malhotra PA. Spatial neglect. *Pract Neurol*. 2015; **15**: 333–9.

Maravita A. Spatial disorders. In: Cappa SF, Abutalebi J, Démonet JF, Fletcher PC, Garrard P, editors. Cognitive neurology: a clinical textbook. Oxford: Oxford University Press; 2008. p. 89–118.

Maxton C, Dineen RA, Padamsey RC, Munshi SK. Don't neglect "neglect" – an update on post stroke neglect. *Int J Clin Pract*. 2013; **67**: 369–78.

Cross References

Alexia; Alloaesthesia; Allokinesia; Asomatognosia; Eastchester clapping test; Extinction; Hemiakinesia; Hypokinesia; Impersistence; Motor neglect

Negro's Sign

Negro has two eponymous signs:

- Cogwheel (jerky) type of rigidity in basal ganglia disorders.
- In both peripheral and central facial paralysis, the eyeball deviates outward and elevates more than normal when the patient attempts to look up due to overaction of the inferior oblique and superior rectus muscles, respectively.

Reference

Ghiglione P, Mutani R, Chiò A. Cogwheel rigidity. *Arch Neurol*. 2005; **62**: 828–30.

Cross References

Bell's palsy; Facial paresis, Facial weakness; Parkinsonism; Rigidity

Neologism

A neologism is a non-word approximating to a real word, produced in spontaneous speech; it is thought to result from an inability to organize phonemes appropriately in the process of speech production. Hence, this is a type of literal or phonemic paraphasia encountered in aphasic syndromes, most usually those resulting from left superior temporal-inferior parietal lobe damage (Wernicke type). A disconnection between stored lexical representations and language output pathways leading to aberrant phoneme activation is a postulated mechanism for neologistic aphasia

(The word "scientist" is said to be a neologism coined in the nineteenth century by William Whewell.)

Reference

Rohrer JD, Rossor MN, Warren JD. Neologistic jargon aphasia and agraphia in primary progressive aphasia. *J Neurol Sci*. 2009; **277**: 155–9.

Cross References

Aphasia; Jargon aphasia; Paraphasia; Schizophasia; Wernicke's aphasia

Neri's Test
- see LASÈGUE'S SIGN

Nerve Thickening
The characterization of a peripheral neuropathy should always include examination to feel if
any nerves are thickened. Good places to palpate for nerve thickening include around the
elbow (ulnar nerve), anatomical snuff box (superficial radial nerves), and head of the fibula
(common peroneal nerve). Nerve thickening may be noted in a variety of conditions, in some
by examination, in others using imaging techniques:

● Leprosy.
● Hereditary motor and sensory neuropathies (HMSN), especially types I, III, and IV
  (Refsum's disease).
● Hereditary neuropathy with liability to pressure palsies (HNLPP)/tomaculous
  neuropathy.
● Neurofibromatosis 1.
● Sarcoidosis.
● Chronic inflammatory demyelinating neuropathy/ophthalmoplegic migraine.
● Nerve tumours (localised).
● Amyloidosis (familial amyloid polyneuropathy, primary systemic amyloidosis): rare.

References
Donaghy M. Enlarged peripheral nerves. *Pract Neurol*. 2003; **3**: 40–5.
Duggins AJ, McLeod JG, Pollard JD, Davies L, Yang F, Thompson EO, Soper JR. Spinal
root and plexus hypertrophy in chronic inflammatory demyelinating polyneuropathy. *Brain*.
1999; **122**: 1383–90.
Cross Reference
Neuropathy

Neuromyotonia
Neuromyotonia is neurogenic muscle stiffness (*cf.* myotonia, myogenic muscle stiffness) which
reflects peripheral nerve hyperexcitability. Clinically this is manifest as muscle cramps and
stiffness, particularly during and after muscle contraction, and as muscular activity at rest
(myokymia, fasciculation). Tendon areflexia and abnormal postures of hands and feet may
also be observed. Sensory features such as paraesthesia, and central nervous system features
(Morvan's syndrome), can occur. A syndrome of ocular neuromyotonia has been described in
which spasms of the extraocular muscles cause a transient heterophoria and diplopia; most
cases follow months to years after cranial irradiation, but some are associated with multiple
sclerosis.
    Neuromyotonia is characterized physiologically by continuous motor unit and muscle
fibre activity which is due to peripheral nerve hyperexcitability; it is abolished by curare (*cf.*
myotonia). Spontaneous firing of single motor units as doublet, triplet, or multiplet discharges with high intraburst frequency (40–300/s) at irregular intervals is the hallmark
finding.
    Neuromyotonia may be associated with autoantibodies directed against presynaptic
voltage-gated K^+ channels. Around 20% of patients have an underlying small-cell lung cancer
or thymoma, suggesting a paraneoplastic aetiology in these patients. Neuromyotonia has also
been associated with mutations within the voltage-gated K^+ ion channel gene.
    Neuromyotonia usually improves with symptomatic treatments such as carbamaza-
epine, phenytoin, lamotrigine, and sodium valproate, in combination if necessary.
Paraneoplastic neuromyotonia often improves and may remit after treatment of the underlying tumour.

References
Dardiotis E, Ralli S. Images in clinical medicine. Paraneoplastic neuromyotonia. *N Engl J Med*. 2015; **372**: e24.
Isaacs H. A syndrome of continuous muscle-fibre activity. *J Neurol Neurosurg Psychiatry*. 1961; **24**: 319–25.
Maddison P. Neuromyotonia. *Clin Neurophysiol*. 2006; **117**: 2118–27.
Menon D, Sreedharan SE, Gupta M, Nair MD. A novel association of ocular neuromyotonia with brainstem demyelination: two case reports. *Mult Scler*. 2014; **20**: 1409–12.
Cross References
Fasciculation; Myokymia; Myotonia; Paramyotonia; Pseudomyotonia; Stiffness

Neuronopathy

Neuronopathies are disorders affecting neuronal cell bodies in the ventral (anterior) horns of the spinal cord or dorsal root ganglia, hence motor and sensory neuronopathies, respectively. Sensory neuronopathy (also known as ganglionopathy, or polyganglionopathy) has a more limited differential diagnosis than neuropathies, including:

- Paraneoplasia: anti-Hu antibody syndrome (although a similar syndrome, presumed paraneoplastic, may occur in the absence of these antibodies).
- Sjögren's syndrome.
- Associated with anti-GD1b ganglioside antibodies.
- Chronic inflammatory demyelinating polyradiculoneuropathy (CIDP).
- HIV.

Anterior horn cell (motor neurone) disorders may be classified as motor neuronopathies, including motor neurone disease (amyotrophic lateral sclerosis), spinal muscular atrophies, and poliomyelitis.

References
Camdessanché JP, Jousserand G, Ferraud K, et al. The pattern of diagnostic criteria of sensory neuronopathy: a case-control study. *Brain*. 2009; **132**: 1723–33.
Ghadiri-Sani M, Larner AJ, Menon RK. Sensory neuronopathy as a possible paraneoplastic syndrome linked with pancreatic cancer. *Br J Hosp Med*. 2016; **77**: 48–9.
Cross Reference
Neuropathy

Neuropathy

Neuropathies are disorders of peripheral nerves. Various clinical patterns of peripheral nerve involvement may be seen:

- *Mononeuropathy*: sensory and/or motor involvement in the distribution of a single nerve.
- *Mononeuropathy multiplex*: simultaneous involvement of two or more nerves, usually in different parts of the body; if due to inflammatory disease, as is often the case, this may be described as mononeuritis multiplex.
- *Polyneuropathy*: a widespread process, predominantly affecting the distal parts of nerves; may be predominantly sensory ("glove and stocking" sensory loss) or motor, with or without concomitant autonomic involvement. It may be helpful to distinguish between polyneuropathies which are either predominantly axonal or demyelinating by means of neurophysiological (EMG/NCS) studies to aid with differential diagnosis.

These clinical patterns may need to be differentiated in practice from disorders affecting the neuronal cell bodies in the ventral (anterior) horns of the spinal cord or dorsal root ganglia (motor and sensory neuronopathies, respectively); and disorders of the nerve roots (radiculopathy) and plexuses (plexopathy). Clinical signs resulting from neuropathies are of lower motor neurone type (wasting, weakness, reflex diminution or loss).

The causes of neuropathy are many. Mononeuropathies often result from local compression (entrapment neuropathy), trauma, or diabetes. Mononeuropathy multiplex often reflects intrinsic inflammation (*e.g.* polyarteritis nodosa, Churg-Strauss syndrome, systemic lupus erythematosus, rheumatoid arthritis, Sjögren's syndrome, cryoglobulinaemia, isolated PNS vasculitis). Polyneuropathies may have genetic, infective, inflammatory, toxic, nutritional, and endocrine aetiologies. Many neuropathies, particularly polyneuropathies in the elderly, especially of sensory axonal type, may remain idiopathic or cryptogenic despite intensive investigation.

References

Dyck PJ, Thomas PK, editors. Peripheral neuropathy. 4th ed. Philadelphia: WB Saunders; 2005.

Mumenthaler M, Schliack H, Mumenthaler M, Goerke H. Peripheral nerve lesions: diagnosis and treatment. New York: Thieme; 1990.

Staal A, van Gijn J, Spaans F. Mononeuropathies: examination, diagnosis and treatment. London: WB Saunders; 1999.

Stewart JD. Focal peripheral neuropathies. 4th ed. Vancouver: JBJ Publishing; 2010.

Cross References

Amyotrophy; Foot drop; Lower motor neurone (LMN) syndrome; Neuronopathy; Plexopathy; Radiculopathy; Wasting; Weakness; Wrist drop

Newspaper Sign
- see FROMENT'S SIGN

Nominal Aphasia
- see ANOMIA

Nuchal Rigidity

Nuchal rigidity refers to neck stiffness, and this term is usually synonymous with meningism, in which case other signs of meningeal irritation are usually present (Kernig's sign, Brudzinski's neck sign). If these other signs are absent, then isolated nuchal rigidity may suggest a foraminal pressure cone. It may also occur in syndromes causing predominantly axial (as opposed to limb) rigidity (*e.g.* progressive supranuclear palsy). In intubated patients, there may be resistance to passive neck movements.

Nuchal rigidity may have better sensitivity (0.3) than either Kernig's or Brudzinski's signs (0.05) in adult patients with meningitis.

Reference

Thomas KE, Hasbun R, Jekel J, Quagliarello VJ. The diagnostic accuracy of Kernig's sign, Brudzinski's sign, and nuchal rigidity in adults with suspected meningitis. *Clin Infect Dis.* 2002; **35**: 46–52.

Cross References

Brudzinski's (neck) sign; Kernig's sign; Meningism; Parkinsonism

Nuchocephalic Reflex

In a standing subject, rapid turning of the shoulders to either left or right (eyes closed to avoid fixation) is associated with bilateral contraction of the cervical musculature so that the head is held in the original position. This nuchocephalic reflex is present in infants and children up to the age of about 4 years. Beyond this age the reflex is inhibited, such that the head is actively turned in the direction of shoulder movement after a time lag of about half a second. If the reflex is present in adults (*i.e.* disinhibited), this has been claimed to be a "regressive" (primitive) sign, indicative of diffuse cerebral dysfunction.

References

Jenkyn LR, Walsh DB, Walsh BT, Culver CM, Reeves AG. The nuchocephalic reflex. *J Neurol Neurosurg Psychiatry*. 1975; **38**: 561–6.

Schott JM, Rossor MN. The grasp and other primitive reflexes. *J Neurol Neurosurg Psychiatry*. 2003; **74**: 558–60.

Cross References

Age-related signs; Primitive reflexes

Numb Chin Syndrome, Numb Cheek Syndrome
- see ROGER'S SIGN

Nyctalopia
Nyctalopia, or night blindness, is an impairment of visual acuity specific to scotopic vision, implying a loss or impairment of rod photoreceptor function. Patients may spontaneously complain of a disparity between daytime and nocturnal vision, in which case acuity should be measured in different ambient illumination. Nyctalopia may be a feature of:

- Retinitis pigmentosa.
- Vitamin A deficiency.
- Cancer-associated retinopathy: most commonly associated with small-cell lung cancer (anti-recoverin antibodies may be detected), though gynaecological malignancy and melanoma have also been associated (with anti-bipolar retinal cell antibodies in the latter).

Since the words nyctalopia and hemeralopia have apparently been used in an opposite sense by many non-English-speaking doctors, the terms "night blindness" and "day blindness" may be preferred to avoid any ambiguity.

Reference
Ohba N, Ohba A. Nyctalopia and hemeralopia: the current usage trend in the literature. *Br J Ophthalmol*. 2006; **90**: 1548–9.

Cross References
Hemeralopia; Retinitis pigmentosa

Nylen-Bárány Manoeuvre
- see HALLPIKE MANOEUVRE, HALLPIKE TEST

Nystagmoid Jerks
- see NYSTAGMUS

Nystagmus
Nystagmus, or talantropia, is an involuntary to-and-fro oscillatory movement of the eyeballs, of which there are many varieties. It is usually bilateral, but occasionally may be unilateral, as in internuclear ophthalmoplegia (INO). The pathophysiological underpinnings are diverse, but all involve brainstem nuclei and tracts which control eye movements and gaze holding, especially the oculomotor (III), trochlear (IV) and abducnes (VI) cranial nerve nuclei, paramedian pontine reticular formation, vestibular nuclei, medial longitudinal fasciculus, central tegmental tract, cerebellar connections to these structures, interstitial nucleus of Cajal, and nucleus prepositus hypoglossi. It is important to distinguish nystagmus from other involuntary eye movements such as square-wave jerks, ocular flutter, and opsoclonus.

The nature of the nystagmus may permit inferences about the precise location of pathology. Observations should be made in the nine cardinal positions of gaze for direction, amplitude and beat frequency of nystagmus. Nystagmus may be abortive or sustained in duration.

Nystagmus may be classified in various ways:

Physiological:

Optokinetic nystagmus (OKN; *e.g.* looking out of a moving railway carriage).

Induced by vestibular stimuli (*e.g.* merry-go-round; caloric testing).

Nystagmoid jerks: in extremes of lateral or vertical gaze (end-point nystagmus, a form of gaze-evoked nystagmus).

Pathological:

Pathological nystagmus may be classified according to direction, wave-form, anatomy/aetiology, or clinical frequency (common, rare).

● *Directional classification of nystagmus*:

Horizontal (common).

Vertical (rare):

Downbeat: seen with structural lesions of the cervico-medullary junction, midline cerebellum and floor of the fourth ventricle, but also with more diffuse cerebellar disease.

Upbeat: of less localising value than downbeat nystagmus, upbeat nystagmus may occur with pontomesencephalic, ponto-medullary, and even caudal medullary lesions (infarct, inflammation); bow-tie nystagmus is probably a variant of upbeat nystagmus.

Torsional: usually accompanies horizontal nystagmus of peripheral vestibular (labyrinthine) origin.

● *Waveform classification of nystagmus*:

Jerk nystagmus:

At least one of the directions of eye movement is slow (slow phase; <40°/s) followed by a rapid, corrective, saccadic movement in the opposite direction (fast phase) for which direction the nystagmus is named. However, since it is the slow phase which is pathological, it is more eloquent concerning anatomical substrate. The intensity of jerk nystagmus may be classified by a scale of three degrees:

1st degree: present when looking in the direction of the fast phase;

2nd degree: present in the neutral position;

3rd degree: present when looking in the direction of the slow phase (*i.e.* present in all directions of gaze).

Pendular or undulatory nystagmus:

In which the movements of the eyes are more or less equal in amplitude and velocity (sinusoidal oscillations) about a central (null) point. This is often congenital, may be conjugate or disconjugate (sometimes monocular), but is not related to concurrent internuclear ophthalmoplegia or asymmetry of visual acuity. Acquired causes include multiple sclerosis and brainstem infarctions.

When studied using oculography, the slow phase of jerk nystagmus may show a uniform velocity ("saw-toothed"), indicative of imbalance in vestibulo-ocular reflex activity. A slow phase with exponentially decreasing velocity (negative exponential slow phase) is ascribed to "leakiness" of a hypothetical neural integrator, a structure which converts eye or head velocity signals into approximations of eye or head position signals (thought to lie in the interstitial nucleus of Cajal in the midbrain for vertical eye movements, and in the nucleus propositus hypoglossi for horizontal eye movements). A slow phase with exponentially increasing velocity (high-gain instability, runaway movements) may be seen in congenital or acquired pendular nystagmus. The pathophysiology of acquired pendular nystagmus is thought to be deafferentation of the inferior olive by lesions of the red nucleus, central tegmental tract, or medial vestibular nucleus.

- *Anatomical/aetiological classification of nystagmus*:
    Peripheral Vestibular:
    > unidirectional (directed to side opposite lesion), and more pronounced when looking in direction of the fast phase (*i.e.* 1st degree), usually with a rotatory component and associated with vertigo. Tends to fatigue, and usually transient (*e.g.* in Hallpike manoeuvre). Nystagmus of peripheral vestibular origin is typically reduced by fixation (hence these patients hold their heads still) and enhanced by removal of visual fixation (in the dark, with Frenzel's lenses).

    Central Vestibular:
    > unidirectional or multidirectional, 1st, 2nd or 3rd degree; typically sustained and persistent. There may be other signs of central pathology (*e.g.* cerebellar signs, upper motor neurone signs). Not affected by removal of visual fixation.

    Cerebellar/brainstem:
    > commonly gaze-evoked due to a failure of gaze-holding mechanisms. It may be unidirectional with a unilateral cerebellar lesion (*e.g.* vascular disease) in which case it typically occurs when the eyes are looking in the direction of the lesion (*cf.* peripheral vestibular nystagmus); multidirectional nystagmus of cerebellar origin may occur in multiple sclerosis, drug/toxin exposure, cerebellar degenerations.

    Congenital:
    > usually horizontal, pendular type nystagmus; worse with fixation, attention, anxiety. It may appear with blindness of childhood onset, or be acquired with neurological disease (multiple sclerosis, mitochondrial disease, Whipple's disease, Pelizaeus-Merzbacher disease).

    Other forms of nystagmus include:
- *Ataxic/Dissociated*:
    > in abducting > > adducting eye, as in internuclear ophthalmoplegia and pseudo-internuclear ophthalmoplegia.
- *Periodic Alternating*:
    > primary position nystagmus, almost always in the horizontal plane, which stops and then reverses direction every minute or so; 4–5 min of observation may be required to see the whole cycle; its localising value is similar to that of downbeat nystagmus.
- *Convergence-retraction* (Körber-Salus-Elschnig syndrome):
    > adducting saccades (medial rectus contraction), occurring spontaneously or on attempted upgaze, often accompanied by retraction of the eyes into the orbits, associated with mesencephalic lesions of the pretectal region (*e.g.* pinealoma).
- *See-saw*:
    > a disconjugate cyclic movement of the eyes, comprising elevation and intorsion of one eye while the other eye falls and extorts, followed by reversal of these movements; may be congenital (*e.g.* with albinism, retinitis pigmentosa) or acquired (mesodiencephalic or lateral medullary lesions, *e.g.* brainstem stroke, head trauma, syringobulbia).

Many types of pathology may cause nystagmus, the most common being demyelination, vascular disease, tumour, neurodegenerative disorders of cerebellum and/or brainstem, metabolic causes (*e.g.* Wernicke-Korsakoff's syndrome), paraneoplasia, drugs (alcohol, phenytoin, barbiturates, sedative-hypnotic drugs), toxins, and epilepsy.

Treatment of nystagmus is usually that of the underlying cause, where possible. Pendular nystagmus may respond to anticholinesterases, consistent with its being a result of cholinergic dysfunction. Periodic alternating nystagmus responds to baclofen, hence the importance of making this diagnosis. See-saw nystagmus may respond to baclofen, clonazepam, or alcohol.

References

Leigh RJ, Zee DS. The neurology of eye movements. 4th ed. New York: Oxford University Press; 2006.

Straube A, Bronstein A, Straumann D; European Federation of Neurologic Societies. Nystagmus and oscillopsia. *Eur J Neurol*. 2012; **19**: 6–14.

Cross References

Caloric testing; Congenital nystagmus; Hallpike manoeuvre, Hallpike test; Internuclear ophthalmoplegia (INO); Myorhythmia; Optokinetic nystagmus (OKN), Optokinetic response; Opsoclonus; Oscillopsia; Palatal myoclonus; Pendular nystagmus; Pseudo-internuclear ophthalmoplegia; Spasmus nutans; Square-wave jerks; Vertigo

O

Obscurations

Visual obscurations are transient losses ("greying out") of vision lasting a few seconds, occurring in the context of raised intracranial pressure (ICP), and especially associated with activities known to elevate ICP, such as coughing, sneezing, bending down, straining at stool, and relieved by their cessation. These symptoms are thought to reflect critical compromise of optic nerve head perfusion and are invariably associated with the finding of papilloedema. Obscurations mandate urgent investigation and treatment to prevent permanent visual loss. Transient visual obscurations may occasionally be due to optic disc drusen.

Cross Reference

Papilloedema

Obtundation

Obtundation is a state of altered consciousness characterized by reduced alertness and a lessened interest in the environment, sometimes described as psychomotor retardation or torpor. An increased proportion of time is spent asleep and the patient is drowsy when awake. Obtundation is a less severe impairment of consciousness than stupor.

Cross References

Coma; Psychomotor retardation; Stupor

Ocular Apraxia

Ocular apraxia, or ocular motor apraxia, is a disorder of voluntary saccade initiation; reflexive saccades and spontaneous eye movements are preserved. Ocular apraxia may be overcome by using dynamic head thrusting, with or without blinking (to suppress vestibulo-ocular reflexes): the desired fixation point is achieved through reflex contraversive tonic eye movements to the midposition following the overshoot of the eyes caused by the head thrust.

The anatomical substrate of ocular apraxia is not certain. Ocular apraxia may occur as a congenital syndrome (in the horizontal plane only: Cogan's syndrome), or in association with various hereditary or metabolic disorders, such as ataxia with ocular apraxia (AOA) types 1 and 2, associated with mutations in the aprataxin and senataxin genes respectively; ataxia telangiectasia (Louis-Bar syndrome); Niemann-Pick disease (mainly vertical plane affected); and Gaucher's disease (horizontal plane only).

Cross References

Apraxia; Saccades

Ocular Bobbing

Ocular bobbing refers to intermittent abnormal vertical eye movements, usually conjugate, consisting of a fast downward movement followed by a slow return to the initial horizontal eye position. The sign has no precise localizing value, but is most commonly associated with intrinsic pontine lesions, *e.g.* infarct, haemorrhage, tumour, central pontine myelinolysis. It has also been described in encephalitis, Creutzfeldt-Jakob disease, and toxic encephalopathies. Its pathophysiology is uncertain but may involve mesencephalic and medullary burst neurone centres. Variations on the theme include:

- Inverse ocular bobbing: slow downward movement, fast return (also known as fast upward ocular bobbing, or ocular dipping).

© Springer International Publishing Switzerland 2016

A.J. Larner, *A Dictionary of Neurological Signs*,

DOI 10.1007/978-3-319-29821-4_15

- Reverse ocular bobbing: fast upward movement, slow return to midposition.
- Converse ocular bobbing: slow upward movement, fast down (also known as slow upward ocular bobbing, or reverse ocular dipping).

References
Bosch EP, Kennedy SS, Aschenbrener CA. Ocular bobbing: the myth of its localizing value. *Neurology*. 1975; **25**: 949–53.
Fisher CM. Ocular bobbing. *Arch Neurol*. 1964; **11**: 543–6.
Mehler MF. The clinical spectrum of ocular bobbing and ocular dipping. *J Neurol Neurosurg Psychiatry*. 1988; **51**: 725–7.
Cross Reference
Ocular dipping

Ocular Dipping
Ocular dipping, or inverse ocular bobbing, consists of a slow spontaneous downward eye movement with a fast return to the midposition. This may be observed in anoxic coma or following prolonged status epilepticus and is thought to be a marker of diffuse, rather than focal, brain damage. Reverse ocular dipping (slow upward ocular bobbing) consists of a slow upward movement followed by a fast return to the midposition.
References
Mehler MF. The clinical spectrum of ocular bobbing and ocular dipping. *J Neurol Neurosurg Psychiatry*. 1988; **51**: 725–7.
Stark JR, Masucci EF, Kurtzke JF. Ocular dipping. *Neurology*. 1984; **34**: 391–3.
Cross Reference
Ocular bobbing

Ocular Flutter
Ocular flutter is an eye movement disorder characterized by involuntary bursts of back-to-back horizontal saccades (almost invariably bidirectional, although rare unidirectional cases are reported) without an intersaccadic interval (*cf.* square-wave jerks). Ocular flutter may be accurately diagnosed with oculography.

The postulated mechanism of ocular flutter is loss of "pause" neuronal inhibition of "burst" neurone function in the paramedian pontine reticular formation (PPRF). A case of ocular flutter with a circumscribed inflammatory pontine lesion involving the PPRF, in which clinical and neuroradiological improvement occurred concurrently, has been reported, supporting the argument that, at least in some cases, PPRF lesions may be associated with ocular flutter. Ocular flutter may occur in association with brainstem infections and as a paraneoplastic or non-paraneoplastic autoimmune phenomenon.
Reference
Schon F, Hodgson TL, Mort D, Kennard C. Ocular flutter associated with a localized lesion in the paramedian pontine reticular formation. *Ann Neurol*. 2001; **50**: 413–6.
Cross References
Opsoclonus; Saccades; Saccadic intrusion, Saccadic pursuit; Square-wave jerks

Ocular Myoclonus
- see MYOCLONUS; PALATAL MYOCLONUS

Ocular Tilt Reaction
The ocular tilt reaction is a postural synkinesis consisting of the triad of:

- ocular torsion.
- lateral head tilt to the same side.
- skew deviation with hypotropia ipsilateral to the direction of head/eye torsion.

The ocular tilt reaction (OTR) is due to disordered function of one utricle or its brainstem connections (vestibular nerve, vestibular nuclei, medial longitudinal fasciculus, interstitial nucleus of Cajal), hence a brainstem otolith-ocular reflex. It has occasionally been reported with cerebellar lesions, and may be under inhibitory cerebellar control. OTR may be tonic, as in the lateral medullary syndrome, or paroxysmal, as in multiple sclerosis.

Reference
Halmagyi GM, Curthoys IS, Brandt T, Dieterich M. Ocular tilt reaction: clinical sign of vestibular lesion. *Acta Otolaryngol Suppl.* 1991; **481**: 47–50.

Cross References
Hypotropia; Lateral medullary syndrome; Skew deviation; Synkinesia, Synkinesis; Tullio phenomenon; Vestibulo-ocular reflexes

Oculocephalic Response
Oculocephalic responses are most commonly elicited in unconscious patients; the head is passively rotated in the horizontal or vertical plane (doll's head maneouvre) and the eye movements are observed. Conjugate eye movement in a direction opposite to that in which the head is turned is indicative of an intact brainstem (intact vestibulo-ocular reflexes). With pontine lesions, the oculocephalic responses may be lost; they disappear after roving eye movements but before caloric responses.

Cross References
Caloric testing; Coma; Doll's eye manoeuvre, Doll's head manoeuvre; Head impulse test; Roving eye movements; Supranuclear gaze palsy; Vestibulo-ocular reflexes

Oculogyric Crisis
Oculogyric crisis is an acute dystonia of the ocular muscles, usually causing upward and lateral displacement of the eye. It is often accompanied by a disorder of attention (obsessive, persistent thoughts: "cognitive dystonia"), with or without dystonic or dyskinetic movements.

It occurs particularly with symptomatic (secondary), as opposed to idiopathic (primary), dystonias, for example post-encephalitic and neuroleptic-induced dystonia, the latter now being the most common cause. This is usually an acute effect of medication but may on occasion be seen as a consequence of chronic therapy (tardive oculogyric crisis). It has also been described in Wilson's disease, neuroleptic malignant syndrome, and organophosphate poisoning. Lesions within the lentiform nuclei have been recorded in cases with oculogyric crisis.

Treatment of acute neuroleptic-induced dystonia is with either parenteral benzodiazepine or an anticholinergic agent such as procyclidine, benztropine, or trihexyphenidyl.

References
Kim JS, Kim HK, Im JH, Lee MC. Oculogyric crisis and abnormal magnetic resonance imaging signals in bilateral lentiform nuclei. *Mov Disord.* 1996; **11**: 756–8.
Leigh RJ, Foley JM, Remler BF, Civil RH. Oculogyric crisis: a syndrome of thought disorder and ocular deviation. *Ann Neurol.* 1987; **22**: 13–7.

Cross References
Dyskinesia; Dystonia

Oculomasticatory Myorhythmia
- see MYORHYTHMIA

Oculomotor (III) Nerve Palsy
Oculomotor (III) nerve palsy produces:

- Ptosis: weakness of levator palpebrae superioris (LPS), ± Müller's muscle.
- Mydriasis: impaired parasympathetic outflow to the pupil ("internal ophthalmoplegia"); most obvious in a well lit room (*cf.* Horner's syndrome).

- Diplopia: weakness of medial rectus (MR), inferior rectus (IR), superior rectus (SR), and inferior oblique (IO) muscles causing the eye to point "down and out" (external ophthalmoplegia); the presence of intorsion confirms integrity of superior oblique muscle/trochlear (IV) nerve function.

These changes may be complete or partial.

Pathological correlates of third nerve palsy may occur anywhere from the brainstem to the orbit:

- Intramedullary (brainstem):

    Nuclear: very rare; SR subnucleus lesion causes bilateral denervation; other clinical signs may be expected, such as pupillary (Edinger-Westphal nucleus) and medial longitudinal fasciculus involvement.

    Fascicular (within substance of midbrain): all muscles or specific muscles involved, + other clinical signs expected, such as contralateral ataxia (Claude's syndrome), hemiparesis (Weber's syndrome).

- Extramedullary:

    Subarachnoid space: peripherally located pupillomotor fibres are often spared by ischaemic lesions, but not by space-occupying lesions (*e.g.* aneurysm), however the distinction ("medical versus surgical") is not absolute.

    Cavernous sinus: oculomotor nerve runs over the trochlear nerve; other ocular motor nerves ± trigeminal nerve are often affected.

    Superior orbital fissure: superior division/ramus to SR, LPS; inferior to MR, IR, IO; selective involvement of rami (divisional palsy) may occur; proptosis with space occupying lesions.

    Orbit: paresis of isolated muscle almost always from orbital lesion or muscle disease.

Oculomotor nerve palsies may be distinguished as "pupil involving" or "pupil sparing", the former implying a "surgical", the latter a "medical" cause, but this distinction only holds for complete palsies. Incomplete palsies are more likely to be of "surgical" origin (*e.g.* posterior communicating artery aneurysm). Neuroimaging is the appropriate management if in doubt about aetiology. Transtentorial (uncal) herniation due to raised intracranial pressure may, particularly in its early stages, cause an oculomotor nerve palsy due to stretching of the nerve, a "false-localising sign".

References
Brazis PW. Subject review: Localization of lesions of the oculomotor nerve: recent concepts. *Mayo Clin Proc.* 1991; **66**: 1029–35.
Coles A. The third cranial nerve. *Adv Clin Neurosci Rehabil.* 2001;**1**(1):20–1.
Cross References
Diplopia; Divisional palsy; "False-localising signs"; Hutchinson's pupil; Mydriasis; Ophthalmoparesis, Ophthalmoplegia; Ptosis; Pupil sparing

Oculovestibular Response
- see CALORIC TESTING; VESTIBULO-OCULAR REFLEXES

"Okay Sign"
- see "PINCH SIGN"

One-and-a-Half Syndrome
The one-and-a-half syndrome consists of ipsilateral horizontal gaze palsy and ipsilateral internuclear ophthalmoplegia, such that the only preserved horizontal eye movement is abduction in one eye; vertical movements and convergence are spared. This results from a

brainstem lesion which involves both the abducens (VI) nerve nucleus or paramedian pontine reticular formation, causing ipsilateral horizontal gaze palsy, and the adjacent medial longitudinal fasciculus, causing internuclear ophthalmoplegia. In young patients this is most often due to demyelination, in the elderly to brainstem ischaemia; brainstem arteriovenous malformation or tumour may also be responsible. Myasthenia gravis may cause a pseudo-one-and-a-half syndrome.

A vertical one-and-a-half syndrome has also been described, characterised by vertical upgaze palsy, and monocular paresis of downgaze, either ipsilateral or contralateral to the lesion.

References
Pierrot-Deseilligny C, Chain F, Serdaru M, et al. The "one-and-a-half" syndrome. Electro-oculographic analyses of five patients with deductions about the physiological mechanisms of lateral gaze. *Brain* 1981; **104**: 665–99.
Wall M, Wray SH. The one-and-a-half syndrome. A unilateral disorder of the pontine tegmentum: a study of 20 cases and a review of the literature. *Neurology*. 1983; **33**: 971–80.
Cross References
Eight-and-a-half syndrome; Gaze palsy; Internuclear ophthalmoplegia (INO)

Onion Peel, Onion Skin
These terms have been used to describe a pattern of facial sensory loss characterised by peri-oral sparing (Dejerine pattern), which is seen with intramedullary or cervicomedullary lesions and with tabes dorsalis. It reflects the somatotopic sensory representation in the spinal nucleus of the trigeminal nerve, with midline face (nose, mouth) represented rostrally and lateral facial sensation represented caudally. The pattern of sensory impairment has also been termed "balaclava helmet".
Reference
Das A, Shinde PD, Kesavadas C, Nair M. Teaching neuroimages: onion-skin pattern facial sensory loss. *Neurology*. 2011; **77**: e45–6.
Cross Reference
Balaclava helmet

Ophthalmoparesis, Ophthalmoplegia
Ophthalmoparesis is a weakness or limitation of eye movements, ophthalmoplegia a paralysis of eye movements. Causes may be central (CNS pathways), or peripheral (cranial nerve nuclei, cranial nerves, neuromuscular junction, extraocular muscles). A distinction is sometimes drawn between:

- *External ophthalmoplegia*: weakness of the extraocular muscles of central, neuromuscular, or myopathic origin, which may be:

    Supranuclear: *e.g.* progressive supranuclear palsy, abetalipoproteinaemia.
    Nuclear, internuclear: *e.g.* internuclear ophthalmoplegia (INO), Möbius syndrome.
    Cranial nerve palsy: oculomotor (III), trochlear (IV), abducens (VI), or combinations thereof.
    Neuromuscular junction: myasthenia gravis.
    Extraocular muscles: *e.g.* oculopharyngeal muscular dystrophy (OPMD), chronic progressive external ophthalmoplegia (CPEO), thyroid ophthalmopathy.

The term "ophthalmoplegia plus" has been used to denote the combination of progressive external ophthalmoplegia with additional symptoms and signs, indicative of brainstem, pyramidal, endocrine, cardiac, muscular, hypothalamic or auditory system involvement, as in mitochondrial disease.

- *Internal ophthalmoplegia*: fixity of the pupil with loss of all pupillary reflexes (iridoplegia) and ciliary apparatus.

Hence in an oculomotor (III) nerve palsy there may be both internal and external ophthalmoplegia.

If structural disease and myasthenia gravis are excluded, then mitochondrial disorder (CPEO) may be responsible for ophthalmoplegia, even if this is not evident on quadriceps muscle biopsy.

Reference
Schaefer AM, Blakely EL, Barron MJ, Griffiths PG, Taylor RW, Turnbull DM. Ophthalmoplegia: when all the tests are negative. *J Neurol Neurosurg Psychiatry*. 2004; **75**: 519. (abstract 020).

Cross References
Diplopia; Internuclear ophthalmoplegia (INO); Miosis; Mydriasis; Oculomotor (III) nerve palsy; Pupillary reflexes; Pupil sparing

Opisthotonos
Opisthotonos is an abnormal posture consisting of arching of the back and extension of the limbs such that the body may be supported just on the head and ankles (*arc de cercle*). Opisthotonos may be seen in:

- Coma; decerebrate rigidity.
- Basilar meningitis.
- Hydrocephalus.
- Structural lesions of the posterior fossa.
- Intermittent tonsillar herniation ("cerebellar fits").
- Acute drug- (neuroleptic-) induced dystonic reaction; or chronic feature of tardive dystonia.
- Tetanus.
- Syncope (especially in children).
- Metabolic disorders: kernicterus, Gaucher's disease (type II).
- Drug-induced: propofol.
- Pseudoseizures.

As in decerebrate rigidity, opisthotonos may reflect unopposed extensor tone from the intact vestibular nuclei released from supratentorial control.

Cross References
Coma; Decerebrate rigidity; Emprosthotonos; Pleurothotonos; Spasm

Oppenheim's Sign
Oppenheim's sign is a variant method for eliciting the plantar respone, by application of heavy pressure to the anterior surface of the tibia, for example with the thumb, and moving it down from the patella to the ankle. Extension of the hallux (upgoing plantar response, Babinski's sign) is pathological. Like Chaddock's sign, Oppenheim's sign always postdates the development of Babinski's sign as a reliable indicator of corticospinal pathway (upper motor neurone) pathology.

References
Pearce JMS. Oppenheim's sign. In: Fragments of neurological history. London: Imperial College Press; 2003. p. 359–61.
Van Gijn J. The Babinski sign: a centenary. Utrecht: Universiteit Utrecht; 1996.

Cross References
Babinski's sign (1); Chaddock's sign; Gordon's sign; Plantar response; Upper motor neurone (UMN) syndrome

Oppenheim's Useless Hand Sign
- see USELESS HAND OF OPPENHEIM

Opsoclonus
Opsoclonus, or saccadomania, is an eye movement disorder characterized by involuntary bursts of polydirectional saccades (sometimes with a horizontal preference) without an intersaccadic interval (*cf.* square-wave jerks). Like ocular flutter, opsoclonus may be accurately characterised with oculography.

Although some normal individuals can voluntarily induce opsoclonus, generally it reflects mesencephalic or cerebellar disease affecting the omnipause cells which exert tonic inhibition on the burst neurones which generate saccades. Recognised causes of opsoclonus include:

- Paraneoplasia: in children with neuroblastoma (Kinsbourne's syndrome); in adults the opsoclonus-myoclonus syndrome ("dancing eyes, dancing feet") is most commonly associated with small-cell lung cancer but it may also occur in association with breast cancer in which case onconeural antibodies (anti-Ri, or type 2 anti-neuronal nuclear antibodies [ANNA-2]) may be detected in serum and CSF.
- Postinfectious: a monophasic disorder following respiratory or gastrointestinal infection; presumably autoimmune.
- Intraparenchymal (especially mesencephalic) lesions, *e.g.* tumour, demyelination, neurosarcoidosis, metabolic/toxic encephalopathy.

Postinfectious opsoclonus generally remits spontaneously. Of the paraneoplastic disorders, opsoclonus associated with lung and breast tumours persists and the patients decline from their underlying illness; neuroblastoma associated opsoclonus may be steroid responsive. Intravenous immunoglobulin (IVIg), clonazepam, and valproate have also been used as symptomatic treatments.

References
Bataller L, Graus F, Saiz A, et al. Clinical outcome in adult onset idiopathic or paraneoplastic opsoclonus-myoclonus. *Brain.* 2001; **124**: 437–43.
Wong A. An update on opsoclonus. *Curr Opin Neurol.* 2007; **20**: 25–31.

Cross References
Ocular flutter; Saccadic intrusion, Saccadic pursuit; Square-wave jerks

Optic Aphasia
Optic aphasia is a visual modality-specific naming disorder. It has sometimes been grouped with associative visual agnosia, but patients with optic aphasia are not agnosic since they can demonstrate recognition of visually-presented stimuli by means other than naming, *e.g.* gesture. Moreover, these patients are not handicapped by their deficit in everyday life, whereas agnosic patients are often functionally blind. Objects that are semantically related can be appropriately sorted, indicating intact semantics. This is not simply anomia, since the deficit is specific to visual stimuli; objects presented in the tactile modality, or by sound, or by spoken definition, can be named. Naming errors are often semantic, and perseverations ("*conduit d'approche*") are common. Perception is intact, evidenced by the ability to draw accurately objects which cannot be named. Reading is poorly performed.

Optic aphasia is associated with unilateral lesions of the left occipital cortex and subjacent white matter.

The neuropsychological explanation of optic aphasia is unclear. It may be a mild type of associative visual agnosia, despite the differences.

References
Beauvois MF. Optic aphasia: a process of interaction between vision and language. *Philos Trans R Soc Lond B Biol Sci.* 1982; **298**: 35–47.
Farah MJ. Visual agnosia: disorders of object recognition and what they tell us about normal vision. Cambridge: MIT Press; 1995.

Marsh EB, Hillis AE. Cognitive and neural mechanisms underlying reading and naming: evidence from letter-by-letter reading and optic aphasia. *Neurocase*. 2005; **11**: 325–37.
Cross References
Anomia; *Conduit d'approche*; Visual agnosia

Optic Ataxia
Optic ataxia is impaired voluntary reaching for a visually presented target, with misdirection and dysmetria. It may resemble cerebellar ataxia. Visual fixation is possible but reaching under visual guidance is impaired. Tactile search with the palm and fingers may be undertaken in searching for an object, using somatosensory cues to compensate for impaired access to visual information. Hence this may be characterised as a modality-specific apraxia, wherein visual information cannot be used to guide goal-directed movements. The disorder is both retinotopic and somatotopic.

Optic ataxia occurs with lesions of posterior parietal cortex: the intraparietal sulcus and regions medial and superior to it; the primary visual cortex is intact. It is one feature, along with psychic paralysis of gaze ("sticky fixation") and simultanagnosia (visual disorientation), of Balint's syndrome in which there is some evidence for parieto-occiptial (and possibly frontal) lobe dysfunction (disconnection).
Reference
Andersen RA, Andersen KN, Hwang EJ, Hauschild M. Optic ataxia: from Balint's syndrome to the parietal reach region. *Neuron*. 2014; **81**: 967–83.
Cross References
Apraxia; Ataxia; Balint's syndrome; Dysmetria; Simultanagnosia; Visual disorientation; Visual form agnosia

Optic Atrophy
Optic atrophy is pallor of the optic nerve head as visualized by ophthalmoscopy. The temporal disc may appear pale in a normal fundus, so that optic atrophy can only be confidently diagnosed when there is also nasal pallor, although temporal pallor may follow damage to the macular fibre bundle with central visual defects.

Optic atrophy may be the consequence of any optic neuropathy which causes optic nerve damage leading to gliotic change of the optic nerve head. Although most often seen with optic nerve pathology, it may be a consequence of pathology in the retina, optic chiasm, or optic tract. "Hemianopic" optic atrophy indicates involvement of the optic tract or lateral geniculate body.

The appearance of optic atrophy is non-specific with respect to aetiology. Recognised causes include:

- Previous optic neuritis.
- Chronic papilloedema.
- Chronic optic nerve compression (see Foster Kennedy syndrome).
- Hereditary: autosomal dominant optic atrophy, autosomal recessive optic atrophy, Leber's hereditary optic neuropathy (LHON), other mitochondrial disorders, Behr's syndrome.
- Macular dystrophies.
- Deficiency: tobacco-alcohol amblyopia; vitamin B_{12} deficiency.
- Drug-induced: *e.g.* ethambutol, isoniazid, chloroquine.
- Glaucoma.

Cross References
Disc swelling; Foster Kennedy syndrome; Papilloedema; Temporal pallor

Optokinetic Nystagmus (OKN), Optokinetic Response
Optokinetic nystagmus (OKN) is familiar to anyone who has watched a railway passenger observing passing telegraph poles from the window of a moving train: OKN is an involuntary rhythmic eye movement induced by observing moving stimuli. In clinical practice a striped

drum serves to test both visual pursuit and saccades. Rotation of the stripe to the left produces leftward pursuit, followed by a compensatory saccade to the right, followed by pursuit to the left of the next stripe, with another compensatory saccade, and so on. Hence, OKN is a physiological nystagmus.

Parietal hemisphere lesions (vascular or neoplastic) typically impair OKN. Testing for OKN may be useful in patients with suspected hysterical visual loss, since OKN cannot occur unless visual function is present; the response is lost in blindness. An internuclear ophthalmoplegia may be made more evident by testing OKN.

Cross References
Cortical blindness; Internuclear ophthalmoplegia (INO); Nystagmus; Saccades; Vestibulo-ocular reflexes

Orator's Hand
- see BENEDICTION HAND

Orofacial Dyspraxia
Orofacial dyspraxia, or buccofacial dyspraxia, is an inability to make voluntary, learned, movements with the orofacial musculature, such as blowing out a match, kissing, licking the lips. Recognised causes of orofacial dyspraxia include:

- a transient accompaniment of Broca's aphasia, conduction aphasia, and transcortical motor aphasia of cerebrovascular origin.
- trauma to pre-Rolandic area just above the Sylvian fissure.
- in some patients with primary non-fluent aphasia; a related but distinct condition of "progressive loss of speech output with orofacial dyspraxia" has also been described.

Clinical and imaging studies show a strong correlation between orofacial dyspraxia and lesions in the frontal operculum; it may also occur with subcortical lesions involving periventricular and/or peristriatal white matter as well as the basal ganglia.

Reference
Tyrrell PJ, Kartsounis LD, Frackowiak RSJ, Findley LJ, Rossor MN. Progressive loss of speech output and orofacial dyspraxia associated with frontal lobe hypometabolism. *J Neurol Neurosurg Psychiatry*. 1991; **54**: 351–7.

Cross References
Apraxia; Speech apraxia

Oromandibular Dystonia
Oromandibular dystonia, including the platysma muscle, may occur spontaneously or emerge with levodopa treatment in some patients with multiple system atrophy (MSA-P type usually), resembling risus sardonicus.

Reference
Khan J, Anwer HM, Eliay E, Heir G. Oromandibular dystonia: differential diagnosis and management. *J Am Dent Assoc*. 2015; **146**: 690–3.

Cross References
Dystonia; Risus sardonicus

Orthostatic Hypotension
Orthostatic hypotension, or postural hypotension, is the finding of a persistent drop in baseline blood pressure (BP) on standing, defined as a fall in systolic BP more than 20 mmHg and in diastolic BP more than 10 mmHg within 3 min of adopting the upright position. Normally there is a drop in blood pressure of lesser magnitude on standing but this is usually quickly compensated for by the baroreceptor reflex. Measuring blood pressure automatically by passive head-up tilt testing (tilt table) is also helpful in diagnosing orthostatic hypotension if the active standing test is negative, and the clinical history is suggestive, or in patients with motor impairment.

Symptoms which may be associated with orthostatic hypotension include exercise-induced or postprandial light-headedness, transient visual loss (usually bilateral), blackouts (syncope), and pain in a "coathanger" distribution across the shoulders. There may be supine hypertension and reversal of the normal circadian blood pressure rhythm (normally lower at night), with an increased frequency of micturition at night. Other features of autonomic dysfunction may be present, including dry eyes and dry mouth (xerophthalmia, xerostomia), a tendency to constipation, and lack of penile erections.

Orthostatic hypotension may be found in:

- Pure autonomic failure (PAF).
- Neurodegenerative disorders such as multiple system atrophy, Parkinson's disease, dementia with Lewy bodies.
- Phaeochromocytoma.
- Other causes of autonomic neuropathy (*e.g.* Guillain-Barré syndrome, amyloidosis).

However, the most common cause of orthostatic hypotension in hospital practice is probably dehydration or overzealous treatment with anti-hypertensive or diuretic agents.

Management of orthostatic hypotension consists of education on factors that influence blood pressure. Non-pharmacological approaches include increased salt and water intake, head-up bed tilt, wearing elastic stockings or a G-suit. Pharmacological therapies include fludrocortisone (first line), and midodrine, ephedrine, or dihydroxyphenylserine (second line). Supine hypertension may also require treatment.

References
Lahrmann H, Cortelli P, Hilz M, Mathias CJ, Struhal W, Tassinari M. EFNS guidelines on the diagnosis and management of orthostatic hypotension. *Eur J Neurol.* 2006; **13**: 930–6.
Mathias CJ, Iodice V, Low DA, Bannister R. Treatment of orthostatic hypotension. In: Mathias CJ, Bannister R, editors. Autonomic failure. A textbook of clinical disorders of the autonomic nervous system. 5th ed. Oxford: Oxford University Press; 2013. p. 569–84.

Cross References
Neuropathy; Parkinsonism; Xerophthalmia, Xerostomia

Orthotonos
- see EMPROSTHOTONOS

Oscillopsia
Oscillopsia is an illusory movement of the environment due to excessive slip of images on the retina ("retinal slip") during active or passive head movement, producing a complaint of blurring, jumping, or oscillation of the visual representation of the environment.

Oscillopsia is most often due to acquired bilateral loss of vestibular function (loss of the vestibulo-ocular reflexes). This may be tested for clinically by:

- recording visual acuity whilst the head is passively shaken horizontally, a drop of three to seven lines of acuity versus performance with the head still suggesting loss of VOR (the dynamic illegible E test);
- by observing the optic disc with an ophthalmoscope as the head is gently shaken, the disc moving with the head if VOR are lost.

Vestibular testing will also demonstrate bilateral loss of vestibular function.

Recognised causes of oscillopsia include:

- acquired nystagmus, *e.g.* pendular nystagmus.
- superior oblique myokymia.
- other ocular oscillations.

Oscillopsia does not occur in congenital nystagmus, nor in opsoclonus, presumably due to the operation of the visual suppression mechanism which normally operates during saccadic eye movements.

Oscillopsia may be treated with clonazepam.

Reference

Straube A, Bronstein A, Straumann D; European Federation of Neurologic Societies. Nystagmus and oscillopsia. *Eur J Neurol*. 2012; **19**: 6–14.

Cross References

Myokymia; Nystagmus; Opsoclonus; Pendular nystagmus; Vestibulo-ocular reflexes

Oscillucusis

Oscillucusis is an abnormal perception of an oscillation in the intensity of ambient sounds, which may occur during a migraine attack.

Reference

Piovesan EJ, Kowacs PA, Werneck LC, Siow C. Oscillucusis and sudden deafness in a migraine patient. *Arq Neuropsiquiatr*. 2003; **61**: 848–50.

Osculation

Osculation or kissing behaviour may be seen as a feature of disinhibition in frontotemporal dementia.

Reference

Mendez MF, Shapira JS. Kissing or "osculation" in frontotemporal dementia. *J Neuropsychiatry Clin Neurosci*. 2014; **26**: 258–61.

Cross Reference

Disinhibition

Osmophobia

Osmophobia, an aversion to smells, may form part of a migraine attack, along with photophobia and phonophobia.

Reference

Wang YF, Fuh JL, Chen SP, Wu JC, Wang SJ. Clinical correlates and diagnostic utilty of osmophobia in migraine. *Cephalalgia*. 2012; **32**: 1180–8.

Cross References

Phonophobia; Photophobia

Overflow

- see DYSTONIA; SYNKINESIA, SYNKINESIS

P

Pagophagia
- see PICA

Palatal Reflex
- see GAG REFLEX

Palatal Tremor
Palatal tremor, also known as palatal myoclonus, is characterized by rhythmic, unilateral or bilateral, palatal contractions which continue during sleep; this may be classified as a focal myoclonic syndrome. A distinction may be made between essential and symptomatic palatal tremor, also known as primary and secondary isolated palatal tremor.

Palatal tremor may be asymptomatic, or there may be a clicking sound in the inner ear, especially in essential palatal tremor. There may be associated contractions of external ocular muscles (oculopalatal myoclonus), larynx, neck, diaphragm (respiratory myoclonus, diaphragmatic flutter, or Leeuwenhoek's disease), trunk, and limbs, which may bring the palatal tremor to attention. Palatal tremor may be accompanied by pendular nystagmus and oscillopsia. A distinct clinical entity of progressive ataxia and palatal tremor (PAPT) has been described.

Palatal myoclonus is associated with lesions interrupting pathways between the red nucleus, inferior olivary nucleus and dentate nucleus (Guillain-Mollaret triangle). Hypertrophy of the inferior olivary nucleus may be evident neuroradiologically (structural or functional imaging) and pathologically. This is a consequence of a lesion in the dentato-olivary pathway which leads to transsynaptic degeneration and hypermetabolism of the olivary nucleus. In PAPT there may be cerebellar atrophy in addition to bilateral olivary hypertrophy.

Although many cases are essential/idiopathic, recognised symptomatic causes of palatal tremor include vascular lesions, trauma, neoplasia, demyelination, epilepsy and, rarely, adult-onset Alexander's disease.

Drug treatment of palatal tremor is often unsuccessful, although reports of benefit with 5-hydroxytryptophan, carbamazepine, sodium valproate, clonazepam, baclofen, and even sumatriptan have appeared. Botulinum toxin injections may also help.

References
Samuel M, Torun N, Tuite PJ, Sharpe JA, Lang AE. Progressive ataxia and palatal tremor (PAPT): clinical and MRI assessment with review of palatal tremors. *Brain*. 2004; **127**: 1252–68.
Zadikoff C, Lang AE, Klein C. The "essentials" of essential palatal tremor: a reappraisal of the noslogy. *Brain*. 2006; **129**: 832–40.

Cross References
Eight-and-a-half syndrome; Myoclonus; Nystagmus; Oscillopsia; Tinnitus; Tremor

Palilalia
Palilalia is a disorder of articulation characterized by the involuntary repetition of syllables within a word, whole words, or phrases, hence a reiterative speech disorder. The term stutter may be used for repetition of single syllables, and the term palilogia has sometimes been used for the repetition of phrases, to distinguish from palilalia. These phenomena may be encountered in:

- Parkinson's disease (along with bradylalia, slowness of speech).
- Progressive supranuclear palsy.

© Springer International Publishing Switzerland 2016
A.J. Larner, *A Dictionary of Neurological Signs*,
DOI 10.1007/978-3-319-29821-4_16

- Tourette syndrome (along with vocal and motor tics).
- Pick's disease, as part of the so-called PES syndrome (palilalia, echolalia, stereotypy) or the PEMA syndrome (palilalia, echolalia, mutism, amimia).
- Late stages of Alzheimer's disease.
- Postencephalitic parkinsonism (von Economo's disease).
- Fahr's disease (bilateral basal ganglia calcification).
- Thalamic/midbrain infarcts.
- Seizure disorders: ictal or post-ictal phenomenon.
- Normal finding in children below the age of about 6 years

In pathological states, palilalia may reflect difficulty in set shifting, as seen in frontal lobe (frontal convexity) syndromes.

References

Landi D, Benvenga A, Quattrocchi CC, et al. Complex epileptic palilalia: a case report. *Seizure*. 2012; **21**: 655–57.

Shin HY, Yoon JH, Lee WY. Palilalia in Parkinson's disease. *J Neurol*. 2009; **256**(Supp 12): S143. (Abstract P403).

Yasuda Y, Akiguchi I, Ino M, Nabatabe H, Kameyama M. Paramedian thalamic and midbrain infarcts associated with palilalia. *J Neurol Neurosurg Psychiatry*. 1990; **53**: 797–9.

Cross References

Bradylalia; Echolalia; Frontal lobe syndromes; Hypomimia; Mutism; Parkinsonism; Stereotypy; Stutter; Tic

Palilogia
- see PALILALIA

Palinacousis, Palinacusis

Palinacousis or palinacusis is a paroxysmal auditory illusion of perseveration or persistence of an external auditory stimulus after it has stopped, a phenomenon also known as auditory perseveration. Although sometimes classified as an illusory experience, musical hallucinations may occur concurrently. Palinacousis may occur as an aura, seizure, or post-ictal phenomenon, and be associated with structural and/or functional pathology in the medial geniculate body or temporal lobe.

Reference

Fields MC, Marcuse LV. Palinacousis. *Handb Clin Neurol*. 2015; **129**: 457–67.

Cross References

Aura; Hallucination; Illusion

Palinopsia

Palinopsia is an illusory visual phenomenon characterized by the persistence or recurrence of visual images immediately after the stimulus has been removed, hence visual perseveration. This is distinct from the physiological after-image. It may be associated with polyopia. The description of the symptom may lead to it being mistaken for diplopia ("pseudodiplopia"). A hallucinatory form of palinopsia has also been described.

Palinopsia occurs most frequently in the context of a left homonymous hemianopia, secondary to right occipitotemporal or occipitoparietal lesions: these may be vascular, neoplastic, metabolic, ictal, or drug- or toxin-induced (*e.g.* carbon monoxide poisoning). Palinopsia has also been described with retinal and optic nerve disease, and occasionally in normal individuals.

Reference

Gersztenkorn D, Lee AG. Palinopsia revamped: a systematic review of the literature. *Surv Ophthalmol*. 2015; **60**: 1–35.

Cross References

Hemianopia; Illusion; Perseveration; Polyopia; Visual perseveration

Pallesthesia

Pallesthesia is the appreciation of vibration sensation; its loss may be described as pallanaesthesia. This may be an age-related sign, or a consequence of peripheral neuropathic disorders.

Cross References

Age-related signs; Vibration

Palmaris Brevis Sign

Palmaris brevis sign may be useful in localising the site of an ulnar nerve lesion. Innervated by the superficial "sensory" division of the ulnar nerve in the wrist (distal canal of Guyon), contraction of the palmaris brevis muscle may be evident with compressive lesions of the deep motor branch of the ulnar nerve which cause intrinsic hand muscle weakness but no sensory loss ("Ramsay Hunt syndrome"): the patient is asked to "contract" the hypothenar eminence with the fifth digit forcibly abducted, and the examiner looks for corrugation of the skin over the eminence. In sensory superficial division ulnar nerve lesions, this sign is lost.

References

Iyer VG. Palmaris brevis sign in ulnar neuropathy 1998. *Muscle Nerve*. 1998; **21**: 675–77.
Larner AJ. Pitfalls in the diagnosis of ulnar neuropathy: remember the deep palmar branch. *Br J Hosp Med*. 2010; **71**: 654–5.

Palmomental Reflex

The palmomental reflex consists of contraction of the mentalis muscle induced by stroking the ipsilateral palm with a blunt object. It may indicate damage to the contralateral paracentral cortex or its connections, but since it is observed in about one quarter of normal adults and is very common in the normal elderly, and may occur in other conditions, both its sensitivity and specificity are low. It may be considered a frontal release sign or primitive reflex, but is less specific than the grasp reflex. Induction of the reflex by stimulation of areas other than the palm is more likely to be associated with cerebral damage.

References

Brodsky H, Vuong KD, Thomas M, Jankovic J. Glabellar and palmomental reflexes in parkinsonian disorders. *Neurology*. 2004; **63**: 1096–8.
Owen G, Mulley GP. The palmomental reflex: a useful clinical sign? *J Neurol Neurosurg Psychiatry*. 2002; **73**: 113–5.

Cross References

Age-related signs; Frontal release signs

Papilloedema

Papilloedema is swelling (oedema) of the optic nerve head due to raised intracranial pressure (*cf.* other causes of disc swelling, which may cause pseudopapilloedema). A number of stages of papilloedema are described: in the acute stage, the only findings may be oedema at the superior and inferior poles of the disc, absence of spontaneous retinal venous pulsation, and enlargement of the blind spot. As papilloedema progresses the whole disc is involved and splinter haemorrhages may be evident at the disc margin. These early stages may be asymptomatic, or may be associated with transient losses of vision (obscurations), often provoked by activities or movements which further raise intracranial pressure, thus compromising retinal perfusion pressure. Enlargement of the blind spot and constriction of the visual field may be evident, but visual acuity is often unimpaired (*cf.* disc swelling due to papillitis). Chronic papilloedema produces gliosis of the optic nerve head and eventually optic atrophy ("sequential optic atrophy") with nerve fibre damage and permanent visual field defects.

A rating scale for papilloedema (Frisén) has been described, but one study found low agreement between reviewers using this scale.

Reference
Sinclair AJ, Burdon MA, Nightingale PG, et al. Rating papilloedema: an evaluation of the Frisén classification in idiopathic intracranial hypertension. *J Neurol*. 2012; **259**: 1406–12.
Cross References
Blind spot; Disc swelling; Obscurations; Optic atrophy; Pseudopapilloedema; Retinal venous pulsation; Scotoma

Paraballismus
- see BALLISM, BALLISMUS; HEMIBALLISMUS

Paradoxical Abdominal Wall Movement, Paradoxical Breathing
The normal movement of the diaphragm (*i.e.* down in inspiration, causing outward abdominal wall movement) may be reversed (paradoxical) in conditions which cause diaphragm weakness (*i.e.* inward abdominal wall movement on inspiration), *e.g.* Guillain-Barré syndrome, acid-maltase deficiency, phrenic nerve injury, hence paradoxical abdominal movement, abdominal paradox, paradoxical breathing, or paradoxical diaphragm movement. This may be detectable clinically or by X-ray screening of the diaphragm. Vital capacity is lower when lying compared to standing. Paradoxical diaphragm movement is a potentially alarming sign since it may indicate incipient respiratory failure.
Reference
Ahmed R, McNamara S, Gandevia S, Halmagyi GM. Paradoxical abdominal wall movement in bilateral diaphragmatic paralysis. *Pract Neurol*. 2012; **12**: 184–6.
Cross Reference
Myopathy

Paradoxical Flexor Reflex
- see GORDON'S SIGN

Paradoxical Head Tilt
- see BIELSCHOWSKY'S SIGN, BIELSCHOWSKY'S TEST

Paradoxical Triceps Reflex
- see INVERTED REFLEXES

Paraesthesia
Paraesthesia (plural: paraesthesiae or paraesthesias) describes an abnormal sensation, often described as a tingling sensation, or likened to "pins and needles" or electricity, pricking, tickling, or even crawling (formication), *i.e.* positive sensory symptoms. The sensation is not pleasant but nor is it painful (*cf.* dysaesthesia). Some patients may describe this sensation as "numbness" or "deadness", in which case care needs to be taken to differentiate it from anaesthesia (*i.e.* a negative phenomenon). Some authorities reserve the term for spontaneous rather than evoked positive sensory phenomena, as a distinction from dysaesthesia.

Paraesthesia is a feature of neuropathy, and may occur in the distribution of a compressed or entrapped nerve, perhaps reflecting the mechanosensitivity of nerves in this situation (*e.g.* Phalen's sign, Tinel's sign), or distally in a "glove and stocking distribution" (acroparaesthesia). Paraesthesia is a more reliable indicator of the diagnosis of neuropathy than pain. Paraesthesia may also be provoked by hyperventilation (especially perioral, hands and feet). Central lesions may also produce paraesthesia (*e.g.* Lhermitte's sign).
Cross References
Anaesthesia; Dysaesthesia; Lhermitte's sign; Phalen's sign; Tinel's sign

Paragrammatism

Paragrammatism is the substitution of morphological elements and function words in the context of fluent speech (*e.g.* in Wernicke's aphasia), as differentiated from agrammatism, the omission of function words and bound morphemes in nonfluent speech (*e.g.* in Broca's aphasia).

Cross References
Agrammatism; Aphasia; Broca's aphasia; Wernicke's aphasia

Paragraphia
- see AGRAPHIA

Parakinesia, Parakinesis
These terms have been used in different ways by different authors, to describe:

- a volitional purposeful act designed to camouflage, mask, or draw attention away from an involuntary movement, such as chorea;
- strange movements of presumed psychogenic origin. In this context, it should be remembered that many movements previously thought to conform to this definition have subsequently been recognised to have an organic basis (*e.g.* tics, klazomania).

The terms are now seldom used, other than to describe the involuntary movement of a paralysed arm following yawning, parakinesia brachialis oscitans.

Reference
Zorzetto FP, Braatz VL, Walusinski O, Teive HA. Parakinesia brachialis oscitans during thrombolytic therapy. *BMJ Case Rep*. 2013; **2013**: pii: bcr2012007079.

Cross References
Chorea, Choreoathetosis; Dyskinesia; Klazomania; Yawning

Paralexia
- see ALEXIA

Paralogia
- see GANSER PHENOMENON, GANSER SYNDROME

Paralysis
Paralysis is a total loss of power to move a body part; equivalent to the suffix -plegia. The use of the word has not been entirely consistent over time, for example James Parkinson (1755–1824) originally used the term *paralysis agitans* to describe the disease which now bears his name. The periodic paralyses are a group of conditions characterized by episodic muscular weakness and stiffness (myotonia) associated with mutations in the skeletal muscle voltage-gated sodium and calcium ion channel genes (channelopathies).

Cross References
Myotonia; Plegia

Paramnesia
Paramnesia is recalling as memories things which have not in fact taken place, hence a distortion of episodic or autobiographical memory. This may be neurological or psychiatric in origin. Relation of paramnesias as the truth occurs in confabulation.

Cross References
Amnesia; Confabulation; Reduplicative paramnesia

Paramyotonia

Paramyotonia describes myotonia induced by cold and exercise. It is similar to myotonia in that muscle does not relax normally following contraction (voluntary, percussion), which may prompt a complaint of muscle aching or stiffness, but differs in that repetitive muscle use (*e.g.* exercise) accentuates the problem, leading to an increased delay in muscle relaxation (worsening stiffness). For example, repeated forced voluntary eyelid closure in a patient with paramyotonia may, after several attempts, lead to a failure of voluntary eyelid opening, the eyes remaining closed for a minute or so. Paramyotonia particularly affects the face and forearms. This type of muscle stiffness may also be sensitive to temperature, being made worse by cooling which may also provoke muscle weakness. Weakness may outlast exposure to cold by several hours.

Neurophysiological studies may assist in the diagnosis of paramyotonia. During the delayed muscle relaxation, electrical activity is not prominent, and after muscle cooling the resting muscle membrane potential may be reduced from around the normal value of -80 mV to around -40 mV, at which point muscle fibres are inexcitable (contracture).

Paramyotonia congenita (Eulenburg's disease) is a channelopathy with mutations affecting the α-subunit of the sodium channel (SCN4A). Mutations in the same gene have been documented in hyperkalaemic periodic paralysis and K^+-aggravated myotonia.

Symptomatic treatment with membrane-stabilizing agents like mexiletine and tocainide, or with the carbonic anhydrase inhibitor acetazolamide, might be tried. Precautions are necessary during general anaesthesia because of the risk of diaphragm myotonia.

References

Ebers GC, George AL, Barchi RL, et al. Paramyotonia congenita and hyperkalaemic periodic paralysis are linked to the adult muscle sodium channel gene. *Ann Neurol.* 1991; **30**: 810–6.

Matthews E, Tan SV, Fialho D, et al. What causes paramytonia in the United Kingdom? Common and new SCN4A mutations revealed. *Neurology.* 2008; **70**: 50–3.

Cross References

Contracture; Myotonia; Paralysis; Warm-up phenomenon

Paraparesis

Paraparesis describes weakness of the lower limbs, short of complete weakness or paralysis (paraplegia). This may result from lesions anywhere from cerebral cortex (frontal, parasagittal lesions) to peripheral nerves, producing either an upper motor neurone (spastic) or lower motor neurone (flaccid) picture. A spinal cord lesion (myelopathy) is probably the most common cause. Paraparesis may be symmetrical or asymmetrical. Recognised causes of paraparesis include:

- *Upper motor neurone lesions*:

    Traumatic section of the cord.

    Cord compression from intrinsic or extrinsic mass lesion, *e.g.* tumour, metastasis, abscess, empyema, haematoma (epidural, subdural).

    Inflammatory lesions: acute transverse myelitis of viral origin, multiple sclerosis, neuromyelitis optica (Devic's syndrome), systemic lupus erythematosus, Behçet's disease, giant cell arteritis (rare).

    Structural lesions: tethered cord syndrome, arteriovenous malformation.

    Metabolic: Hereditary spastic paraplegia (HSP), adrenoleukodystrophy (X-ALD), subacute combined degeneration of the cord (usually mild).

- *Lower motor neurone lesions*:

    Acute or chronic neuropathies (Guillain-Barré syndrome, chronic inflammatory demyelinating polyradiculoneuropathy).

Reference
Jacob A, Larner AJ. Diseases of the spinal cord. In: Cox TM, et al., editors. Oxford textbook of medicine. 6th ed. Oxford: Oxford University Press; 2016. in press.
Cross References
Flaccidity; Myelopathy; Paraplegia; Spasticity

Paraphasia
Paraphasias are a feature of aphasias (disorders of language), particularly (but not exclusively) fluent aphasias resulting from posterior dominant temporal lobe lesions (*cf.* anterior lesions which tend to produce non-fluent aphasias with agrammatism).

Paraphasias refer to a range of speech output errors, both phonological and lexical, including substitution, addition, duplication, omission and transposition of linguistic units, affecting letters within words, letters within syllables, or words within sentences. Paraphasic errors may be categorised as:

- *Phonemic* or *literal*:
    Errors involve individual phonemes; impaired phonology (*i.e.* sound based) causing approximations to real words; nonwords resulting from phonemic paraphasia may be referred to as neologisms. Phonemic paraphasias may be encountered in Broca's aphasia and conduction aphasia, when the patient may recognise them to be errors, and Wernicke's aphasia.
- *Formal*:
    Target word is replaced by another word that is phonemically similar.
- *Morphemic*:
    Errors involving word stems, suffixes, prefixes, inflections and other parts of words.
- *Verbal*:
    Errors involving whole words. These may be further classified as:
    Semantic or *categoric*: substitution of a different exemplar from the same category (*e.g.* "orange" for "apple"; *paradigmatic*) or of a thematically related word (*e.g.* "sit" for "chair"; *syntagmatic*). Verbal paraphasias showing both semantic and phonemic resemblance to the target word are called *mixed* errors. These types may be observed in patients with Wernicke's aphasia, who often seem unaware of their paraphasias due to a failure of self-monitoring of output.

Cross References
Aphasia; Broca's aphasia; Conduction aphasia; Jargon aphasia; Neologism; Schizophasia; Transcortical aphasias; Wernicke's aphasia

Paraplegia
Paraplegia is a total weakness (paralysis) of the lower limbs (*cf.* paraparesis). This may result from lower motor neurone lesions involving multiple nerve roots and/or peripheral nerves (*e.g.* paraparetic Guillain-Barré syndrome) producing a flaccid, areflexic paraplegia; but more commonly it is due to upper motor neurone lesions interrupting corticospinal pathways (corticospinal tract, vestibulospinal tract, reticulospinal tracts, and other extrapyramidal pathways), most usually in the spinal cord. The latter may acutely produce a flaccid areflexic picture ("spinal shock"), but later this develops into an upper motor neurone syndrome (hypertonia, clonus, hyperreflexia, loss of superficial reflexes [*e.g.* abdominal, cremasteric reflexes] and Babinski's sign) with possible lower motor neurone signs at the level of the lesion; bladder involvement is common (urinary retention). Because of the difficulty in distinguishing whether an acute paraplegia is of LMN or UMN origin, imaging to exclude

potentially reversible cord compression is mandatory. Recognised causes of paraplegia of upper motor neurone origin include:

- traumatic section of the cord.
- cord compression.
- inflammatory lesions: acute transverse myelitis of viral origin, multiple sclerosis, neuro-myelitis optica (Devic's syndrome).
- ischaemic lesions; anterior spinal artery syndrome, venous infarction of the cord.

In paraplegia of upper motor neurone origin, enhanced flexion defence reflexes ("flexor spasms") may occur, producing hip and knee flexion, ankle and toe dorsiflexion. Eventually such flexor responses may become a fixed flexion deformity with secondary contractures ("paraplegia in flexion"). Prevention of this situation may be possible by avoiding spasms, which are often provoked by skin irritation or ulceration, bowel constipation, bladder infection, and poor nutrition. Physiotherapy and pharmacotherapy with agents such as baclofen, dantrolene and tizanidine may be used; botulinum toxin injections may be helpful for focal spasticity. "Paraplegia in extension", with extension at the hip and knee, may be seen with incomplete or high spinal cord lesions.

Cross References
Abdominal reflexes; Areflexia; Babinski's sign (1); Clonus; Contracture; Cremasteric reflex; Flaccidity; Hyperreflexia; Hypertonia, Hypertonus; Lower motor neurone (LMN) syndrome; Myelopathy; Paraparesis; Spasticity; Upper motor neurone (UMN) syndrome; Urinary retention

Parapraxia, Parapraxis
Although these terms may be used in common parlance as synonymous with a "Freudian slip", slips which Freud himself referred to as *Fehlleistungen* ("faulty actions" or "misperformances"), in neurological practice they have a different meaning, referring to one of the cardinal symptoms of ideomotor apraxia: a combination of deficient action selection with errors of sequencing of actions and spatial orientation errors. Parapraxic errors include:

- Perseveration: repetition of movements.
- Substitution: of one movement for another (*e.g.* patient shows tongue when asked to close eyes).
- Surplus movements.
- Verbal overflow: explaining a movement rather than performing it.
- Omission: incomplete movements.
- *Conduit d'approche*: several attempts to perform the correct movement.
- Body part as object.

Reference
Klein R, Mayer-Gross W. The clinical examination of patients with organic cerebral disease. London: Cassell; 1957. p. 39.
Cross References
Apraxia; Body part as object; *Conduit d'approche*; Perseveration

Paratonia
Paratonia (or paratonic rigidity, or *gegenhalten*, or oppositional rigidity) is a variable resistance to passive movement of a limb when changing its posture or position, which is evident in both flexor and extensor muscles (as in rigidity, but not spasticity), which seems to increase further with attempts to encourage the patient to relax, such that there is a resistance to any applied movement (German: to counter, stand ones ground). However, this is not a form of impaired muscle relaxation akin to myotonia and paramyotonia. For instance, when lifting the legs by placing the hands under the knees, the legs may be held extended at the knees

despite encouragement on the part of the examiner for the patient to flex the knees. The degree of resistance is said to depend on the speed of movement (as in spasticity). Generally, tendon reflexes are normal, plantar responses downgoing, and there is no clonus. A Paratonia Assessment Instrument has been described.

Paratonia is a sign of bilateral frontal lobe dysfunction, especially mesial cortex and superior convexity (premotor cortex, area 6). It may be related to executive dysfunction and planning impairments. It is not uncommon in otherwise healthy elderly individuals with diffuse frontal lobe cerebrovascular disease, and may also be seen in neurodegenerative disorders such as Alzheimer's disease.

Reference
Hobbelen JS, Koopmans RT, Verhey FR, Habraken KM, de Bie RA. Diagnosing paratonia in the demented elderly: reliability and validity of the Paratonia Assessment Instrument (PAI). *Int Psychogeriatr*. 2008; **20**: 840–52.

Cross References
Frontal release signs; Myotonia; Paramyotonia; Rigidity; Spasticity

Paresis
Paresis denotes a degree of weakness which is less than total paralysis (−plegia), which may be of upper or lower motor neurone origin. Various prefixes denote the location of such weakness, *e.g.* hemiparesis, monoparesis, ophthalmoparesis, paraparesis, quadriparesis.

Since localised pain may inhibit voluntary muscular exertion, apparent weakness in such circumstances may be labelled "algesic pseudoparesis".

Cross References
Lower motor neurone (LMN) syndrome; Paralysis; Plegia; Upper motor neurone (UMN) syndrome; Weakness

Parinaud's Syndrome
Parinaud's syndrome, also sometimes known as the dorsal midbrain syndrome, the periaqueductal grey matter syndrome, or the pretectal syndrome, consists of the following features:

• Eye movements:

> Paralysis of vertical gaze, especially upgaze: Bell's phenomenon may be spared.
> Loss of convergence; convergence spasm may cause slow abduction ("midbrain pseudo-sixth").
> Skew deviation.
> Convergence-retraction nystagmus (Körber-Salus-Elschnig syndrome); sometimes downbeat nystagmus.

• Eyelids:

> Lid retraction (Collier's "tucked lid" sign) or ptosis (ventral extension of lesion).

• Pupils:

> Mydriasis.

This constellation of signs results from dorsal midbrain lesions, such as pineal tumours, which affect the pretectum and posterior commissure and so interfere with conjugate eye movements in the vertical plane. The key anatomical substrates, damage to which causes the syndrome, are probably the interstitial nucleus of Cajal and the nucleus of the posterior commissure and their projections.

References
Keane JR. The pretectal syndrome: 206 patients. *Neurology*. 1990; **40**: 684–90.
Ouvrier R. Henri Parinaud (1844–1905). *J Neurol*. 2011; **258**: 1571–2.
Parinaud H. Paralysie des mouvements associés des yeux. *Archives de Neurologie Paris*. 1883; **5**: 145–72.

Pierrot-Deseilligny C, Chain F, Gray M, et al. Parinaud's syndrome. *Brain*. 1982; **105**: 667–96.

Cross References
Collier's sign; Light-near pupillary dissociation; Nystagmus; Supranuclear gaze palsy

Parkinsonism
Parkinsonism describes a clinical syndrome characterized by the presence of some or all of the following features; there is overlap with so-called akinetic-rigid syndromes in which these features predominate:

- Akinesia, hypokinesia (*sine qua non*).
- Rigidity: consistent (leadpipe) or jerky (cogwheeling; Negro's sign).
- Bradykinesia.
- Tremor, usually at rest, of frequency 3.5–7.0 Hz, "pill rolling" type; there may sometimes be an additional action component to the tremor, and very occasionally there is exclusively an action tremor. "Re-emergent tremor" is also described.
- Stooped posture: forward flexion of trunk, flexion of knees, elbows; "simian posture".
- Impaired postural reflexes, with or without a history of falls; propulsion, retropulsion.
- Mask-like facies, poverty of spontaneous facial expression (hypomimia).
- Reduced blink rate (this may be a particular feature of progressive supranuclear palsy).
- Hypophonic, monotonic voice (hypokinetic dysarthria).
- Widened palpebral fissure (Stellwag's sign).
- Hypometria.
- Seborrhea.
- Sialorrhoea.
- Festinant (shuffling) gait.
- Micrographia.
- Dystonic postures, *e.g.* striatal toe.
- Apraxia.
- Akathisia.
- Cognitive impairment (usually of frontal-subcortical type).
- Hallucinations: minor (*anwesenheit*; passage type), or formed, visual > auditory. Insight into the non-reality of these experiences may be retained, hence may be described as "pseudohallucinations" rather than hallucinations.
- Autonomic dysfunction, especially orthostatic hypotension.

Conventionally parkinsonism is viewed as a disorder of the extrapyramidal system producing "extrapyramidal signs", although this term has limitations: despite the fact that some of the cardinal features of parkinsonism (bradykinesia, rigidity, postural instability, tremor) result from pathology in the basal ganglia, particularly affecting dopaminergic pathways, other features may reflect cortical involvement, at least in part (*e.g.* apraxia, micrographia).

The incidence of parkinsonism increases dramatically with age; it is also associated with an increased risk of death, particularly in the presence of a gait disturbance.

The differential diagnosis of parkinsonism is broad, and includes:

- Idiopathic Parkinson's disease.
- Dementia with Lewy bodies.
- Multiple system atrophy.
- Progressive supranuclear palsy (Steele-Richardson-Olszewski syndrome).
- Corticobasal degeneration, cortical basal ganglionic degeneration.
- Drug-induced parkinsonism (*e.g.* neuroleptics, MPTP).
- Toxin-induced parkinsonism (*e.g.* carbon monoxide, manganese).
- Wilson's disease (hepatolenticular degeneration); non-Wilsonian hepatocerebral degeneration.

- Neuroleptic malignant syndrome.
- Normal pressure hydrocephalus.
- "Arteriosclerotic parkinsonism", resulting from multiple subcortical infarcts.
- Huntington's disease, especially juvenile onset type (Westphal variant).
- Post-encephalitic parkinsonism (encephalitis lethargica, von Economo's disease).
- Dementia pugilistica, post-traumatic parkinsonism.
- Systemic lupus erythematosus.
- Sjögren's syndrome.
- Hypoparathyroidism.
- Parkinsonism-dementia complex of Guam.

Obsessive slowness also enters the differential diagnosis but typical parkinsonian features (akinesia, rigidity) are not present in this condition.

It is crucial not to miss the diagnosis of Wilson's disease, although rare, since in the early stages this disorder is reversible with copper chelation therapy; hence copper and caeruloplasmin should be checked in all patients with young-onset (under age 40 or 50 years) parkinsonism (and dystonia).

Response to levodopa therapy is only reliably seen in idiopathic Parkinson's disease, although some patients with multiple system atrophy or progressive supranuclear palsy may benefit. The features particularly responsive in Parkinson's disease are bradykinesia and rigidity; tremor is less reliably helped.

References
Bennett DA, Beckett LA, Murray AM, et al. Prevalence of parkinsonian signs and associated mortality in a community population of older people. *New Engl J Med*. 1996; **334**: 71–6.
Gardner-Thorpe C. James Parkinson 1755–1824. Exeter: A Wheaton & Co. Ltd; 1987. [Includes facsimile of Parkinson's book on the shaking palsy].
Gibb WRG, Lees AJ. The relevance of the Lewy body to the pathogenesis of idiopathic Parkinson's disease. *J Neurol Neurosurg Psychiatry*. 1988; **51**: 745–52.

Cross References
Apraxia; Blinking; Bradykinesia; Dysarthria; Dystonia; Hypokinesia; Hypomimia; Hypophonia; Mask-like facies; Micrographia; Orthostatic hypotension; Postural reflexes; Rigidity; Seborrhoea; Sialorrhoea; Striatal toe; Supranuclear gaze palsy; Tremor

Parosmia
Parosmia is a false smell, *i.e.* the subjective sensation of a smell which does not exist (*i.e.* an hallucination). Such smells are usually unpleasant (cacosmia), may be associated with a disagreeable taste (cacogeusia), and may be difficult for the patient to define. Causes include purulent nasal infections or sinusitis, and partial recovery following transection of olfactory nerve fibres after head injury. Transient parosmia may presage epileptic seizures of temporal lobe cortical origin (olfactory aura), particularly involving the medial (uncal) region. The symptom may also be common amongst the normal population.

Reference
Nordin S, Brämerson A, Millqvist E, Bende M. Prevlance of parosmia: the Skövde population-based studies. *Rhinology*. 2007; **45**: 50–3.

Cross References
Aura; Cacogeusia; Seizures

Parry-Romberg Syndrome
Parry-Romberg syndrome describes hemifacial atrophy, a thinning of subcutaneous tissues on one side of the face which may also involve muscle and bone (causing enophthalmos), and sometimes brain, in which case neurological features (hemiparesis, hemianopia, focal epileptic seizures, cognitive impairment) may also be present.

The clinical heterogeneity of hemifacial atrophy probably reflects pathogenetic heterogeneity. The syndrome may result from maldevelopment of autonomic innervation or vascular supply, or as an acquired feature following trauma, or a consequence of linear scleroderma (morphoea), in which case a *coup de sabre* may be seen.

References
Larner AJ, Bennison DP. Some observations on the aetiology of hemifacial atrophy ("Parry-Romberg syndrome"). *J Neurol Neurosurg Psychiatry*. 1993; **56**: 1035–6.
Stone J. Parry-Romberg syndrome: a global survey of 205 patients using the Internet. *Neurology*. 2003; **61**: 674–6.

Cross References
Coup de sabre; Enophthalmos; Hemianopia; Hemiparesis

Past-pointing
- see DYSMETRIA

Patellar Reflex
- see REFLEXES

Pathological Crying, Pathological Laughter
Pathological laughter and pathological crying (PLC), or forced laughter and crying, also referred to as involuntary emotional expression disorder, have been defined as reflecting an incongruence of mood (subjective feeling) and expression or affect ("objective", observed), such that patients laugh involuntarily though not happy, or cry though not sad. There may be a sense that the patient is struggling against these displays of emotion, in contrast to the situation in other forms of emotional lability where there is said to be congruence of mood and affect, although sudden fluctuations and exaggerated emotional expression are common to both, suggesting a degree of overlap.

PLC is ascribed to a loss (release) of the normal inhibition of the motor component of facial expression (*i.e.* cortical-subcortical disinhibition). PLC may occur in the context of a pseudobulbar palsy ("pseudobulbar affect") but not invariably so. PLC has been reported in:

- Multiple sclerosis: crying > laughing; related to cognitive impairment (more extensive brain involvement, but not brainstem).
- Alzheimer's disease.
- Stroke: PLC may be the harbinger of brainstem stroke or a feature of anterior choroidal artery territory infarctions; rarely a feature of TIAs.
- Motor neurone disease.
- Head injury.
- Gelastic epilepsy.
- Traumatic brain injury.

A Pathological Laughter and Crying Scale has been developed. Suggested treatments for PLC include amitriptyline, levodopa, amantadine, and serotonin reuptake inhibitors such as fluoxetine and citalopram.

References
Larner AJ. Crying spells as symptoms of a transient ischaemic attack. *J Neurol Neurosurg Psychiatry*. 2000; **68**: 800–1.
Robinson RG, Parikh RM, Lipsey JR, Starkstein SE, Price TR. Pathological laughter and crying following stroke: validation of a measurement scale and a double-blind treatment study. *Am J Psychiatry*. 1993; **150**: 286–93.
Wild B, Rodden FA, Grodd W, Ruch W. Neural correlates of laughter and humour. *Brain*. 2003; **126**: 2121–38.

Cross References
Automatism; Emotionalism, Emotional lability; *Fou rire prodromique*; Pseudobulbar palsy

Peduncular Hallucinosis
Peduncular hallucinosis is a rare syndrome characterised by hallucinations and brainstem symptoms. Hallucinations are vivid and naturalistic. Brainstem findings include oculomotor disturbances, dysarthria, ataxia, and impaired arousal. Episodic memory impairments also occur. Pathology may be in the midbrain, thalamus and pons.
Reference
Benke T. Peduncular hallucinosis. A syndrome of impaired reality monitoring. *J Neurol.* 2006; **253**: 1561–71.
Cross Reference
Hallucination

"Peek Sign"
One of the eye signs of myasthenia gravis: on attempted forced eye closure, orbicularis oculi may fatigue such that the patient "peeks" through the partially open palpebral fissure.

Peliopsia
Peliopsia or pelopsia is a form of metamorphopsia characterised by the misperception of objects as being closer to the observer than they really are (*cf.* porropsia, teliopsia).
Cross References
Metamorphopsia; Porropsia

Pelvic Thrusting
Pelvic thrusting may be a feature of epileptic seizures of frontal lobe origin; occasionally it may occur in temporal lobe seizures. Pelvic thrusting also occurs in pseudoseizures, particularly those of the "thrashing" variety.
     Choreiform disorders may involve the pelvic region causing thrusting or rocking movements.
Reference
Geyer JD, Payne TA, Drury I. The value of pelvic thrusting in the diagnosis of seizures and pseudoseizures. *Neurology.* 2000; **54**: 227–9.
Cross References
Automatism; Chorea, Choreoathetosis; Seizure

Pendular Nystagmus
Pendular or undulatory nystagmus is charactrerised by eye movements which are more or less equal in amplitude and velocity (sinusoidal oscillations) about a central (null) point. In acquired causes such as multiple sclerosis, this may produce oscillopsia and blurred vision. Treatment options include gabapentin and memantine.
Reference
Starck M, Albrecht H, Pöllmann W, Dieterich M, Straube A. Acquired pendular nystagmus in multiple sclerosis: an examiner-blind cross-over treatment study of memantine and gabapentin. *J Neurol.* 2010; **257**: 322–7.
Cross References
Nystagmus; Oscillopsia

Percussion Myotonia
Percussion myotonia is the myotonic response of a muscle to a mechanical stimulus, *e.g.* when struck with a tendon hammer. For example, a blow to the thenar eminence may produce involuntary and sustained flexion of the thumb. This response, which may be seen in myotonic dystrophy, reflects the impaired muscle relaxation which characterises myotonia.
Reference
Barroso FA, Nogues MA. Images in clinical medicine. Percussion myotonia. *New Eng J Med.* 2009; **360**: e13.

Cross Reference
Myotonia

Periodic Alternating Nystagmus
Periodic alternating nystagmus is a horizontal jerk nystagmus, which damps or stops for a few seconds and then reverses direction. Eye movements may need to be observed for up to 5 min to see the whole cycle. Periodic alternating nystagmus may be congenital (idiopathic infantile, associated with a number of genetic loci) or acquired, if the latter then its localising value is similar to that of downbeat nystagmus (with which it may coexist), especially for lesions at the cervico-medullary junction (*e.g.* Chiari malformation). Treatment of the associated lesion may be undertaken, otherwise periodic alternating nystagmus usually responds to baclofen, hence the importance of correctly identifying this particular form of nystagmus.

References
Halmagyi GM, Rudge P, Gresty MA, et al. Treatment of periodic alternating nystagmus. *Ann Neurol.* 1980; **8**: 609–11.
Thomas MG, Crosier M, Lindsay S, et al. The clinical and molecular genetic features of idiopathic infantile periodic alternating nystagmus. *Brain.* 2011; **134**: 892–902.

Cross Reference
Nystagmus

Periodic Respiration
Periodic respiration is a cyclical waxing and waning of the depth and rate of breathing (Cheyne-Stokes breathing or respiration), over about 2 min, the crescendo-decrescendo sequence being separated by central apnoeas. A so-called variant Cheyne-Stokes pattern has hypopnoeas rather than apnoeas.

Periodic respiration may be observed in unconscious patients with lesions of the deep cerebral hemispheres, diencephalon, or upper pons, or with central or tonsillar brain herniation; it has also been reported in multiple system atrophy. Prolonged circulatory time (congestive heart failure) and hypoxaemia (*e.g.* at altitude) may also cause periodic respiration, but with a shorter cycle.

Reference
Pearce JMS. Cheyne-Stokes respiration. In: Fragments of neurological history. London: Imperial College Press; 2003. p. 355–8.

Cross References
Coma

Periphrasis
- see CIRCUMLOCUTION

Perseveration
Perseveration refers to any continuation or recurrence of activity without appropriate stimulus (*cf.* intrusions). Perseverations may be repeated motor behaviours (*e.g.* drawing, writing, applause sign) or speech. These are viewed as a failure to inhibit a previous response pattern. Sensory perseveration is also described, *e.g.* palinopsia in the visual system. A number of varieties of perseveration have been described, associated with lesions in different areas of the brain:

- "*Stuck-in-set*":
    Inappropriate maintenance of a current category or framework; thought to reflect a deficit in executive function; associated with frontal lobe (especially frontal convexity) damage, which is associated with an inert, apathetic pattern of behaviour, rather than the disinhibited pattern associated with orbitofrontal damage.

- "*Recurrent*":

  Unintentional repetition of a previous response to a subsequent stimulus; thought to represent an abnormal post-facilitation of a memory trace; associated with posterior left (dominant) hemisphere damage; commonly seen in aphasics, Alzheimer's disease; this overlaps with "intrusions".

- "*Continuous*":

  Inappropriate prolongation or repetition of a current behaviour without interruption; thought to represent a deficit of motor output; associated with basal ganglia damage.

References
Hudson AJ. Perseveration. *Brain*. 1968; **91**: 571–82.
Sandson J, Albert ML. Varieties of perseveration. *Neuropsychologia*. 1984; **22**: 715–32.
Cross References
Aphasia; Applause sign; Dysexecutive syndrome; Frontal lobe syndromes; Intrusion; Logoclonia; Palinopsia

Personification of Paralysed Limbs
Critchley drew attention to the tendency observed in some hemiplegic patients to give their paralysed limbs a name or nick-name and to invest them with a personality or identity of their own. This sometimes follows a period of anosognosia and may coexist with a degree of anosodiaphoria; it is much more commonly seen with left hemiplegia. A similar phenomenon may occur with amputated limbs, and it has been reported in the context of functional limb weakness.
References
Critchley M. Personification of paralysed limbs in hemiplegics. *BMJ*. 1955; **ii**: 284–6.
Critchley M. The divine banquet of the brain and other essays. New York: Raven Press; 1979. p. 104–5, 116–7.
Larner AJ. Critchley revisited: personification of a neurologically dysfunctional limb. *Adv Clin Neurosci Rehabil*. 2010; **10**(2): 28.
Cross References
Anosodiaphoria; Anosognosia

Pes Cavus
Pes cavus is a high-arched foot due to equinus (plantar flexion) deformity of the first ray with secondary changes in the other rays (*i.e.* deformity is more evident on the medial side of the foot in most cases). Hammer toes may also be present.

  This may be due to imbalance of muscular forces during development, which may be a consequence of neurological disease. The precise pattern may differ with cause, involving the muscles of either the lower leg (*e.g.* strong peroneus longus, weak peroneus brevis and tibialis anterior) or the foot (selective denervation of lumbricals in Charcot-Marie-Tooth disease type 1A).

  Pes cavus may be associated with disease of genetic origin, *e.g.* hereditary motor and sensory neuropathy (HMSN, Charcot-Marie-Tooth syndrome), hereditary spastic paraparesis, Friedreich's ataxia, Marfan's syndrome; or be due to an early neurological insult, *e.g.* cerebral palsy, paralytic poliomyelitis. Familial pes cavus without other neurological signs has also been reported (a *forme fruste* of HMSN?).

  Surgical treatment of pes cavus may be necessary, especially if there are secondary deformities causing pain, skin breakdown, or gait problems.
Reference
Berciano J, Gallardo E, Garcia A, Pelayo-Nero AL, Infante J, Combarros O. New insights into the pathophysiology of pes cavus in Charcot-Marie-Tooth disease type 1A duplication. *J Neurol*. 2011; **258**: 1594–602.

Cross References
Claw foot; Hammer toes

"Petite Madeleines Phenomenon"
- see PROUST PHENOMENON

Phalen's Sign
Phalen's sign is present when tingling (paraesthesia) is experienced in the distribution of the median nerve when the wrist is held in forced flexion (90° for 30–60 s; Phalen's maneouvre). Patients may volunteer that they experience such symptoms when carrying heavy items such as shopping bags which puts the hand in a similar posture. Hyperextension of the wrist ("reverse Phalen's manoeuvre") may also reproduce symptoms.

These are signs of compression of the median nerve at the wrist (carpal tunnel syndrome). Like other provocative tests (*e.g.* Tinel's sign), the sensitivity and specificity of Phalen's sign for this diagnosis are variable (10–91 %, and 33–86%).

The pathophysiology of Phalen's sign is probably the lower threshold of injured nerves to mechanical stimuli, as for Tinel's sign and Lhermitte's sign.

References
D'Arcy CA, McGee S. Does this patient have carpal tunnel syndrome? *JAMA*. 2000; **283**: 3110–7.
Hi ACF, Wong S, Griffith J. Carpal tunnel syndrome. *Pract Neurol*. 2005; **5**: 210–7.

Cross References
Durkan's compression test; "Flick sign"; Lhermitte's sign; Paraesthesia; Tinel's sign

"Phantom Alloaesthesia"
- see ALLOAESTHESIA

"Phantom Boarder Sign"
- see "MIRROR SIGN"; MISIDENTIFICATION SYNDROMES

Phantom Chromatopsia
This term has been coined to refer to the complaint of patients who are blind or nearly so that a colour, usually golden or purple, enlarges to invade the entire visual field. This is presumably cortical in origin, and has been described as an hallucination. "Phantom vision" may describe a similar phenomenon.

Reference
Zeki S. A vision of the brain. Oxford: Blackwell Science; 1993. p. 278, 279.

Cross References
Erythropsia; "Monochromatopsia"; Phantom vision

Phantom Limb
Phantom limbs, or ghost limbs, describe the subjective report of the awareness of a non-existing or deafferented body part in a mentally otherwise competent individual. The term was coined by Weir Mitchell in the nineteenth century, but parts other than limbs (either congenitally absent or following amputation) may be affected by phantom phenomena, such as lips, tongue, nose, eye, penis, breast and nipple, teeth, and viscera. Phantom phenomena are perceived as real by the patient, may be subject to a wide range of sensations (pressure, temperature, tickle, pain), and are perceived as an integral part of the self. Such "limbless perception" is thought to reflect the mental representation of body parts generated within the brain (body schema), such that perception is carried out without somatic peripheral input. Reorganisation of cortical connections following amputation may explain phantom phenomena such as representation of a hand on the chest or face, for which there is also evidence from functional brain imaging.

References
Halligan PW. Phantom limbs: the body in mind. *Cogn Neuropsychiatry*. 2002; **7**: 251–68.
Melzack R. Phantom limbs. *Sci Am*. 1992; **266**: 120–6.
Ramachandran VS, Hirstein W. The perception of phantom limbs. *Brain*. 1998; **121**: 1603–30.
Cross Reference
Asomatognosia

Phantom Vision
This name has been given to visual hallucinations following eye enucleation, by analogy with somaesthetic sensation experienced in a phantom limb after amputation. Similar phenomena may occur after acute visual loss, and may overlap with phantom chromatopsia. Unformed or simple hallucinations are more common than formed or complex hallucinations.
References
Cohn R. Phantom vision. *Arch Neurol*. 1971; **25**: 468–71.
Lepore FE. Spontaneous visual phenomena with visual loss. *Neurology*. 1990; **40**: 444–7.
Cross References
Hallucination; Phantom chromatopsia; Phantom limb

Phantosmia
This term has sometimes been used to describe olfactory hallucinations.

Pharyngeal Reflex
- see GAG REFLEX

Phonagnosia
Phonagnosia is an inability to recognise familiar voices in the absence of hearing impairment, hence a form of auditory agnosia. The patient can recognise and understand words and sentences (*cf*. pure word deafness). Phonagnosia is the equivalent in the auditory domain of prosopagnosia in the visual domain. The neuroanatomical substrate is thought to be right parietal lobe pathology.
Reference
Biederman I, Herald S, Xu X, Amir O, Shilowich B. Phonagnosia, a voice homologue to prosopagnosia. *J Vision*. 2015; **15**(12): 1206.
Cross References
Agnosia; Prosopagnosia; Pure word deafness

Phonemic Disintegration
Phonemic disintegration refers to an impaired ability to organise phonemes, the smallest units in which spoken language may be sequentially described, resulting in substitutions, deletions and misorderings of phonemes. Phonemic disintegration is relatively common in aphasic disorders, including Broca's aphasia, conduction aphasia, and transcortical motor aphasia. Isolated phonemic disintegration is rare. The neural substrate may be primary motor cortex of the left inferior precentral gyrus and subjacent white matter, with sparing of Broca's area.
References
Larner AJ, Robinson G, Kartsounis LD, et al. Clinical-anatomical correlation in a selective phonemic speech production impairment. *J Neurol Sci*. 2004; **219**: 23–9.
Taubner RW, Raymer AM, Heilman KM. Frontal-opercular aphasia. *Brain Lang*. 1999; **70**: 240–61.
Cross References
Aphasia; Aphemia; Broca's aphasia

Phonetic Disintegration
- see APHEMIA; SPEECH APRAXIA

Phonophobia
Phonophobia is a dislike, or fear, of sounds, especially loud sounds, often experienced during a migraine headache at the same time as photophobia and osmophobia.
Cross References
Hyperacusis; Photophobia

Phosphene
Phosphenes are percepts in one modality induced by an inappropriate stimulus, *e.g.* when pressure is applied to the eyeball, the mechanical stimulus may induce the perception of light (Newton investigated his own vision in this way, stimulating the back of his eye with a bodkin). The perception of flashes of light when the eyes are moved has been reported in optic neuritis, presumably reflecting the increased mechanosensitivity of the demyelinated optic nerve fibres; this is suggested to be the visual equivalent of Lhermitte's sign. Eye gouging to produce phosphenes by mechanical stimulation of the retina is reported in Leber's congenital amaurosis. Noise-induced visual phosphenes have also been reported, and may be equivalent to auditory-visual synaesthesia.
References
Bolognini N, Convento S, Fusaro M, Vallar G. The sound-induced phosphene illusion. *Exp Brain Res.* 2013; **231**: 469–78.
Davis FA, Bergen D, Schauf C, McDonald I, Deutsch W. Movement phosphenes in optic neuritis: a new clinical sign. *Neurology.* 1976; **26**: 1100–4.
Lessell JB, Cohen MM. Phosphenes induced by sound. *Neurology.* 1979; **29**: 1524–6.
Cross References
Auditory-visual synaesthesia; Gaze-evoked phenomena; Lhermitte's sign; Photism; Synaesthesia

Photic Sneeze Reflex
- see SNEEZING

Photism
Photisms are transient positive visual phenomenon, such as geometrical shapes or brightly coloured spectral phenomena, occurring in the context of epilepsy, migraine, or in blind visual fields (hence overlapping with photopsia). Auditory-visual synaesthesia may also be described as sound-induced photism.
Cross References
Auditory-visual synaesthesia; Photopsia

Photophobia
Photophobia is an abnormal intolerance of light, often experienced with eye pain. It is associated with a wide range of causes, and may result from both peripheral and central mechanisms:

- Anterior segment eye disorders: uveitis, glaucoma, cataract.
- Vitreo-retinal disorders: retinitis pigmentosa.
- Optic neuropathies: optic neuritis.
- Intracranial disease: migraine, meningitis and other causes of meningeal irritation, central photophobia (possibly associated with a thalamic lesion), dazzle.
- Physiological photophobia: sudden exposure to light after light deprivation.

Cross References
Dazzle; Meningism; Retinitis pigmentosa

Photopsia
Photopsias are simple visual hallucinations consisting of flashes of light which often occur with a visual field defect. They suggest dysfunction in the inferomedial occipital lobe, such as migraine or an epileptogenic lesion.

Cross References
Aura; Hallucination; Photism

Physical Duality
Physical duality describes a rare somaesthetic metamorphopsia occurring as a migraine aura
in which individuals feel as though they have two bodies.
Cross Reference
Metamorphopsia

Piano-Playing Fingers
- see PSEUDOATHETOSIS

Pica
Pica, or pagophagia, is a morbid craving for unusual or unsuitable food in association with
iron deficiency. It has also been reported in tuberous sclerosis. Sufferers risk infection from
contaminated foods.
References
Larner AJ. Neurological signs: geophagia (geophagy) and pica (pagophagia). *Adv Clin
Neurosci Rehabil.* 2009; **9**(4): 20.
Von Garnier C, Stunitz H, Decker M, Battegay E, Zeller A. Pica and refractory iron defi-
ciency anaemia: a case report. *J Med Case Rep.* 2008; **2**: 324.
Cross Reference
Geophagia, Geophagy

"Picture Sign"
The "picture sign" is present when a patient believes that individuals seen on the television
screen are actually present in the external world; indeed they may be reported to emerge from
the television set into the room. This may occur as part of the cognitive disturbance of
Alzheimer's disease or dementia with Lewy bodies, or as part of a psychotic disorder. Like the
"mirror sign", the "picture sign" may be classified as a misidentification phenomenon.
Cross References
"Mirror sign"; Misidentification syndromes

"Picture Within a Picture" Sign
Following a right parieto-occipital infarction, a patient complained of seeing people moving
about in the left lower quadrant of the visual field whilst vision was normal in the remainder
of the visual field, a phenomenon labelled as the "picture within a picture" sign. This has been
categorized as a visual release hallucination.
Reference
Benegas MN, Liu GT, Volpe NJ, Galetta SL. "Picture within a picture" visual hallucinations.
Neurology. 1996; **47**: 1347–8.

Pied En Griffe
- see CLAW FOOT

"Pie-In-The-Sky" Defect
This name has sometimes been given to the superior homonymous quadrantanopia ending
sharply at the vertical midline due to a temporal lobe lesion interrupting Meyer's loop, that
part of the optic radiation coursing through the temporal lobe.
Cross Reference
Quadrantanopia

"Pill Rolling"
- see PARKINSONISM; TREMOR

"Pinch Sign"

The "pinch sign", or "okay sign", is an inability to make a small circle ("form the letter O", divers' okay sign) by approximating the distal phalanges of the thumb and index finger, due to weakness of flexor digitorum profundus in the index finger and flexor pollicis longus in the thumb as a consequence of median nerve lesions in the forearm, *e.g.* anterior interosseous neuropathy, pronator teres syndrome. This results in a pinching posture of thumb and index finger. The "straight thumb sign" may also be present.

Cross References

Froment's sign; "Straight thumb sign"

Pinhole Test

Impairments in visual acuity due to refractory defects (changes in shape of the globe or defects in the transparent media of the eye) may be improved or corrected by looking through a pinhole which restricts vision to the central beam of light.

Pisa Syndrome

- see PLEUROTHOTONOS

Plantar Grasp Reflex

- see GRASP REFLEX

Plantar Response

The plantar response is most commonly elicited by stroking the sole of the foot with a blunt object. The first response of the hallux is the critical observation, which may be facilitated by having ones line of vision directly above the axis of the toe. The normal response after maturation of the corticospinal tracts (*i.e.* after about 3 years of age) is for the big toe to flex. An extensor response of the big toe in an adult (Babinski's sign) is a reliable sign of upper motor neurone pathology. This may or may not be accompanied by fanning (abduction) of the other toes (fan sign, *signe de l'éventail*), but this does not constitute part of the sign and in isolation has no clinical value.

Use of the terminology "negative Babinski's sign" or "negative Babinski response" to mean "flexor plantar response" is incorrect and should not be used. This normal plantar response is a superficial cutaneous reflex, analogous to abdominal and cremasteric reflexes, whereas the pathological response is often accompanied by activity in other flexor muscles. In some individuals the toes do not move at all, in which case the response is labelled as "mute" or absent. Assessment of the response may be confounded by withdrawal of the foot in ticklish individuals. Stroking the lateral border of the dorsum of the foot rather than the sole has been advocated.

The plantar response may be elicited in a variety of other ways which are not in routine clinical use. Of these, perhaps the most frequently used are Chaddock's sign (application of a stimulus in a circular direction around the external malleolus, or the lateral aspect of the foot from heel to little toe) and Oppenheim's sign (application of heavy pressure to the anterior surface of the tibia from patella to ankle). If the plantar response thus elicited is upgoing, this suggests a spread of the "receptive field" of the reflex. Babinski's sign is the earliest to occur in the presence of upper motor neurone pathology.

It is often difficult to form a definite judgment on the plantar response and reproducibility is also questionable. A study of 24 experienced clinicians invited to examine plantar responses "blind" found that the interobserver percentage agreement beyond chance was on average only 16.7% (95% confidence interval [CI] 0.4–33%); intraobserver percentage agreement was a little better (average 59.6%; CI 39.6–79.6%). There remains a persistent belief, particularly amongst trainees, that an experienced neurologist can make the plantar response go which ever way s/he chooses.

Differentiation of the Babinski sign from the striatal toe seen in parkinsonian syndromes may need to be made.

References

Maher J, Reilly M, Daly L, Hutchinson M. Plantar power: reproducibility of the plantar response. *BMJ*. 1992; **304**: 482.

Van Gijn J. The Babinski sign: a centenary. Utrecht: Universiteit Utrecht; 1996.

Van Munster CEP, Weinstein HC, Uitdehaag BMJ, van Gijn J. The plantar reflex: additional value of stroking the lateral border of the foot to provoke an upgoing toe sign and the influence of experience. *J Neurol*. 2012; **259**: 2424–8.

Cross References

Abdominal reflexes; Babinski's sign (1); Chaddock's sign; Gordon's sign; Oppenheim's sign; Reflexes; Striatal toe, Upper motor neurone (UMN) syndrome

Platysma Sign

"Platysma sign" has been used to describe weakness of platysma, which may be seen in the context of central hemiparesis or in high cervical cord lesions, since innervation of the muscle comes from both the seventh cranial nerve and from the high cervical cord (C3).

Reference

Ogawa Y, Sakakibara R. Platysma sign in high cervical lesion. *J Neurol Neurosurg Psychiatry*. 2005; **76**: 735.

Plegia

Plegia means stillness, implying a complete weakness (or paralysis in common parlance), as in monoplegia, diplegia, ophthalmoplegia, paraplegia, quadriplegia, cardioplegia. Hence plegia denotes more severe weakness than paresis.

Cross References

Paresis; Weakness

Pleurothotonos

Pleurothotonos describes lateral flexion of the trunk due to spasm in paraspinal musculature. It may occur as one form of tonic spasm in tetanus.

Pisa syndrome is a truncal dystonia characterised by twisting and bending of the upper thorax, with involuntary flexion of the neck and head, to one side. Tilting symptoms occurring bilaterally may be labelled as "metronome Pisa syndrome". It may be seen in extrapyramidal disorders such as Parkinson's disease and multiple system atrophy, or as a rare extrapyramidal side effect caused by neuroleptic medications, or by cholinesterase inhibitors in Alzheimer's disease patients. Hence some form of cholinergic-dopaminergic imbalance would seem to be involved in pathogenesis. Other than discontinuing or adjusting medication, no specific treatment has been described.

Reference

Michel SF, Oscar AC, Correa TE, Alejandro PL, Micheli F. Pisa syndrome. *Clin Neuropharmacol*. 2015; **38**: 135–40.

Cross References

Dystonia; Emprosthotonos; Opisthtonos

Plexopathy

Lesions confined to the brachial, lumbar, or sacral plexi may produce a constellation of motor and sensory signs (weakness, reflex diminution or loss, sensory loss) which cannot be ascribed to single or multiple roots (radiculopathy) or peripheral nerves (neuropathy). Lesions may involve the whole plexus (panplexopathy):

- Brachial: C5-T1
- Lumbar: L2-L4
- Sacral: L5-S3

or be partial, *e.g.* upper trunk of brachial plexus (C5-C6), producing "waiter's tip" posture (as for C5/C6 root avulsion); lower trunk of brachial plexus (C8-T1; as for C8/T1 root avulsion).

Neurophysiological studies may be helpful in distinguishing plexopathy from radiculopathy: sensory nerve action potentials (SNAPs) are reduced or absent in plexopathies because the lesion is located distal to the dorsal root ganglion (DRG), whereas SNAPs are normal in radiculopathies because the lesion is proximal to the DRG. EMG shows sparing of paraspinal muscles in a plexopathy because the lesion is, by definition, distal to the origin of the dorsal primary rami (*cf.* radiculopathy). Coexistence of radiculopathy and plexopathy may invalidate these simple rules.

- Recognised causes of brachial plexopathy include:

    Trauma: upper plexus: Dejerine-Klumpke paralysis ("waiter's tip" posture): lower plexus: Erb Duchenne paralysis (claw hand).
    Inflammation/Idiopathic: brachial neuritis, neuralgic amyotrophy.
    Malignant infiltration, *e.g.* carcinoma of lung (Pancoast), breast, +/− Horner's syndrome; pain a significant symptom.
    Post-radiation (*e.g.* after radiotherapy for malignant breast cancer with axillary spread; myokymic discharges may be seen on EMG).
    Tomaculous neuropathy.
    Hereditary neuropathy with liability to pressure palsies (HNLPP).

    Neurogenic thoracic outlet syndrome (rare): cervical rib or C7 transverse process or fibrous band compressing the lower trunk; may be surgically remediable.
- Recognised causes of lumbosacral plexopathy include:

    Compression; *e.g.* iliopsoas haematoma (anticoagulation, haemophilia), abscess (tuberculosis); abdominal aortic aneurysm; pregnancy (fetal head in the second stage of labour).
    Neoplasia (direct spread > metastasis).
    Trauma (rare; *cf.* brachial plexopathy).
    Post-radiation.
    Vasculitis (mononeuritis multiplex much commoner).
    Idiopathic.

Imaging with MRI is superior to CT for defining structural causes of plexopathy.

References
Chad DF. Nerve root and plexus disorders. In: Bogousslavsky J, Fisher M, editors. Textbook of neurology. Boston: Butterworth-Heinemann; 1998. p. 491–506.
Taylor BV, Kimmel DW, Krecke KN, Cascino TL. Magnetic resonance imaging in cancer-related lumbosacral plexopathy. *Mayo Clin Proc.* 1997; **72**: 823–9.
Cross References
Amyotrophy; Claw hand; Horner's syndrome; Myokymia; Nerve thickening; Neuropathy; Radiculopathy; "Waiter's tip" posture

Polyganglionopathy
- see NEUROPATHY

Polymyoclonus
- see MYOCLONUS

Polyneuropathy
- see NEUROPATHY

Polyopia
Polyopia, or polyopsia, or multiplication of images, is a visual illusory phenomenon in which a single target is seen as multiple images, most usually double but sometimes higher multiples (*e.g.* entomopia), persisting when looking away from the object. This may be likened to

"echoes" of the image, and eye movement may produce a trailing effect. Polyopia may be related to palinopsia.

Polyopia may occur as part of the visual aura of migraine, and has also been associated with occipital and occipito-parietal lesions, either bilateral or confined to the non-dominant hemisphere, and with drug abuse. It has also been described in disease of the retina and optic nerve, and occasionally in normal individuals.

The pathophysiology is unknown; suggestions include a defect of visual fixation or of visual integration; the latter may reflect pure occipital cortical dysfunction.

Reference
Pomeranz HD, Lessell S. Palinopsia and polyopia in the absence of drugs or cerebral disease. *Neurology*. 2000; **54**: 855–9.

Cross References
Entomopia; Illusion; Palinopsia

"Popeye Arms"
In facioscapulohumeral (FSH) muscular dystrophy, the deltoid muscle is normally well preserved, whilst biceps and triceps are weak and wasted, giving rise to an appearance of the upper limbs sometimes labelled as "Popeye arms" or "chicken wings".

Cross Reference
Winging of the scapula

Poriomania
Poriomania is a name sometimes given to prolonged wandering as an epileptic automatism, or a fugue state of nonconvulsive status epilepticus.

Reference
Mayeux R, Alexander MP, Benson DF, et al. Poriomania. *Neurology*. 1979; **29**: 1616–9.

Cross References
Automatism; Fugue; Seizures

Porropsia
Porropsia, or teliopsia, is a form of metamorphopsia characterised by the misperception of objects as farther away from the observer than they really are (*cf.* peliopsia)

Cross References
Metamorphopsia; Peliopsia

Positional Manoeuvres
- see HALLPIKE MANOEUVRE, HALLPIKE TEST; HEAD IMPULSE TEST; VESTIBULO-OCULAR REFLEXES

Post-tetanic Potentiation
- see AUGMENTATION; FACILITATION

Postural Hypotension
- see ORTHOSTATIC HYPOTENSION

Postural Reflexes
Postures such as standing are largely reflex in origin, dependent upon involuntary muscle contraction in anti-gravity muscles. Interference with such reflex activity impairs normal standing. Postural and righting reflexes depend on the integration of labyrinthine, proprioceptive, exteroceptive, and visual stimuli, mostly in the brainstem but also involving the cerebral cortex. However, abnormalities in these reflexes are of relatively little diagnostic value except in infants.

One exception is extrapyramidal disease (parkinsonism, Huntington's disease, but not idiopathic dystonia) in which impairment or loss of postural reflexes may be observed. In the "pull test" the examiner stands behind the patient, who is standing comfortably, and pulls briskly on the shoulders; if balance is normal, the patient takes a step back; with impaired postural reflexes, this may provoke repetitive steps backwards (retropulsion, festination) or even *en bloc* falling, due to the failure of reflex muscle contraction necessary to maintain equilibrium. Pushing the patient forward may likewise provoke propulsion or festination, but this manoeuvre is less safe since the examiner will not be placed to catch the patient should they begin to topple over.

Parkinson's disease patients have a characteristic pattern of muscle activation during the pull test which is not reversed after levodopa treatment.

Reference
Schestatsky P, Gomes-Araujo T, Gamarra A, Mello-Rieder C. Neurophysiological study of pull test in patients with Parkinson's disease and controls. *J Neurol*. 2011; **258**(Suppl 1): S29. (abstract O229).

Cross References
Dystonia; Festinant gait, Festination; Parkinsonism; Proprioception; "Rocket sign"

Potomania
Potomania, or beer potomania, refers to excess drinking of beer (or cider) which may result in dilutional hyponatraemia if the diet is concurrently poor in salt and protein. This is a recognized association of central pontine myelinolysis.

Reference
Odier C, Nguyen DK, Panisset M. Central pontine and extrapontine myelinolysis: from epileptic and other manifestations to cognitive prognosis. *J Neurol*. 2010; **257**: 1176–80.

Pourfour Du Petit Syndrome
Pourfour du Petit syndrome is characterized by mydriasis, widening of the palpebral fissure (eyelid retraction), exophthalmos, hyperhidrosis (*i.e.* inverse or reverse Horner's syndrome, sympathetic overactivity), flushing and increased intraocular pressure due to irritation of the sympathetic chain in the neck.

Reference
Al-Ansari A, Walters RJL. Case report: Pourfour du Petit syndrome in a patient with migraine. *J Neurol Neurosurg Psychiatry*. 2015; **86**: e4. doi:10.1136/jnnp-2015-312379.76.

Cross Reference
Horner's syndrome

Pouting, Pout Reflex
The pout reflex consists of a pouting movement of the lips elicited by lightly tapping orbicularis oris with a finger or tendon hammer, or by tapping a spatula placed over the lips. This myotactic stretch reflex is indicative of a bilateral upper motor neurone lesion, which may be due to cerebrovascular small vessel ischaemic disease, motor neurone disease, or multiple sclerosis. It differs from the snout reflex, which refers to the reflex elicited by constant pressure on the philtrum. Hence the pout reflex is a phasic response, the snout reflex a tonic response.

Reference
Rossor M. Snouting, pouting and rooting. *Pract Neurol*. 2001; **1**: 119–21.

Cross References
Frontal release signs; Primitive reflexes

"Prayer Sign"
An inability to oppose fully the palmar surfaces of the digits with the hands held in the praying position, the so-called "prayer sign", may be caused by ulnar neuropathy (*main en griffe*), Dupuytren's contracture, diabetic cheiroarthropathy, and camptodactyly.

Cross References
Camptodactyly; "Table top" sign

Prehensile Thumb Sign
- see FROMENT'S SIGN

Presbyastasis
Presbyastasis, or the disequilibrium of ageing, is a condition of elderly patients who present with imbalance and disequilibrium that cannot be ascribed to a particular disease state or single causative factor (*e.g.* vestibular disease, visual impairment, peripheral neuropathy). It is thought that abnormalities in sensory input, CNS sensory processing, control mechanisms for balance, and a decreased range of movement and strength may all contribute to symptoms. White matter changes on brain MRI have been associated with the condition. Vestibular rehabilitation therapy and avoidance of vestibular suppressant medications may be helpful.
Reference
Belal A, Glorig A. Disequilibrium of ageing (presbyastasis). *J Laryngol Otol.* 1986; **100**: 1037–41.
Cross References
Age-related signs; Astasia-abasia

Presbycusis
Presbycusis is a progressive sensorineural hearing loss, especially for high frequencies, developing with increasing age, which may reduce speech discrimination. It is thought to be due to age-related attrition of hair cells in the organ of Corti and/or spiral ganglion neurones.
Reference
Gates GA, Mills JH. Presbycusis. *Lancet.* 2005; **366**: 1111–20.
Cross Reference
Age-related signs

Presbyopia
Presbyopia is progressive far-sightedness which is increasingly common with increasing age, thought to be due to an age-related impairment of accommodation.
Cross Reference
Age-related signs

Prèsque Vu
- see DÉJÀ VU

Pressure Provocation Test
This is one of the provocative tests for carpal tunnel syndrome: it is positive if paraesthesia in the distribution of the median nerve develops when pressure is exerted on the palmar aspect of the patient's wrist at the level of the carpal tunnel for 60 s. It is sometimes referred to as the carpal compression test or Durkan's compression test.
References
D'Arcy CA, McGee S. Does this patient have carpal tunnel syndrome? *JAMA.* 2000; **283**: 3110–7.
Hi ACF, Wong S, Griffith J. Carpal tunnel syndrome. *Pract Neurol.* 2005; **5**: 210–7.
Cross References
Durkan's compression test; "Flick sign"; Phalen's sign; Tinel's sign

Prevost's Sign
Also known as Vulpian's sign, this refers to the acute and transient gaze palsy in a frontal lesion (*e.g.* infarct) which is towards the side of the lesion and away from the concurrent hemiparesis. The eyes can be brought to the other side with the oculocephalic manoeuvre or caloric testing. In contrast, thalamic and basal ganglia haemorrhages produce forced deviation of the eyes to the side contralateral to the lesion (wrong-way eyes).

Priapism

Priapism is an unintended, sustained, and usually painful erection of the penis unrelated to sexual activity. It may occur with intramedullary spinal cord lesions (*e.g.* multiple sclerosis) which damage the lumbosacral erection centres, and has also been reported with lumbar canal spinal stenosis. There are also non-neurological causes, such as haematological conditions (sickle cell anaemia, polycythaemia rubra vera) which may cause intrapenile thromboses.

Primitive Reflexes

Reflexes which are normally found in infancy but which disappear with brain maturation during childhood may be labelled as "primitive reflexes" if they re-emerge in adulthood as a consequence of pathological states. Many of these reflexes are seen with frontal lobe pathology (*e.g.* grasp, pout/snout, palmomental, rooting, corneomandibular) and hence may also be known as "frontal release signs". However, the term "primitive reflex" could equally apply to Babinski's sign which is not necessarily frontal in origin.

References

Paulson G, Gottlieb G. Developmental reflexes: the reappearance of foetal and neonatal reflexes in aged patients. *Brain*. 1968; **91**: 37–52.

Schott JM, Rossor MN. The grasp and other primitive reflexes. *J Neurol Neurosurg Psychiatry*. 2003; **74**: 558–60.

Cross References

Babinski's sign (1); Corneomandibular reflex; Frontal release signs; Grasp reflex; Palmomental reflex; Pout reflex; Rooting reflex

Procerus Sign

A focal dystonia of the procerus muscle, denoted the procerus sign, has been suggested to contribute to the "astonished", "worried" or "reptile-like" facial expression typical of progressive supranuclear palsy, which may also be characterised by reduced blinking, lid retraction, and gaze palsy. All these features contrast with the hypomimia of Parkinson's disease. It has also been described in corticobasal degeneration.

References

Romano S, Colosimo C. Procerus sign in progressive supranuclear palsy. *Neurology*. 2001; **57**: 1928.

Shibasaki Warabi Y, Nagao M, Bandoh M, Kanda T, Hirai S. Procerus sign in corticobasal degeneration. *Intern Med*. 2002; **41**: 1217–8.

Cross References

Blinking; Dystonia; Hypomimia; Parkinsonism

Pronator Drift

Pronator drift describes a gradual pronation of the forearm observed when the arms are held straight forward, palms up, with the eyes closed. It suggests a contralateral corticospinal tract lesion and may be accompanied by downward drift of the arm and flexion of the fingers and/ or elbow. It reflects the relative weakness of supinators versus pronators in the arm with a pyramidal lesion, in addition to the relative weakness of extensors versus flexors. It may be an early sign of corticospinal tract dysfunction.

Cross References

Forearm and finger rolling, Upper motor neurone (UMN) syndrome; Weakness

Proprioception

Proprioception sensation, or joint position sense, is knowledge about ones position in space, originating from sensory receptors in skin, muscle, and viscera. Proprioceptive information is carried within the dorsal columns of the spinal cord (more reliably so than vibration sensation, though not necessarily exclusively). Lesions affecting this part of the cord, particularly in the cervical region (*e.g.* subacute combined degeneration of the cord due to vitamin B_{12} deficiency, tabes dorsalis), lead to impairments of proprioception with sparing of spinothalamic sensations (pin-prick, temperature) producing a dissociated sensory loss. Impairment of proprioception leads to sensory ataxia which may manifest clinically with pseudoathetosis or pseudochoreoathetosis (also seen in useless hand of Oppenheim) and with a positive Romberg's sign.

Reference
Gilman S. Joint position sense and vibration sense. *J Neurol Neurosurg Psychiatry*. 2002; **73**: 473–7.

Cross References
Ataxia; Dissociated sensory loss; Myelopathy; Pseudoathetosis; Pseudochoreoathetosis; Rombergism, Romberg's sign; Useless hand of Oppenheim; Vibration

Proptosis
Proptosis is forward displacement of the eyeball, an exaggerated degree of exophthalmos. There may be lower lid retraction. Proptosis may be assessed clinically by standing directly behind the patient and gradually tipping the head back, observing when the globe of the eyeball first comes into view; this is most useful for asymmetric proptosis. An exophthalmometer may be used to measure proptosis.

Once established, it is crucial to determine whether the proptosis is axial or non-axial. Axial proptosis reflects increased pressure within or transmitted through the cone of extraocular muscles (*e.g.* thyroid ophthalmopathy, cavernous sinus thrombosis), whereas non-axial proptosis suggests pressure from an orbital mass outside the cone of muscles (*e.g.* orbital lymphoma, pseudotumour, mucocele). Pulsatile axial proptosis may occur in caroticocavernous fistula, in which case there may be a bruit audible by auscultation over the eye. Venous angioma of the orbit may cause an intermittent proptosis associated with straining, bending, coughing or blowing the nose.

Dedicated orbital CT or MRI, the latter with fat-suppression sequences and intravenous gadolinium contrast, may be required to detect intraorbital masses.

Middle cranial fossa tumours may cause pressure on the veins of the cavernous sinus with secondary intraorbital venous congestion causing a "false-localising" proptosis.

Cross References
Exophthalmos; "False-localising signs"; Lid retraction

Propulsion
- see FESTINANT GAIT, FESTINATION; POSTURAL REFLEXES

Prosopagnosia
Prosopagnosia is a form of visual agnosia characterized by an inability to recognize human faces or equivalent stimuli. This may be developmental, or acquired loss of recogntion (hence, a retrograde defect) and inability to learn new faces (anterograde defect). As with more pervasive visual agnosia, prosopagnosia may be characterised as:

- *apperceptive*: due to faulty perceptual analysis of faces; or
- *associative*: a semantic defect in recognition.

Familiar individuals may be recognized by their voices or clothing or hair; hence, the defect may be one of visually triggered episodic memory. It is important to note that the defect is not limited solely to faces; it may encompass animals ("zooagnosia"), or cars.

Prosopagnosia is often found in association with a visual field defect, most often a left superior quadrantanopia or even hemianopia, although for the diagnosis of prosopagnosia to be made this should not be sufficient to produce a perceptual deficit. Alexia and achromatopsia may also be present, depending on the exact extent of the underlying lesion.

Anatomically, prosopagnosia occurs most often in association with bilateral occipitotemporal lesions involving the inferior and mesial visual association cortices in the lingual and fusiform gyri, sometimes with subjacent white matter. Unilateral non-dominant (right) hemisphere lesions have occasionally been associated with prosopagnosia, and a syndrome of progressive prosopagnosia associated with selective focal atrophy of the right temporal lobe has been reported. Involvement of the periventricular region on the left side may explain accompanying alexia, and disconnection of the inferior visual association cortex (area V4) may explain achromatopsia.

Pathological causes of prosopagnosia include:

- Cerebrovascular disease: by far the most common cause.
- Tumour, *e.g.* glioma, extending from one hemisphere to the other via the splenium of the corpus callosum.
- Epilepsy (paroxysmal prosopagnosia), due to bilateral foci or spread from one occipital focus to the contralateral hemisphere.
- Focal right temporal lobe atrophy: possibly a non-dominant hemisphere form of semantic dementia.
- Herpes simplex encephalitis, usually as part of an extensive amnesic syndrome (although memory impairment may put this outwith the operational criteria for an agnosia).

A developmental (or "congenital") form of prosopagnosia suggests that facial recognition is a separate neuropsychological function, since acquired pathologies do not respect functional boundaries.

References
Evans JJ, Heggs AJ, Antoun N, Hodges JR. Progressive prosopagnosia associated with selective right temporal lobe atrophy. A new syndrome? *Brain*. 1995; **118**: 1–13.
Farah MJ. Visual agnosia: disorders of object recognition and what they tell us about normal vision. Cambridge: MIT Press; 1995.
Larner AJ. Lewis Carroll's Humpty Dumpty: an early report of prosopagnosia? *J Neurol Neurosurg Psychiatry*. 2004; **75**: 1063.
Nunn JA, Postma P, Pearson R. Developmental prosopagnosia: should it be taken at face value? *Neurocase*. 2001; **7**: 15–27.

Cross References
Achromatopsia; Agnosia; Alexia; Hemianopia; Phonagnosia; Quadrantanopia; Visual agnosia; Zooagnosia

Prosopoplegia
- see BELL'S PALSY; FACIAL PARESIS, FACIAL WEAKNESS

Proust Phenomenon
The Proust phenomenon, named after the author Marcel Proust (1871–1922), is the observation that particular odours may trigger reminders of autobiographical memories. There is some experimental evidence that olfactory stimuli can cue autobiographical memories more effectively than cues from other sensory modalities. The "petite madeleines phenomenon" has been used to describe sudden triggering of memories in individuals with amnesia due to thalamic infarction.

References
Lucchelli F, Muggia S, Spinnler H. The "Petites Madeleines" phenomenon in two amnesic patients: sudden recovery of forgotten memories. *Brain*. 1995; **118**: 167–83.
Toffolo MB, Smeets MA, van den Hout MA. Proust revisited: odours as triggers of aversive memories. *Cogn Emot*. 2012; **26**: 83–92.

Cross Reference
Amnesia

Proximal Limb Weakness
Weakness affecting predominantly the proximal limb musculature (shoulder abductors and hip flexors) is a pattern frequently observed in myopathic and dystrophic muscle disorders and neuromuscular junction transmission disorders, much more so than predominantly

distal weakness (the differential diagnosis of which encompasses myotonic dystrophy, distal myopathy of Miyoshi type, desmin myopathy, and, rarely, myasthenia gravis). Some neuropathic disorders may also cause a predominantly proximal weakness (*e.g.* Guillain-Barré syndrome). Age of onset and other clinical features may help to narrow the differential diagnosis:

- painful muscles may suggest an inflammatory cause (polymyositis, dermatomyositis);
- fatiguability may suggest myasthenia gravis (although lesser degrees of fatigue may be seen in myopathic disorders);
- weakness elsewhere may suggest a specific diagnosis (*e.g.* face in facioscapulohumeral muscular dystrophy, diaphragm in acid-maltase deficiency);
- cachexia points to underlying malignant disease;
- calf pseudohypertrophy suggests Duchenne or Becker muscular dystrophy;
- autonomic features and post-tetanic potentiation of reflexes occur in Lambert-Eaton myasthenic syndrome.

Investigations including blood creatine kinase, neurophysiology, and muscle biopsy may be required to determine exact diagnosis. Differential diagnosis includes:

- Myopathies:
  - Inflammatory: polymyositis, dermatomyositis.
  - Progressive muscular dystrophies: Duchenne, Becker, limb-girdle, facioscapulo-humeral (FSH).
  - Metabolic: acid maltase deficiency; thyroid dysfunction, Cushing's syndrome.
  - Non-metastatic feature of malignant disease.
  - Drug-induced: alcohol, steroids.
- Neuromuscular junction transmission disorders:
  - Myasthenia gravis.
  - Lambert-Eaton myasthenic syndrome.
- Neuropathy:
  - Guillain-Barré syndrome.

Cross References
Facilitation; Fatigue

Pruritus
Pruritus or itch may be a consequence of dermatologocial disorders or may be neuropathic in origin. Itch may share similar neural pathways as pain. Recognized neurological causes of pruritus include some peripheral neuropathies, multiple sclerosis, neuromyelitis optica, and Creutzfeldt-Jakob disease.

References
Cohen OS, Chapman J, Lee H, et al. Pruritus in familial Creutzfeldt-Jakob disease: a common symptom associated with central nervous system pathology. *J Neurol.* 2011; **258**: 89–95.
Davidson S, Giesler GJ. The multiple pathways for itch and their interactions with pain. *Trends Neurosci.* 2010; **33**: 550–8.
Elsone L, Townsend T, Mutch K, et al. Neuropathic pruritus (itch) in neuromyelitis optica. *Mult Scler.* 2013; **19**: 475–9.

Pseudo-Abducens Palsy
- see ABDUCENS (VI) NERVE PALSY

Pseudoachromatopsia

Pseudoachromatopsia is failure on tests of colour vision (*e.g.* pseudoisochromatic plates) which is not due to central or peripheral achromatopsia, for example due to visual neglect.

Cross References

Achromatopsia; Neglect

Pseudoagnosia

- see AGNOSIA

Pseudo-Argyll Robertson Pupil

A pseudo-Argyll Robertson pupil shows light-near dissociation of pupillary reactions but, unlike the "true" Argyll Robertson pupil, there is no miosis or pupil irregularity. Indeed the pupil may be dilated (mydriasis) and resemble a Holmes-Adie pupil. The latter may be differentiated on the basis of its response to dilute (0.2%) pilocarpine: Holmes-Adie pupil results from a peripheral lesion and shows denervation supersensitivity, constricting with dilute pilocarpine, whereas the pseudo-Argyll Robertson pupil results from a central lesion and does not respond. Pseudo-Argyll Robertson pupil has been reported in:

- diabetes mellitus.
- multiple sclerosis.
- Wernicke's encephalopathy (thiamine deficiency).
- neurosarcoidosis.
- tumour.
- haemorrhage.
- aberrant oculomotor (III) nerve regeneration.
- spinocerebellar ataxia type 1 (SCA1).

Cross References

Argyll Robertson pupil; Holmes-Adie pupil, Holmes-Adie syndrome; Miosis; Mydriasis

Pseudoathetosis

Pseudoathetosis is the name given to athetoid-like movements, most usually of the outstretched fingers ("piano-playing fingers") and hands, resulting from sensory ataxia (impaired proprioception), worse with the eyes closed. There may also be chorea-like movements, hence pseudochoreoathetosis. Causes include any interruption to the anatomical pathway mediating proprioception, most often lesions in the dorsal cervical cord (*e.g.* multiple sclerosis, subacute combined degeneration of the cord due to vitamin B_{12} deficiency or nitrous oxide overuse), but also lesions of the large (myelinated) peripheral nerve fibres, and of the parietal lobe.

References

Ghika J, Bogousslavsky J. Spinal pseudoathetosis: a rare, forgotten syndrome, with a review of old and recent descriptions. *Neurology*. 1997; **49**: 432–7.

Lo YL, See S. Images in clinical medicine. Pseudoathetosis. *N Engl J Med*. 2010; **363**: e29.

Spitz M, Costa Machado AA, Carvalho Rdo C, et al. Pseudoathetosis: report of three patients. *Mov Disord*. 2006; **21**: 1520–2.

Cross References

Athetosis; Chorea, Choreoathetosis; Proprioception; Pseudochoreoathetosis

Pseudo-Babinski Sign

Pseudo-Babinski sign is the name given to dystonic extension of the great toe on stroking the sole of the foot, as when trying to elicit Babinski's sign, with which this may be confused, although pseudo-Babinski responses persist for longer, and spontaenous extension of the toe, striatal toe, may also be present. Pseudo-Babinski signs may normalise after dopaminergic treatment in dopa-responsive dystonia.

Reference
Horstink MWIM, Haaxma C, Bloem BR. Babinski, pseudo-Babinski, and dystonia. *Arch Neurol.* 2007; **64**: 1207–9.
Cross References
Babinski sign (1); Striatal toe

Pseudobitemporal Hemianopia
- see HEMIANOPIA

Pseudobulbar Affect
- see EMOTIONALISM, EMOTIONAL LABILITY; PATHOLOGICAL CRYING, PATHOLOGICAL LAUGHTER; PSEUDOBULBAR PALSY

Pseudobulbar Palsy
Pseudobulbar palsy, or spastic bulbar palsy, describes bilateral upper motor neurone lesions affecting fibres passing to the cranial nerve nuclei (*cf.* bulbar palsy). This leads to a variety of clinical features, including:

- difficulty with speech: spastic dysarthria, dysphonia.
- difficulty with swallowing: dysphagia.
- brisk jaw jerk and pout reflex; there may be trismus.
- gag reflex may be depressed or exaggerated.
- slow, spastic, tongue movements.

There may be associated emotional lability, or pathological laughter and crying ("pseudobulbar affect"), and a gait disorder with *marche à petit pas*. There are otherwise few signs in the limbs, aside from brisk reflexes and upgoing plantar responses (Babinski's sign).
Recognised causes of pseudobulbar palsy include:

- Motor neurone disease (in which there may be coincident bulbar palsy).
- Multiple sclerosis.
- Bilateral internal capsule lacunar infarctions, widespread small vessel ischaemic disease (Binswanger's disease).
- Progressive supranuclear palsy: pseudobulbar palsy was part of the initial description of this condition by Steele, Richardson, and Olszewski.
- Congenital childhood suprabulbar palsy (Worster-Drought syndrome; perisylvian syndrome).

Pseudobulbar affect may respond to serotonin reuptake inhibitors.
Cross References
Babinski's sign (1); Bulbar palsy; Dysarthria; Dysphagia; Dysphonia; Emotionalism, Emotional lability; Gag reflex; Jaw jerk; *Marche à petit pas*; Pathological crying, Pathological laughter; Trismus; Upper motor neurone (UMN) syndrome

Pseudochoreoathetosis
Pseudochoreoathetosis is a name which has been given to choreoathetoid type involuntary movements, including dystonic movements, which result from a loss or impairment of proprioception. These may be observed with lesions anywhere along the proprioceptive pathways, including parietal cortex, thalamus (there may be associated ataxic hemiparesis and hemihypoaesthesia), spinal cord, dorsal root ganglia (neuronopathy), and mononeuropathy.
References
Dineen JM, Greenberg SA. Pseudochoreoathetosis in sensory ataxic variant of Guillain-Barré syndrome. *Muscle Nerve.* 2014; **50**: 300–1.

Kim JW, Kim SH, Cha JK. Pseudochoreoathetosis in four patients with hypesthetic ataxic hemiparesis in a thalamic lesion. *J Neurol.* 1999; **246**: 1075–9.
Sharp FR, Rando TA, Greenberg SA, Brown L, Sagar SM. Pseudochoreoathetosis. Movements associated with loss of proprioception. *Arch Neurol.* 1994; **51**: 1103–9.
Cross References
Ataxic hemiparesis; Chorea, Choreoathetosis; Dystonia; Proprioception; Pseudoathetosis; Useless hand of Oppenheim

Pseudodementia

The term pseudodementia has been used by some authors to describe cognitive impairments which result from affective disorders, most commonly anxiety and depression. The terms "dementia syndrome of depression" and "depression-related cognitive dysfunction" have also been used. The pattern of cognitive deficits in individuals with depression most closely resembles that seen in so-called subcortical dementia, with bradyphrenia, attentional and executive deficits. In addition there may be evident lack of effort and application, frequent "No" or "Don't know" answers, approximate answers (Ganser phenomenon, *vorbereiden*), and evidence of mood disturbance (tearfulness). Memory loss for recent and distant events may be equally severe (*cf.* temporal gradient of memory loss in dementia, *e.g.* due to Alzheimer's disease). A 22-item checklist to help differentiate pseudodementia from Alzheimer's disease has been described, based on clinical history, behaviour and mental status.

The recognition of pseudodementia is important since the deficits are often at least partially reversible with appropriate treatment with antidepressant medications. However, it should be borne in mind that depression is sometimes the presenting symptom of an underlying neurodegenerative dementing disorder such as Alzheimer's disease. Psychomotor retardation in dementia syndromes may also be mistaken for depression. Longitudinal assessment may be required to differentiate between these diagnostic possibilities.

References
Andrews C. Pseudodementia responding to antidepressant therapy. *Prog Neurol Psychiatry.* 2002; **6**(1): 26.
Kiloh L. Pseudodementia. *Acta Psychiatr Scand.* 1961; **37**: 336–51.
Roose SP, Devanand DP. The interface between dementia and depression. London: Martin Dunitz; 1999.
Wells CE. Pseudodementia. *Am J Psychiatry.* 1979; **136**: 895–900.
Cross References
Attention; Bradyphrenia; Dementia; Ganser phenomenon; Psychomotor retardation

Pseudodiplopia
- see PALINOPSIA

Pseudo-Foster Kennedy Syndrome
- see FOSTER KENNEDY SYNDROME

Pseudohallucination

The term pseudohallucination has been used in different ways. In the European psychopathological tradition, it may refer simply to vivid visual imagery, whereas in the American arena it may refer to hallucinations that are recognised for what they are, *i.e.* the patient has insight into their non-real nature. The term "non-psychotic hallucinations" has also been proposed for these phenomena. Some patients with dementia with Lewy bodies certainly realise that their visual hallucinations do not correspond to external reality, and similar experiences may occur with dopamine agonist treatment. Pseudohallucinations may fall along a continuum of perceptual disorders.

References
van der Zwaard R, Polak M. Pseudohallucinations: a pseudoconcept? A review of the validity of the concept, related to associate symptomatology. *Compr Psychiatry.* 2001; **42**: 42–50.

Wearne D, Genetti A. Pseudohallucinations versus hallucinations: wherein lies the difference? *Australas Psychiatry*. 2015; **23**: 254–7.
Cross References
Charles Bonnet syndrome; Hallucination

Pseudohypertrophy
- see CALF HYPERTROPHY; MUSCLE HYPERTROPHY

Pseudo-Internuclear Ophthalmoplegia
Pseudo-internuclear ophthalmoplegia (pseudo-INO) describes a disorder of eye movements with impaired adduction in one eye and horizontal nystagmus in the abducting eye (*i.e.* signs as seen in an internuclear ophthalmoplegia) but without an intrinsic brainstem lesion. This sign may be seen in:

- Myasthenia gravis (a diagnosis which is always worthy of consideration in a patient with an "isolated INO") due to extraocular muscle weakness.
- Brainstem compression due to subdural haematoma with transtentorial herniation.
- Cerebellar mass lesion.
- Guillain-Barré syndrome, Miller Fisher syndrome.
- Thyroid ophthalmopathy.
- Orbital pseudotumour.

The preservation of rapid saccades despite restriction of eye movements in myasthenia gravis may result from selective sparing of pale global muscle fibres which generate high-speed movements.
References
Glaser JS. Myasthenic pseudo-internuclear ophthalmoplegia. *Arch Ophthalmol*. 1966; **75**: 363–6.
Khanna S, Liao K, Kaminski HJ, Tomsak RL, Joshi A, Leigh RJ. Ocular myasthenia revisited: insights from pseudo-internuclear ophthalmoplegia. *J Neurol*. 2007; **254**: 1569–74.
Cross References
Internuclear ophthalmoplegia (INO); One-and-a-half syndrome

Pseudomyotonia
The term pseudomyotonia has been used in various ways:

- It may be used to describe the clinical appearance of myotonia (slow muscular relaxation after contraction) in the absence of myotonic discharges on electromyography. Pseudomyotonia is most commonly observed as the slow-relaxing or "hung-up" tendon reflexes (Woltman's sign) of hypothyroidism, although other causes are described.
- Pseudomyotonia has also been used to describe difficulty opening the hand in cervical osteoarthritis, although muscle relaxation is normal; finger flexion on attempted extension has been explained as due to aberrant axonal regeneration of the C7 root.
- The term pseudomyotonia has also been used to describe neuromyotonia and myokymia (as, for example, in Isaacs syndrome), to distinguish it from myotonia.

References
Coers C, Teleman-Toppet N, Durdu J. Neurogenic benign fasciculations, pseudomyotonia, and pseudotetany. A disease in search of a name. *Arch Neurol*. 1981; **38**: 282–7.
Satoyoshi E, Doi Y, Kinoshita M. Pseudomyotonia in cervial root lesions with myelopathy. A sign of the misdirection of regenerating nerve. *Arch Neurol*. 1972; **27**: 307–13.
Cross References
Myotonia; Neuromyotonia; Woltman's sign

Pseudo-One-and-a-Half Syndrome
Pseudo-one-and-a-half syndrome is the eye movement disorder of one-and-a-half syndrome without a brainstem lesion. Myasthenia gravis and Guillain-Barré syndrome are recognised causes.
Reference
Davis TL, Lavin PJ. Pseudo one-and-a-half syndrome with ocular myasthenia. *Neurology*. 1989; **39**: 1553.
Cross Reference
One-and-a-half syndrome

Pseudopapilloedema
Pseudopapilloedema is the name given to elevation of the optic disc that is not due to oedema (*i.e.* intracranial pressure is not raised). There may or may not be visible drusen (hyaline bodies). In distinction to oedematous disc swelling, the nerve fibre layer is not hazy and the underlying vessels are not obscured; however, spontaneous retinal venous pulsation is usually absent, and haemorrhages may be seen, so these are not reliable distinguishing features. Visual acuity is usually normal, but visual field defects (most commonly in the inferior nasal field) may be found.
Cross References
Disc swelling; Papilloedema; Retinal venous pulsation

Pseudoparesis
- see PARESIS; WEAKNESS

Pseudoptosis
Ptosis, drooping of the eyelid, may need to be differentiated from pseudoptosis or functional ptosis. This may result simply from a redundant tarsal skin fold, especially in older patients, or be a functional condition. Frontalis underactivity may be a clinical indicator of the latter diagnosis (*cf.* compensatory overactivity of frontalis with other causes of ptosis, *e.g.* myasthenia gravis).

The term pseudoptosis has also been used in the context of hypotropia; when the non-hypotropic eye fixates, the upper lid follows the hypotropic eye and appears ptotic, disappearing when fixation is with the hypotropic eye.
References
Hop JW, Frijns CJ, van Gijn J. Psychogenic pseudoptosis. *J Neurol*. 1997; **244**: 623–4.
Stone J. Pseudo-ptosis. *Pract Neurol*. 2002; **2**: 364–5.
Cross Reference
Ptosis

Pseudoradicular Syndrome
Thalamic lesions may sometimes cause contralateral sensory symptoms in an apparent radicular (*e.g.* C8) distribution. If associated with perioral sensory symptoms this may be known as the cheiro-oral syndrome.
Reference
Kim JS. Restricted acral sensory syndrome following minor stroke: further observations with special reference to differential severity of symptoms among individual digits. *Stroke*. 1994; **25**: 2497–502.
Cross Reference
"False-localising signs"

Pseudo-Von Graefe's Sign
Pseudo-von Graefe's sign is involuntary retraction or elevation of the upper eyelid (*cf.* von Graefe's sign), medial rotation of the eye, and pupillary constriction seen on attempted downgaze or adduction of the eye. This constellation of findings is said to be a lid-gaze synkinesis

following aberrant axonal regeneration after an oculomotor (III) nerve palsy, usually of traumatic or chronic compressive rather than ischaemic origin.
Cross References
Lid retraction; Synkinesia, Synkinesis; Von Graefe's sign

Psychic Akinesia
- see ATHYMHORMIA

Psychic Blindness
- see VISUAL AGNOSIA

Psychic Paralysis of Gaze
- see BALINT'S SYNDROME; OCULAR APRAXIA

Psychomotor Retardation
Psychomotor retardation is a slowness of thought (bradyphrenia) and movement (bradykinesia) seen in psychiatric disorders, particularly depression, or as a consequence of drug use (*e.g.* multiple analgesic, sedative, hypnotic medications). It may be confused with the akinesia of parkinsonism and with states of abulia or catatonia. Psychomotor retardation may also be a feature of the "subcortical" type of dementia, or of impairments of arousal (obtundation).
Cross References
Abulia; Akinesia; Catatonia; Dementia; Obtundation; Parkinsonism

Psychomotor Signs
- see FRONTAL RELEASE SIGNS

Ptarmus
- see SNEEZING

Ptosis
Ptosis, or blepharoptosis, is the name given to drooping of the eyelid. This may be due to mechanical causes such as aponeurosis dehiscence, or neurological disease, in which case it may be congenital or acquired, partial or complete, unilateral or bilateral, fixed or variable, isolated or accompanied by other signs, *e.g.* miosis in a Horner's syndrome; diplopia in myasthenia gravis; mydriasis and downward and outward deviation of the eye in an oculomotor (III) nerve palsy.

Ptosis may result from pathology in a variety of locations: brainstem disease involving the oculomotor (III) nerve; anywhere along the oculosympathetic autonomic pathway causing a Horner's syndrome; or cortical disease (*e.g.* infarction) reflecting hemispheric control of the eyelid (probably bilaterally represented).

When considering the cause of ptosis, the differential diagnosis is broad. Recognised neurological causes include:

- Congenital:
    Cranial nerve dysinnervation disorder.
    Congenital Horner's syndrome.
    Oculomotor-trigeminal (or trigeminal-levator) synkinesis: Marcus Gunn jaw-winking phenomenon, or inverse Marcus Gunn phenomenon (ptosis on jaw opening).
- Neurogenic:
    Supranuclear lesion:
        Hemiparesis: due to cortical infarct; ptosis usually ipsilateral, incomplete.

Duane syndrome: ptosis on eye adduction, due to supranuclear levator inhibition; usually with family history.

Oculomotor (III) nerve:

Hypertension, diabetes mellitus: ptosis often complete; in a superior divisional third nerve palsy partial ptosis is associated with superior rectus weakness only.

Compressive lesion (*e.g.* posterior communicating artery aneurysm): ptosis usually incomplete; ptosis may be present with subarachnoid haemorrhage.

Guillain-Barré syndrome.

Facial paresis.

- Neuromuscular junction:

  Myasthenia gravis: ptosis variable, bilateral or unilateral.

  Excessive botulinum toxin, *e.g.* given for treatment of blepharospasm.
- Myogenic: ptosis usually bilateral:

  Mitochondrial disease (CPEO).
  Myotonic dystrophy.
  Oculopharyngeal muscular dystrophy (OPMD).

Local, ophthalmological causes should also be considered, such as age-related aponeurosis dehiscence, trauma, thyroid eye disease, lid inflammation (chalazion), and lymphoma. Pseudoptosis (*q.v.*) enters the differential diagnosis.

Enhanced ptosis, worsening of ptosis on one side when the other eyelid is held elevated in a fixed position, may be demonstrated in myasthenia gravis and Lambert Eaton myasthenic syndrome.

References

Ahmad K, Wright M, Lueck CJ. Ptosis. *Pract Neurol*. 2011; **11**: 332–40.

Caplan LR. Ptosis. *J Neurol Neurosurg Psychiatry*. 1974; **37**: 1–7.

Cross References

Blepharospasm; Curtaining; Diplopia; Divisional palsy; Enhanced ptosis; Ewart phenomenon; Horner's syndrome; Ice pack test; Jaw winking; Miosis; Mydriasis; Pseudoptosis; Pupil sparing; Synkinesia, Synkinesis

Ptyalism

- see SIALORRHOEA

Pulfrich Phenomenon

The Pulfrich phenomenon is the observation that a pendulum swinging from side to side appears to traverse a curved trajectory. This is a stereo-illusion resulting from latency disparities in the visual pathways, most commonly seen as a consequence of slowed conduction in a demyelinated optic nerve following unilateral optic neuritis. A tinted coloured lens in front of the good eye can alleviate the symptom (or induce it in the normally sighted).

References

McGowan G, Ahmed TY, Heron G, Diaper C. The Pulfrich phenomenon; clumsiness and collisions which can be ameliorated. *Pract Neurol*. 2011; **11**: 173–6.

Rushton D. Use of the Pulfrich pendulum for detecting abnormal delay in the visual pathways in multiple sclerosis. *Brain*. 1975; **98**: 283–96.

Cross References

Phosphene; Relative afferent pupillary defect (RAPD)

"Pull Test"

- see POSTURAL REFLEXES

Punding

Punding describes repetitive pointless behaviours, with a compulsive flavour to them, carried on for long periods of time to the exclusion of other activities. It is frequently related to previous occupation or hobbies but is seldom pleasurable (writing a book might be an example?). It occurs in Parkinson's disease but the incidence is low (1.4% in one study). It is thought to be related to dopaminergic stimulation, and may be associated with impulse control disorders such as pathological gambling and hypersexuality.

References

O'Sullivan SS, Evans AH, Lees AJ. Punding in Parkinson's disease. *Pract Neurol.* 2007; **7**: 397–9.

Spencer AH, Rickards H, Fasano A, Cavanna AE. The prevalence and clinical characteristics of punding in Parkinson's disease. *Mov Disord.* 2011; **26**: 578–86.

Cross References

Gambling; Hypersexuality

Pupillary Reflexes

Two pupillary reflexes, first described by Robert Whytt (1714–1766) and sometimes known as Whytt's reflex, are routinely examined in clinical practice:

- *Light reflex*:

  The eye is illuminated directly and the reaction (constriction) observed; the consensual light reflex is observed by illuminating the contralateral eye. In an eye with poor visual acuity, a relative afferent pupillary defect may be observed using the "swinging flashlight test". The afferent pathway subserving the light reflex is optic nerve to thalamus, brainstem, and Edinger-Westphal nucleus, with the efferent limb (pupillomotor parasympathetic fibres) in the oculomotor (III) nerve. The contralateral (consensual) response results from fibres crossing the midline in the optic chiasm and in the posterior commissure at the level of the rostral brainstem.

  Paradoxical constriction of the pupil in darkness (Flynn phenomenon) has been described.

- *Accommodation reflex*:

  This is most conveniently examined by asking the patient to look into the distance, then focus on a near object (sufficiently close to necessitate convergence of the visual axes) when pupil constriction should occur (accommodation-convergence synkinesis). The afferent pathways subserving this response are less certain than for the light reflex, and may involve the occipital cortex, although the final (efferent) pathway via Edinger-Westphal nucleus and oculomotor (III) nerve is common to both accommodation and light reflexes.

In comatose patients, fixed dilated pupils may be observed with central diencephalic herniation, whereas midbrain lesions produce fixed midposition pupils.

A dissociation between the light and accommodation reactions (light-near pupillary dissociation, *q.v.*) may be observed.

Reference

Kawasaki A. Approach to the patient with abnormal pupils. In: Biller J, editor. Practical neurology. 2nd ed. Philadelphia: Lippincott Williams & Wilkins; 2002. p. 135–46.

Cross References

Argyll Robertson pupil; Ciliospinal response; Cortical blindness; Flynn phenomenon; Light-near pupillary dissociation; Miosis; Mydriasis; Relative afferent pupillary defect (RAPD); Swinging flashlight sign

Pupil Sparing
Oculomotor (III) nerve lesions may be pupil sparing (normal response to light) or pupil-involving (mydriasis, loss of light reflex). The latter situation usually implies a "surgical" cause of oculomotor nerve palsy (*e.g.* posterior communicating artery aneurysm), especially if extraocular muscle function is relatively preserved. Pupil sparing suggests a "medical" cause (*e.g.* diabetes mellitus, hypertension) especially if the palsy is otherwise complete (complete ptosis, eye deviated downwards and outwards). This disparity arises because pupillomotor fibres run on the outside of the oculomotor nerve, and are relatively spared by ischaemia but are vulnerable to external compression. However, the distinction is not absolute; imaging for an aneurysm (by means of spiral CT, MRA, or catheter angiography) may be necessary if the clinical scenario leaves room for doubt.
Cross References
Oculomotor (III) nerve palsy; Ophthalmoparesis, Ophthalmoplegia; Ptosis; Pupillary reflexes

Pure Word Blindness
- see ALEXIA

Pure Word Deafness
The term word deafness was first used by Henry Charlton Bastian in 1869 (as was word blindness). Pure word deafness is a rare condition characterized by an inability to comprehend and discriminate spoken language, despite adequate hearing as measured by audiometry, and with preserved spontaneous speech, reading, reading comprehension, and writing (*i.e.* no aphasia, alexia, or agraphia). Lip reading may assist in the understanding of others who sometimes seem to the patient as though they are speaking in a foreign language. Patients can copy and write spontaneously, follow written commands, but cannot write to dictation. Word repetition tasks are impaired. There may be associated amusia, depending on the precise location of cerebral damage.

Pure word deafness has been variously conceptualised as a form of auditory agnosia or a subcortical sensory aphasia.

Pure word deafness is most commonly associated with bilateral lesions of the temporal cortex or subcortical lesions whose anatomical effect is to damage the primary auditory cortex or isolate it (*e.g.* from Wernicke's area) through lesions of the auditory radiation; unilateral lesions producing this syndrome have been reported. Very rarely pure word deafness has been associated with bilateral brainstem lesions at the level of the inferior colliculi.
References
Meyer B, Kral T, Zentner J. Pure word deafness after resection of a tectal plate glioma with preservation of wave V of brain stem auditory evoked potentials. *J Neurol Neurosurg Psychiatry*. 1996; **61**: 423–4.
Roberts M, Sandercock P, Ghadiali E. Pure word deafness and unilateral right temporoparietal lesions: a case report. *J Neurol Neurosurg Psychiatry*. 1987; **50**: 1708–9.
Tanaka Y, Yamadori A, Mori E. Pure word deafness following bilateral lesions. A psychophysical analysis. *Brain*. 1987; **110**: 381–403.
Cross References
Agnosia; Amusia; Aphasia; Auditory agnosia

Pursuit
Pursuit, or smooth pursuit, eye movements hold the image of a moving target on the fovea, or during linear self motion, *i.e.* they stabilize the gaze. This is dependent upon vestibulo-ocular reflexes and visually-mediated reflexes. Impaired ("broken") pursuit may result from occipital lobe lesions, and may be abolished by bilateral lesions, and may co-exist with some forms of congenital nystagmus.
References
Gaymard B, Pierrot-Deseilligny C. Neurology of saccades and smooth pursuit. *Curr Opin Neurol*. 1999; **12**: 13–9.

Leigh RJ, Zee DS. The neurology of eye movements. 4th ed. New York: Oxford University Press; 2006. p. 188–240.
Cross References
Nystamgus; Saccades; Saccadic intrusion, Saccadic pursuit

Pyramidal Decussation Syndrome
Pyramidal decussation syndrome is a rare crossed hemiplegia syndrome, with weakness of one arm and the contralateral leg (hemiplegia cruciata) without involvement of the face, due to a lesion within the pyramid below the decussation of corticiospinal fibres destined for the arm but above that for fibres destined for the leg.
Cross Reference
Hemiplegia cruciata

Pyramidal Signs, Pyramidal Syndrome, Pyramidal Weakness
- see HEMIPARESIS; UPPER MOTOR NEURONE (UMN) SYNDROME; WEAKNESS

Q

Quadrantanopia

Quadrantanopia (or quadrantanopsia), a defect in one quarter of the visual field, suggests an optic radiation lesion. Occipital lobe pathology is the most common cause of both inferior and superior quadrantanopias, although temporal lobe pathology damaging Meyer's loop typically must be considered with a superior homonymous quadrantanopia ("pie-in-the-sky" defect). Parietal lobe lesions may produce inferior quadrantic defects, usually accompanied by other localising signs. Damage to extrastriate visual cortex (areas V2 and V3) has also been suggested to cause quadrantanopia; concurrent central achromatopsia favours this localisation.

References

Horton JC, Hoyt WF. Quadrantic visual field defects. A hallmark of lesions in extrastriate (V2/V3) cortex. *Brain*. 1991; **114**: 1703–8.

Jacobson DM. The localizing value of quadrantanopia. *Arch Neurol*. 1997; **54**: 401–4.

Cross References

Achromatopsia; Hemianopia; "Pie-in-the-sky" defect; Visual field defects

Quadriparesis, Quadriplegia

Quadriparesis or quadriplegia (tetraparesis, tetraplegia) refers to weakness, partial or total, respectively, of all four limbs which may be of upper motor neurone or, less commonly, lower motor neurone type (*e.g.* in Guillain-Barré syndrome).

- Lower motor neurone, and some acute upper motor neurone, pathologies produce a flaccid quadriparesis/quadriplegia with areflexia; urinary retention may be present.
- Upper motor neurone lesions, particularly if chronic, produce a spastic quadriparesis with hypertonia, sustained clonus, hyperreflexia, loss of abdominal and cremasteric reflexes, and bilateral Babinski's sign. As with hemiplegia, upper motor neurone quadriplegia may result from lesions of the corticospinal pathways anywhere from motor cortex to cervical cord via the brainstem, but is most commonly seen with brainstem and upper cervical cord lesions. In such circumstances, respiration may be affected. There may also be enhanced flexion defence reflexes ("flexor spasms") which may develop over time into a fixed flexion deformity with secondary contractures ("paraplegia in flexion"). Incomplete or high spinal cord lesions may evolve to "paraplegia in extension".

Cross References

Hemiparesis; Paraplegia

Quadrupedalism

Quadrupedalism, facultative quadrupedal locomotion (walking on all fours), has been observed as part of a recessive cerebellar hypoplastic syndrome associated with cerebellar ataxia and learning disability in consanguineous families in Turkey, the Uner Tan syndrome, which is genetically heterogeneous. The hypothesis that this gait pattern is an example of "devolution", an atavistic expression of quadrupedal primate ancestry, has been challenged by biomechanical analysis suggesting that the gait shows lateral sequence and not the diagonal sequence-quadrupedal gait typical of other primates.

© Springer International Publishing Switzerland 2016
A.J. Larner, *A Dictionary of Neurological Signs*,
DOI 10.1007/978-3-319-29821-4_17

References
Shapiro LJ, Cole WG, Young JW, Raichlen DA, Robinson SR, Adolph KE. Human quadrupeds, primate quadrupedalism, and Uner Tan syndrome. *PLoS One*. 2014; **9**(7): e101758.
Tan U. Uner tan syndrome: history, clinical evaluations, genetics, and the dynamics of human quadrupedalism. *Open Neurol J*. 2010; **4**: 78–89.

R

Rabbit Syndrome

The rabbit syndrome is a rest tremor of perioral and nasal muscles. It has been associated with both antipsychotic drug therapy and idiopathic Parkinson's disease and is therefore presumably related to deficient dopaminergic neurotransmission. No specific investigations are required, but a drug history, including over-the-counter medication, is crucial. The condition may be confused with edentulous dyskinesia if there is accompanying tremor of the jaw and/or lip, or with tardive dyskinesia. Drug-induced rabbit syndrome may remit with drug withdrawal but not always. Appropriate treatment of Parkinson's disease may also improve the involuntary movements. Anticholinergics may be tried.

Reference

Catena M, Fagiolini A, Consoli G, et al. The rabbit syndrome: state of the art. *Curr Clin Pharmacol.* 2007; **2**: 212–6.

Cross Reference

Parkinsonism

Raccoon Eyes, Raccoon Sign

"Raccoon eyes" refers to an appearance of bilateral periorbital ecchymosis (bruising, blepharohaematoma), appearing 48–72 h after an anterior basal skull fracture. This sign is reported to have high positive predictive value for skull base fracture (unilateral 90%, bilateral 70%).

Reference

Pretto Flores L, De Almeida CS, Casulari LA. Positive predictive values of selected clinical signs associated with skull base fractures. *J Neurosurg Sci* 2000; **44**: 77–82.

Cross Reference

Battle's sign

Radiculopathy

A radiculopathy is a disorder of spinal nerve roots. Radicular sensory symptoms may include sensory diminution or loss in the corresponding dermatome, paraesthesia, and pain; motor symptoms may include lower motor neurone type weakness with reflex diminution or loss in the corresponding myotome. Radiculopathies may be single or multiple (polyradiculopathy, *e.g.* cauda equina syndrome, chronic inflammatory demyelinating polyradiculoneuropathy [CIDP]). There may be concurrent myelopathy, typically of extrinsic or extramedullary type.

Most radiculopathies are in the lumbosacral region (60–90%), followed by the cervical region (5–30%). Electrophysiological studies may be helpful in distinguishing radiculopathy from a neuropathy or plexopathy: sensory nerve action potentials (SNAPs) are normal for intrathecal root lesions, and EMG shows involvement of paraspinal muscles. Recognised causes of radiculopathy include:

- Structural lesions:

    Compression: disc protrusion: cervical (especially C6, C7), lumbar (L5, S1) >>> thoracic; bony metastases; spondylolisthesis; fracture; infection.

    Root avulsion, *e.g.* C5/C6, "waiter's tip" posture; C8/T1, claw hand ± Horner's syndrome.

© Springer International Publishing Switzerland 2016

A.J. Larner, *A Dictionary of Neurological Signs*,

DOI 10.1007/978-3-319-29821-4_18

- Diabetic polyradiculopathy: lumbosacral (= diabetic amyotrophy, also known as diabetic lumbar sacral plexopathy, proximal diabetic neuropathy, Bruns-Garland syndrome; especially involves L2–L4); thoraco-abdominal (truncal neuropathy).
- Neoplasia: with meningeal symptoms, due to spread from carcinoma of breast or lung, melanoma, non-Hodgkin's lymphoma, leukaemia.
- Infection: HIV (CMV late in the course), *Borrelia* (Lyme disease), syphilis (tabes dorsalis), herpes zoster (thoracic > cervical > lumbosacral; sensory >> motor), leprosy.
- Demyelination: Guillain-Barré syndrome, CIDP.

Painful radiculoneuropathy (possibly with CSF pleocytosis) should prompt consideration of:

- Herpes zoster.
- CMV (immunocompromised patient).
- Lyme disease.
- Malignant infiltration.
- Sarcoidosis.
- Vasculitis.
- Diabetes.

Reference
Feldman EL, Grisold W, Russell JW, Zifko U. Atlas of neuromuscular disease. A practical guideline. Vienna: Springer; 2005. p. 117–39.
Cross References
Cauda equina syndrome; Dermatomal sensory loss; Lasègue's sign; Myelopathy; Neuropathy; Paraesthesia; Plexopathy; Reflexes; "Waiter's tip" posture; Weakness

Raynaud's Phenomenon
Raynaud's phenomenon consists of intermittent pallor or cyanosis, with or without suffusion and pain, of the fingers, toes, nose, ears, or jaw, in response to cold or stress. It may be observed by asking the patient to put their hands in cold water.
    Raynaud's phenomenon may occur in Raynaud's disease (idiopathic, primary) or Raynaud's syndrome (secondary, symptomatic). Recognised causes of the latter include:

- connective tissue disease, especially systemic sclerosis;
- cervical rib or thoracic outlet syndromes;
- vibration white finger;
- hypothyroidism;
- uraemia.

Associated symptoms should be sought to ascertain whether there is an underlying connective tissue disorder (*e.g.* rash, arthralgia, myalgia, calcium deposits in the skin, dysphagia). History of use of power tools should be sought (vibration white finger). The differential diagnosis includes causalgia.
    For Raynaud's syndrome, the treatment is that of the underlying cause where possible. For Raynaud's disease, and Raynaud's syndrome where there is no effective treatment of the underlying cause, non-drug treatment encompasses life style adjustment to avoid precipitants, and use of heated gloves. Drug therapy includes oral vasodilators (calcium channel blockers, ACE inhibitors), antioxidants (probucol), prostacyclin analogues (bolus, infusions). Beta-blockers should be avoided.
Reference
Bowling JCR, David PM. Raynaud's disease. *Lancet.* 2003; **361**: 2078–80.

Rebound Phenomenon
This is one feature of the impaired checking response seen in cerebellar disease, along with dysdiadochokinesia and macrographia. It may be demonstrated by observing an overshoot of the outstretched arms when they are released suddenly after being pressed down by the examiner, or suddenly releasing the forearm flexed against resistance so that it hits the chest (Stewart-Holmes sign). Although previously attributed to hypotonia, it is more likely a reflection of asynergia between agonist and antagonist muscles.
Cross References
Asynergia; Ataxia; Cerebellar syndromes; Dysdiadochokinesia; Dysmetria; Hypotonia; Hypotonus; Macrographia

Recruitment
Recruitment, or loudness recruitment, is the phenomenon of abnormally rapid growth of loudness with increase in sound intensity, which is encountered in patients with sensorineural (especially cochlear sensory) hearing loss. Thus patients have difficulty with sounds of low to moderate intensity ("Speak up, doctor!") but intense sounds are uncomfortably loud ("There's no need to shout, doctor!"). Speech discrimination is relatively unimpaired in conductive hearing loss.
"Recruitment" may also be used to refer to pathological "spread" of tendon reflexes, implying broadening of their receptive field.
Cross Reference
Reflexes

Recurrent Utterances
The recurrent utterances of global aphasia, sometimes known as verbal stereotypies, stereotyped aphasia, or monophasia, are reiterated words or syllables produced by patients with profound non-fluent aphasia (*e.g.* Broca's original case, Leborgne, who could only repeat "tan, tan", by which name he was known). The poet Charles Baudelaire (1821–1867) may have been reduced to a similar state following a stroke. Recurrent utterances have been thought to reflect the limited linguistic abilities of the non-dominant hemisphere.
References
Dieguez S, Bogousslavsky J. Baudelaire's aphasia: from poetry to cursing. In: Bogousslavsky J, Hennerici MG, editors. Neurological disorders in famous artists, part 2. Basel: Karger; 2007. p. 121–49.
Hale S. The man who lost his language. A case of aphasia (Revised edition). London: Jessica Kingsley; 2007.
Cross Reference
Aphasia

Red Ear Syndrome
The red ear syndrome is characterized by brief attacks of reddening of the external ear associated with burning pain. The syndrome may be associated with migraine or trigeminal autonomic cephalalgias, or with upper cervical spine pathology (irritation of the C3 nerve root) or temporomandibular joint dysfunction. Some patients may benefit from migraine prophylactic treatments.
References
Lambru G, Miller S, Matharu MS. The red ear syndrome. *J Headache Pain.* 2013; **14**: 83.
Lance JW. The red ear syndrome. *Neurology.* 1996; **47**: 617–20.

Reduplicative Paramnesia
Reduplicative paramnesia is a delusion in which patients believe familiar places, objects, individuals, or events to be duplicated. The syndrome is probably heterogeneous and bears some resemblance to the Capgras delusion as described in the context of some psychiatric disorders.

Reduplicative paramnesia is more commonly seen with right (non-dominant) hemisphere damage; frontal, temporal and limbic system damage has been implicated. This may occur transiently as a consequence of cerebrovascular disease, following head trauma, or even after migraine attacks, or more persistently in the context of neurodegenerative disorders such as Alzheimer's disease.

References
Benson DF, Gardner H, Meadows JC. Reduplicative paramnesia. *Neurology*. 1976; **26**: 147–51.
Politis M, Loane C. Reduplicative paramnesia: a review. *Psychopathology*. 2012; **45**: 337–43.
Cross References
Capgras delusion; Delusion; Paramnesia

Reflexes
Reflex action – a sensory stimulus provoking an involuntary motor response – is a useful way of assessing the integrity of neurological function, since disease in the afferent (sensory) limb, synapse, or efferent (motor) limb of the reflex arc may lead to reflex dysfunction, as may changes in inputs from higher centres.

Different types of reflex may be distinguished. Muscle tendon reflexes (or, as some authors prefer, myotatic or myotactic reflexes) may be either tonic (in response to a static applied force: "stretch reflex") or phasic (in response to a brief applied force, for example a blow from a tendon hammer to the muscle tendon). The latter are of particular use in clinical work because of their localising value (see Table). However, there are no reflexes between T2 and T12, and thus for localisation one is dependent on sensory findings, or occasionally cutaneous (skin or superficial) reflexes, such as the abdominal reflexes.

Reflex	Root value
Jaw jerk	Trigeminal (V) nerve
Supinator (Brachioradialis, Radial)	C5, C6
Biceps	C5, C6
Triceps	C7
Finger flexion (Digital)	C8, T1
Abdominal	T7–T12
Cremasteric	L1, L2
Knee (Patellar)	L3, L4
Hamstring	L5, S1
Ankle (Achilles)	(L5) S1 (S2)
Bulbocavernosus	S2, S3, S4
Anal	S4, S5

Tendon reflex responses are usually graded on a five point scale:

–	absent (areflexia; as in lower motor neurone syndromes, such as peripheral nerve or anterior horn cell disorders; or acute upper motor neurone syndromes, *e.g.* "spinal shock").
±	reduced (hyporeflexia); present only with reinforcement (*e.g.* Jendrassik's manoeuvre).
+	normal.
++	brisk normal.
+++	pathologically brisk (hyperreflexia, as in upper motor neurone syndromes).

Reflex "spread", or "recruitment" of reflexes, for example a finger jerk seen when eliciting the supinator or biceps jerk, is suggestive of corticospinal pathway (upper motor neurone) pathology, producing an enlarged receptive field for the reflex response. Concurrent disruption of the local reflex arc may result in inverted reflexes.

Reflex responses may vary according to the degree of patient relaxation or anxiety (precontraction). Moreover, there is interobserver variation in the assessment of tendon reflexes (as with all clinical signs). A biasing effect of prior knowledge upon reflex assessment has been recorded.

There is also a class or "primitive", "developmental", or "psychomotor" reflexes, present in neonates but disappearing with maturity but which may re-emerge with ageing or cerebral (especially frontal lobe) disease, hence sometimes known as "frontal release signs".

References
Dick JPR. The deep tendon and the abdominal reflexes. *J Neurol Neurosurg Psychiatry*. 2003; **74**: 150–3.
Stam J, van Crevel H. Reliability of the clinical and electromyographic examination of tendon reflexes. *J Neurol*. 1990; **237**: 427–31.

Cross References
Age-related signs; Areflexia; Crossed adductor reflex; Facilitation; Frontal release signs; Hyperreflexia; Hyporeflexia; Inverted reflexes; Jendrassik's manoeuvre; Lower motor neurone (LMN) syndrome; Primitive reflexes; Pupillary reflexes; Upper motor neurone (UMN) syndrome; Woltman's sign. See also specific (named) reflexes

Relative Afferent Pupillary Defect (RAPD)
An afferent pupillary defect (APD), or relative afferent pupillary defect (RAPD), is an abnormal pupillary response in which the normally equal direct and consensual pupillary reflexes are asymmetric, the direct response being less than the consensual.

This response discrepancy may be rendered particularly evident by performing the "swinging flashlight" test. The pupils are alternately illuminated every 2–3 s in a darkened room. Quickly moving the light to the diseased side may produce pupillary dilatation (Marcus Gunn pupil). Subjectively patients may note that the light stimulus seems less bright in the affected eye.

RAPD suggests asymmetric optic nerve pathology, such as optic neuritis or tumour, causing a conduction defect; indeed this is the most sensitive sign of optic nerve pathology. Although visual acuity may also be impaired in the affected eye, and the disc may appear abnormal on fundoscopy, this is not necessarily the case. Since RAPD depends on asymmetry of optic nerve conduction, no defect may be observed if both optic nerves are affected.

RAPD has also been described with lesions of the retina, optic chiasm, optic tract (contralateral), brachium of the superior colliculus and pretectal nucleus (in the latter two situations without visual impairment).

References
Broadway DC. How to test for a relative afferent pupillary defect (RAPD). *Community Eye Health*. 2012; **25**: 58–9.
Chen CJ, Scheufele M, Sheth M, Torabi A, Hogan N, Frohman EM. Isolated relative afferent pupillary defect secondary to contralateral midbrain compression. *Arch Neurol*. 2004; **61**: 1451–3

Cross References
Amblyopia; Marcus Gunn pupil, Marcus Gunn sign; Pupillary reflexes; Swinging flashlight sign

Religiosity
- see HYPERRELIGIOSITY

Remote Atrophy
- see ATROPHY; "FALSE-LOCALISING SIGNS"

Retinal Venous Pulsation

Venous pulsation is evident in the normal retina when observed with an ophthalmoscope, particularly at the margin of the disc. It results from fluctuations in the pressure gradient between intraocular pressure and cerebrospinal fluid pressure. Because CSF pressure is lower in the sitting than the recumbent position, it may be anticipated that retinal venous pulsation is more likely to be detected in the sitting position.

Spontaneous retinal venous pulsation is expected to be lost when intracranial pressure rises. The presence of spontaneous retinal venous pulsation indeed has high sensitivity and positive predictive value for the exclusion of raised intracranial pressure as measured at lumbar puncture, but the specificity of the sign is low, such that the presence of pulsation does not exclude raised intracranial pressure. Moreover its absence cannot be relied upon to indicate raised intracranial pressure.

Reference

Wong SH, White RP. The clinical validity of the spontaneous retinal venous pulsation. *J Neuroophthalmol.* 2013; **33**: 17–20.

Cross References

Papilloedema; Pseudopapilloedema

Retinitis Pigmentosa

Retinitis pigmentosa, or tapetoretinal degeneration, is a generic name for inherited retinal degenerations characterized clinically by typical appearances on ophthalmoscopy, specifically peripheral pigmentation of "bone-spicule" type, arteriolar attenuation, and eventual unmasking of choroidal vessels and optic atrophy.

Despite the name, there is no inflammation; the pathogenetic mechanism may be apoptotic death of photoreceptors. This process may be asymptomatic in its early stages, but may later be a cause of nyctalopia (night blindness), and produce a mid-peripheral ring scotoma on visual field testing.

A variety of genetic causes of isolated retinitis pigmentosa have been partially characterized:

- autosomal recessive: linked to chromosome 1q.
- X-linked: Xp11, Xp21.
- autosomal dominant: 3q, 6p, 8.

At least some of these are related to mutations in the gene for the rod cell protein rhodopsin.

In most cases, patients with retinitis pigmentosa have no associated systemic or extraocular abnormalities, but there are a number of multisystem disorders in which it occurs:

- Abetalipoproteinaemia (Bassen-Kornzweig syndrome; HARP syndrome).
- Alström's syndrome.
- Cockayne syndrome.
- Friedreich's ataxia.
- Lawrence-Moon-Bardet-Biedl syndrome.
- Mitochondrial disorders (*e.g.* Kearns-Sayre syndrome and NARP [neurogenic weakness, ataxia, and retinitis pigmentosa]).
- Neuronal ceroid lipofuscinosis.
- Peroxisomal disorders, Refsum's disease.
- Usher's disease.

Reference

Dryja TP. Retinitis pigmentosa. In: Scriver CR, Beaudet al, Sly WS, Valle D, editors. The metabolic and molecular basis of inherited disease. New York: McGraw-Hill; 1995. p. 4297–309.

Cross References

Nyctalopia; Optic atrophy; Scotoma

Retinopathy

Retinopathy is a pathological process affecting the retina, with changes observable on ophthalmoscopy; dilatation of the pupil aids observation of the peripheral retina. Common causes include:

- Diabetes mellitus: various abnormalities may occur, in both insulin-dependent (IDDM) and non-insulin dependent (NIDDM) patients. "Background" diabetic retinopathy is manifest as microaneuryms, dot and blot haemorrhages, hard exudates, and diffuse retinal oedema, all of which may be asymptomatic. Oedema and hard exudates at the macula are a common cause of visual impairment. Proliferative retinopathy is characterized by neovascularisation of the disc due to retinal hypoxia, typically in IDDM, with the risk of vitreous haemorrhage, traction retinal detachment and irreversible visual loss. Laser treatment of new vessels is the treatment of choice.
- Hypertension: hypertensive retinopathy may cause arteriolar constriction, with the development of cotton-wool spots; and abnormal vascular permeability causing flame-shaped haemorrhages, retinal oedema and hard exudates; around the fovea, the latter may produce a macular star. Optic disc swelling may be seen in malignant hypertension. Arteriosclerosis, thickening of vessel walls with prolonged hypertension, may cause changes at arteriovenous crossings ("AV nipping"). Systemic hypertension is associated with an increased risk of branch retinal vein and central retinal artery occlusion.
- Drug-induced, *e.g.* antimalarials (chloroquine); chlorpromazine.
- Retinitis pigmentosa.
- Serous retinopathy or chorioretinopathy: leakage of fluid into the subretinal space, causing unilateral sudden non-progressive visual loss.
- Cancer-associated retinopathy: arteriolar narrowing, optic atrophy.
- "Salt and pepper" retinopathy of Kearns-Sayre syndrome (mitochondrial disorder).

An electroretinogram (ERG) may be helpful in confirming the presence of a retinopathic disorder.

Cross References

Maculopathy; Retinitis pigmentosa; Scotoma

Retrocollis

Retrocollis is an extended posture of the neck. Progressive supranuclear palsy (PSP; Steele-Richardson-Olszewski syndrome) is commonly associated with retrocollis (*cf.* antecollis in multiple system atrophy). Retrocollis may also be a feature of cervical dystonia (torticollis), advanced Parkinson's disease, and of kernicterus.

References

Kashihara K, Imamura T. Frequency and clinical correlates of retrocollis in Parkinson's disease. *J Neurol Sci.* 2013; **324**: 106–8.

Papapetropoulos S, Baez S, Zister J, Sengun C, Singer C. Retrocollis: classification, clinical phenotype, treatment outcomes and risk factors. *Eur Neurol.* 2008; **59**: 71–5.

Cross References

Antecollis; Dystonia; Parkinsonism; Torticollis

Retropulsion, Retropulsion Test

- see FESTINANT GAIT, FESTINATION; POSTURAL REFLEXES

Reverse Horner's Syndrome

- see POURFOUR DU PETIT SYNDROME

Reverse Lhermitte's Sign

- see LHERMITTE'S SIGN

Reverse Ocular Bobbing
- see OCULAR BOBBING

Reverse Ocular Dipping
- see OCULAR DIPPING

Reverse Phalen's Manoeuvre
- see PHALEN'S SIGN

"Reverse Ptosis"
- see HORNER'S SYNDROME; PTOSIS

Reverse Sensory Geste
Whereas a sensory trick (or *geste antagoniste*) transiently reverses the severity of dystonia, reverse sensory geste worsens it, for example in cervical dystonia (torticollis).
Reference
Asmus F, von Coelln R, Boertlein A, Gasser T, Mueller J. Reverse sensory geste in cervical dystonia. *Mov Disord.* 2009; **24**: 297–300.
Cross References
Dystonia; Sensory tricks; Torticollis

Reverse Straight Leg Raising
- see FEMORAL STRETCH TEST

Revilliod's Sign
Revilliod's sign is an acquired inability to wink. This is a sign, possibly early, of corticobulbar disease.

Riddoch's Phenomenon
Riddoch's phenomenon is the dissociation of the perception of static and kinetic visual stimuli (statokinetic dissociation). This phenomenon does not have particular localizing value, since it may occur with both occipital and anterior visual pathway lesions.
Reference
Zeki S, Ffytche DH. The Riddoch syndrome: insights into the neurobiology of conscious vision. *Brain.* 1998; **121**: 25–45.
Cross References
Akinetopsia; Visual agnosia

Right-Left Disorientation
Right-left disorientation is an inability to say whether a part of the body is on the right or left side, or to use a named lateralised body part to command. This may occur in association with acalculia, agraphia, and finger agnosia, collectively known as the Gerstmann syndrome. Although all these features are dissociable, their concurrence indicates a posterior parietal dominant hemisphere lesion involving the angular and supramarginal gyri.
Cross References
Acalculia; Agraphia; Autotopagnosia; Finger agnosia; Gerstmann syndrome

Rigidity
Rigidity describes an increased resistance to the passive movement of a joint which is constant throughout the range of joint displacement and not related to the speed of joint movement; resistance is present in both agonist and antagonist muscles. In these particulars,

rigidity differs from spasticity. Rigidity also needs to be differentiated from stiffness. Rigidity may be described as:

- *consistent*: "leadpipe rigidity"; or
- *jerky*: "cogwheel rigidity" or Negro's sign, when a rhythmic fluctuation (*i.e.* tremor), like a ratchet or cogwheel, is superimposed on the background of sustained rigidity (NB cogwheeling, reflecting underlying tremor, may occur in the absence of rigidity, *e.g.* in essential tremor; cogwheeling and rigidity are dissociable).

The presence of rigidity may be made more obvious by reinforcing manoeuvres (*e.g.* clenching and relaxing the contralateral fist, performing mental arithmetic), a finding variously known as activated rigidity, or Froment's sign, or synkinesis (but note that both Froment's sign and synkinesis have other meanings too). However, this may occur in some normal subjects; it is most helpful in the diagnosis of Parkinson's disease if unilateral. Rigidity may also be demonstrated using Wartenberg's pendulum test.

Rigidity is a feature of parkinsonism and may co-exist with any of the other clinical features of extrapyramidal system disease, but particularly akinesia (akinetic-rigid syndrome); both are associated with loss of dopamine projections from the substantia nigra to the putamen. Rigidity is a feature of pathology within the basal ganglia.

The pathophysiology of rigidity is thought to relate to overactivity of tonic stretch reflexes in the spinal cord due to excessive supraspinal drive to spinal cord α-motor neurones following loss of descending inhibition as a result of basal ganglia dysfunction. In other words, there is a change in the sensitivity of the spinal interneurons, which control α-motor neurons, due to defective supraspinal control. Hence rigidity is a positive or release symptom, reflecting the operation of intact suprasegmental centres. The physiological correlate of this is the increased EMG activity found in rigid muscles with increased 1A afferent fibre activity, suggesting maintained α-γ linkage. In support of this, pyramidotomy has in the past been shown to produce some relief of rigidity.

Rigidity in Parkinson's disease may be lessened by treatment with levodopa preparations. The techniques of modern stereotactic neurosurgery may also be helpful, particularly stimulation of the subthalamic nucleus, although both thalamotomy and pallidotomy may also have an effect.

The term rigidity has also been used clinically in other ways, for example to describe:

- posturing associated with coma: decorticate or decerebrate, flexor and extensor posturing respectively;
- a lack of mental flexibility, particularly evident in patients with frontal lobe dysfunction.

References

Curra A, Agostino R, Berardelli A. Neurophysiology of Parkinson's disease, levodopa-induced dyskinesias, dystonia, Huntington's disease and myoclonus. In: Beal MF, Lang AE, Ludolph A, editors. Neurodegenerative diseases. Neurobiology, pathogenesis and therapeutics. Cambridge: Cambridge University Press; 2005. p. 227–50 [at 234–235].
Ghiglione P, Mutani R, Chiò A. Cogwheel rigidity. *Arch Neurol*. 2005; **62**: 828–30.
Meara RJ, Cody FWJ. Relationship between electromyographic activity and clinically assessed rigidity studied at the wrist joint in Parkinson's disease. *Brain*. 1992; **115**: 1167–80.

Cross References

Decerebrate rigidity; Decorticate rigidity; Froment's sign; Frontal lobe syndromes; Parkinsonism; Stiffness; Synkinesia, Synkinesis; Tremor; Wartenberg's pendulum test

Rindblindheit
- see CORTICAL BLINDNESS

Ring Scotoma
- see ANNULAR SCOTOMA; SCOTOMA

Rinne's Test
Rinne's test is one of the tuning fork tests (512 Hz fork preferred), which is used to define whether there is a conductive element to hearing loss. The patient is asked to compare the loudness of a vibrating tuning fork held at the external auditory meatus (air conduction; AC) with the loudness of the fork held against the mastoid process (bone conduction; BC); concurrent masking of the other ear, for example by rubbing the tragus, is advised. Normally air conduction is louder (AC > BC). If bone conduction sounds louder (BC > AC), then this is indicative of a conductive hearing loss. In sensorineural hearing loss, AC and BC are diminished to a similar extent, and air conduction remains louder (AC > BC).
Reference
Miyamoto RT, Wynne MK. Approach to the patient with hearing loss. In: Biller J, editors. Practical neurology. 2nd ed. Philadelphia: Lippincott Williams & Wilkins; 2002. p. 206–26.
Cross References
Schwabach test; Weber's test

Rising Sign
- see BABINSKI'S TRUNK-THIGH TEST

Risus Sardonicus
Risus sardonicus ("sardonic smile") due to spasm of the facial musculature is a classic feature of the neuromuscular syndrome of tetanus, now exceptionally rarely seen in developed nations. Risus sardonicus may also occur in the context of dystonia, more usually symptomatic (secondary) than idiopathic (primary) dystonia.
Cross References
Dystonia; Oromandibular dystonia; Spasm

Robot Syndrome
- see ATHYMHORMIA

"Rocket Sign"
The so-called "rocket sign" is a toppling backwards, after jumping to the feet from the sitting position, due to postural instability, seen in progressive supranuclear palsy (PSP) and ascribed to frontal lobe dysfunction. A history of falls due to postural instability in the first year after disease onset is one of the mandatory inclusion criteria for the diagnosis of PSP.
Cross References
Parkinsonism; "Wheelchair sign"

Roger's Sign
Roger's sign, or the numb chin syndrome, is an isolated neuropathy affecting the mental branch of the mandibular division of the trigeminal (V) nerve, causing pain, swelling, and numbness of the lower lip, chin and mucous membrane inside the lip. This is usually a sign of metastatic spread of cancer to the jaw, with poor overall prognsosis.

Hypoaesthesia involving the cheek, upper lip, upper incisors and gingiva, due to involvement of the infraorbital portion of the maxillary division of the trigeminal nerve ("numb cheek syndrome") is also often an ominous sign, resulting from recurrence of squamous cell carcinoma of the face infiltrating the nerve.
References
Acarin N. Roger's sign. Chin neuropathy. *Med Clin (Barc)*. 1985; **84**: 546.

Campbell WW Jr. The numb cheek syndrome: a sign of infraorbital neuropathy. *Neurology*. 1986; **36**: 421–3.
Kheder A, Hoggard N, Hickman SJ. Neurological red flag: the numb chin. *Pract Neurol*. 2014; **14**: 258–60.
Roger H, Paillas J. Le signe du mentonnier (parasthésie et anesthésie unilatérale) révélateur d'un processus néoplasique métastatique. *Rev Neurol (Paris)*. 1937; **2**: 751–2.

"Rolex" Sign
Apparent malfunction of self-winding (Rolex) watches, which depend on movement of the arm, may occur when they are worn on a hypokinetic, rigid arm; this may be the first sign of a parkinsonian syndrome.
Cross References
Parkinsonism; Wartenberg's pendulum test

Rombergism, Romberg's Sign
Romberg's sign is adjudged present (or positive) when there is a dramatic increase in unsteadiness, sometimes with falls, after eye closure in a patient standing comfortably (static Romberg's test). Before asking the patient to close his or her eyes, it is advisable to position ones arms in such a way as to be able to catch the patient should they begin to fall. Patients may fall forward immediately on eye closure ("sink sign"). These phenomena result from sensory ataxia (*i.e.* loss of proprioception from the feet), which occurs most commonly with posterior column spinal cord disease: Romberg's sign may be seen in tabes dorsalis.

A modest increase in sway on closing the eyes may be seen in normal subjects, and patients with cerebellar ataxia, frontal lobe ataxia, and vestibular disorders (toward the side of the involved ear); on occasion these too may produce an increase in sway sufficient to cause falls. Hence, Romberg's test is not specific. Posturography is an attempt to quantify the Romberg test.

Large amplitude sway without falling, due to the patient clutching hold of the physician, has been labelled "psychogenic Romberg's sign", an indicator of functional stance impairment.

Heel-toe (tandem) walking along a straight line is sometimes known as the dynamic Romberg's test.
References
Lanska DJ, Goetz CG. Romberg's sign: development, adoption, and adaptation in the 19th century. *Neurology*. 2000; **55**: 1201–6.
Schiffter R. Moritz Heinrich Romberg (1795–1873). *J Neurol*. 2010; **257**: 1409–10.
Cross References
Ataxia; Functional weakness and sensory disturbance; Howship-Romberg sign; Parry-Romberg syndrome; Proprioception; Tandem walking

Roos Test
Roos test, or the elevated arm stress test, may be helpful in the diagnosis of vascular thoracic outlet syndrome, along with Adson's test. The arm is held above the head with the elbow extended and the hand exercised. Development of numbness, pain and paraesthesia, along with pallor of the hand, supports the diagnosis of vascular thoracic outlet syndrome.
Cross Reference
Adson's test

Rooting Reflex
The rooting reflex is a turning of the head towards a tactile stimulus on the face or an object approaching the mouth, a normal response in infants which is lost during childhood. Its presence in adults is indicative of diffuse premotor frontal disease, this being a primitive reflex or frontal release sign.

Reference
Rossor M. Snouting, pouting and rooting. *Pract Neurol*. 2001; **1**: 119–21.
Cross References
Age-related signs; Frontal release signs; Primitive reflexes

Rosenbach's Sign
- see ABDOMINAL REFLEXES

Ross's Syndrome
- see HOLMES-ADIE PUPIL, HOLMES-ADIE SYNDROME

"Round the Clock" Weakness
- see SEQUENTIAL PARESIS

"Round the Houses" Sign
This name has been proposed for the inability of patients with progressive supranuclear palsy to produce pure vertical saccades along a straight line in the visual midline. Full vertical excursions are still present, but only accomplished by saccades moving the eyes in a lateral arc ("round the houses").
Reference
Quinn N. The "round the houses" sign in progressive supranuclear palsy. *Ann Neurol*. 1996; **40**: 951.

Roving Eye Movements
Roving eye movements consist of slow drifting movements of the eyes from side to side; the eyelids are closed and there may be slight divergence of the ocular axes. Roving eye movements may be seen in normal sleep, but also in comatose patients in whom they are indicative of an intact brainstem (*e.g.* the early diencephalic stage of central herniation) but are otherwise non-localising. As coma deepens, roving eye movements are lost before the movements provoked by the oculocephalic (doll's head) manoeuvre (oculocephalic reflexes, vestibulo-ocular reflexes), or the caloric tests. Roving eye movements cannot be mimicked, hence their presence excludes psychiatric coma or pseudocoma.
Reference
Posner JB, Saper CB, Schiff ND, Plum F. Plum and Posner's diagnosis of stupor and coma. 4th ed. Oxford: Oxford University Press; 2007. p. 70–1.
Cross References
Caloric testing; Coma; Vestibulo-ocular reflexes

Rubral Tremor
- see HOLMES' TREMOR; TREMOR

S

Saccades

Saccades, or saccadic eye movements, are rapid, ballistic, yoked movements of the eyes which bring the gaze to a new location in visual space. These movements may be performed voluntarily (tested clinically by asking the patient to "Look to your left, keeping your head still", *etc.*) or reflexively, *i.e.* in response to an object of potential interest within the visual field (tested clinically by asking the patient to shift gaze from one of examiner's hands to another). Internuclear ophthalmoplegia may be revealed when testing in this way for saccadic eye movements.

A number of parameters may be observed, including latency of saccade onset, saccadic amplitude, and saccadic velocity. An anti-saccadic task (*i.e.* suppression of saccades to a novel visual stimulus) may be used to assess ease of saccade suppression.

Of these indices, saccadic velocity is the most important in terms of localization value, since it depends on burst neurones in the brainstem (paramedian pontine reticular formation for horizontal saccades, rostral interstitial nucleus of the medial longitudinal fasciculus for vertical saccades). Assessment of saccadic velocity may be of particular diagnostic use in parkinsonian syndromes. In progressive supranuclear palsy slowing of vertical saccades is an early sign (suggesting brainstem involvement; horizontal saccades may be affected later), whereas vertical saccades are affected late (if at all) in corticobasal degeneration.

Saccade latency involves cortical and basal ganglia circuits. In corticobasal degeneration, increased saccade latency is the more typical finding, perhaps reflective of cortical involvement, than slow saccade velocity. Difficulty in initiating saccades may be described as ocular (motor) apraxia.

Saccde amplitude involves basal ganglia and cerebellar circuits. Saccadic hypometria, with a subsequent correctional saccade, may be seen in extrapyramidal disorders such as Parkinson's disease; saccadic hypermetria or overshoot may be seen in cerebellar disorders.

Anti-saccades involve frontal lobe structures. Anti-saccades may be poorly suppressed in Huntington's disease. In Alzheimer's disease, patients may make reflex saccades towards a target in an anti-saccadic task (visual grasp reflex).

References

Carpenter R. The saccadic system: a neurological microcosm. *Adv Clin Neurosci Rehabil.* 2004; **4**(1): 6–8.

Gaymard B, Pierrot-Deseilligny C. Neurology of saccades and smooth pursuit. *Curr Opin Neurol.* 1999; **12**: 13–9.

Leigh RJ, Riley DE. Eye movements in parkinsonism: it's saccadic speed that counts. *Neurology.* 2000; **54**: 1018–9.

Cross References

Internuclear ophthalmoplegia (INO); Ocular apraxia; Ocular flutter; Opsoclonus; Parkinsonism; Saccadic intrusion, Saccadic pursuit; Square-wave jerks

Saccadic Intrusion, Saccadic Pursuit

Saccadic intrusions are inappropriate saccades which interfere with visual fixation (static, or during motor pursuit: saccadic pursuit, broken pursuit). Several types of saccadic intrusion are described, including ocular flutter, opsoclonus, and square-wave jerks. Saccadic (cogwheel) pursuit is normal in infants and may be a non-specific finding in adults; however, it may be seen in Huntington's disease.

© Springer International Publishing Switzerland 2016
A.J. Larner, *A Dictionary of Neurological Signs*,
DOI 10.1007/978-3-319-29821-4_19

Cross References
Ocular flutter; Opsoclonus; Pursuit; Saccades; Saccadic intrusion, Saccadic pursuit; Square-wave jerks

Saccadomania
- see OPSOCLONUS

Sacral Sparing
Sacral sparing is the preservation of pain and temperature sensation in sacral dermatomes when there is sensory loss in the legs and trunk. This is a late, unusual, but diagnostic feature of a spinal cord lesion, usually an intrinsic (intramedullary) lesion but sometimes an extra-medullary compression. Spastic paraparesis below the level of the lesion due to corticospinal tract involvement is invariably present by this stage of sacral sparing.

Sacral sparing is explained by the lamination of fibres within the spinothalamic tract: ventrolateral fibres (of sacral origin), the most external fibres, are involved later than the dorsomedial fibres (of cervical and thoracic origin) by an expanding central intramedullary lesion (*e.g.* glioma, ependymoma, syringomyelia).

Although sacral sparing is rare, sacral sensation should always be checked in any patient with a spastic paraparesis.
Cross References
Dissociated sensory loss; Myelopathy; Paraparesis

Saddle Anaesthesia
- see ANAESTHESIA; CAUDA EQUINA SYNDROME

Saturday Night Palsy
- see WRIST DROP

Savant Syndrome
Savant syndrome, previously known as "idiot savant syndrome", refers to individuals with developmental learning disability yet displaying skills at a level inconsistent with their general intellectual functioning. The outstanding ability may be feats of memory (recalling names), calculation (especially calendar calculation), music, or artistic skills, often in the context of autism or pervasive developmental disorder. Obsolete classification of such abilities as super-lative technical skill, hypermnesia, "calculating idiots", and calendar artists has been super-seded by interest in how the disparities between these and general intellectual abilities come about, and whether this is some form of "release" phenomenon. Occasionally, skills such as artistic ability may emerge in the context of neurodegenerative disease (Alzheimer's disease, frontotemporal lobar degeneration).
References
Critchley M. The divine banquet of the brain and other essays. New York: Raven Press; 1979. pp. 172–7.
Hughes JR. The savant syndrome and its possible relationship to epilepsy. *Adv Exp Med Biol.* 2012; **724**: 332–43.
Treffert DA. Savant syndrome: realities, myths and misconceptions. *J Autism Dev Disord.* 2014; **44**: 564–71.

Scanning Speech
Scanning speech describes a motor speech disorder (*i.e.* a dysarthria) comprising slow, delib-erate, dysprosodic, monotonic verbal output. It may be confused with non-fluent aphasia (Broca's aphasia).

Scanning speech was originally considered a feature of cerebellar disease in multiple scle-rosis (after Charcot), and the term is often used with this implication. However, cerebellar disease typically produces an ataxic dysarthria (variable intonation, interruption between

syllables, "explosive" speech) which is somewhat different to scanning speech. Scanning speech correlates with midbrain lesions, often after recovery from prolonged coma.
Cross References
Asynergia; Aphasia; Broca's aphasia; Cerebellar syndromes; Dysarthria

Scapula Alata
- see WINGING OF THE SCAPULA

Schizophasia
This term has been used to describe the language disorder in schizophrenia, which may be characterised by paraphasias and neologisms, loose connections between thoughts, tangential thinking, and delusional intrusions. A formal analysis of schizophrenic patients' speech has suggested expressive semantic abnormality with spared naming. The resulting output may be unintelligible, and may resemble Wernicke's aphasia.
Reference
Oh TM, McCarthy RA, McKenna PJ. Is there a schizophasia? A study applying the single case approach to formal thought disorder in schizophrenia. *Neurocase*. 2002; **8**: 233–44.
Cross References
Delusion; Neologism; Paraphasia; Wernicke's aphasia

Schwabach Test
In the Schwabach test, a vibrating tuning fork is held against the patient's mastoid process, as in Rinne's test, until it is no longer audible. The examiner then places the tuning fork over his/her own mastoid, hence comparing bone conduction with that of the patient. If still audible to the examiner (presumed to have normal hearing), a sensorineural hearing loss is suspected, whereas in conductive hearing loss the test is normal.
Cross References
Rinne's test

Scoliosis
- see KYPHOSCOLIOSIS

Scotoma
A scotoma is a localised area of impaired vision within an otherwise normal visual field. Mapping of the defect may be performed manually by confrontation testing or by using an automated system. In addition to the peripheral field, the central field should also be tested, with the target object moved around the fixation point. A central scotoma may be picked up in this way, or a more complex defect such as a centrocaecal scotoma in which both the macula and the blind spot are involved. Infarction of the occipital pole will produce a central visual loss, as will optic nerve inflammation.

Scotomata may be absolute (no perception of form or light) or relative (preservation of form, loss of colour). Blindsight may fall into the latter category. A scotoma may be physiological, as in the blind spot or angioscotoma, or pathological, reflecting disease anywhere along the visual pathway from retina and choroid to visual cortex. Various types of scotoma may be detected:

- Central scotoma.
- Centrocaecal or caecocentral scotoma.
- Arcuate scotoma.
- Annular or ring scotoma.
- Junctional scotoma.
- Junctional scotoma of Traquair.
- Peripapillary scotoma (enlarged blind spot).

Cross References
Altitudinal field defect; Angioscotoma; Blindsight; Blind spot; Central scotoma, Centrocaecal scotoma; Hemianopia; Junctional scotoma, Junctional scotoma of Traquair; Maculopathy; Papilloedema; Quadrantanopia; Retinitis pigmentosa; Retinopathy; Visual field defects

Scratch Collapse Test
The scratch collapse test is a provocative test used to assess peripheral nerve compression, for example from entrapment in the carpal or cubital tunnel. The seated patient is asked to resist bilateral shoulder external rotation with elbows flexed; the area of suspected nerve compression is then lightly scratched, following which the resistance to external shoulder rotation is immediately retested. A momentary loss of shoulder external rotation resistance (*i.e.* "collapse") on the affected side is considered a positive test; the effect lasts only briefly.

References
Cheng CJ, Mackinnon-Patterson B, Beck JL, Mackinnon SE. Scratch collapse test for evaluation of carpal and cubital tunnel syndrome. *J Hand Surg*. 2008; **33**: 1518–24.
Sollero CE, Maranhao Filho P. Scratch collapse test: a new clinical test for peripheral nerve compression. *Arq Neuropsiquiatr*. 2015; **73**: 64.

Cross References
Tinel sign

"Scratch Test"
The "scratch test", or "direction of scratch" test, examines perception of the direction (up or down) of a scratch applied to the anterior shin (for example, with the sharp margin of a paper clip). It has been claimed as a reliable test of posterior column function of the spinal cord. Errors in this test correlate with central conduction times and vibration perception threshold.

References
Hankey GJ, Edis R. The utility of testing tactile perception of direction of scratch as a sensitive clinical sign of posterior column dysfunction in spinal cord disorders. *J Neurol Neurosurg Psychiatry*. 1989; **52**: 395–8.
Motoi Y, Matsumoto H, Kaneshige Y, Chiba S. A reappraisal of "direction of scratch" test: using somatosensory evoked potentials and vibration perception. *J Neurol Neurosurg Psychiatry*. 1992; **55**: 509–10.

Cross References
Proprioception; Vibration

Seborrhoea
Seborrhoea describes greasiness of the skin which may occur in extrapyramidal disorders, particularly Parkinson's disease.

Cross References
Parkinsonism

Seelenblindheit
- see VISUAL AGNOSIA

Seizures
Seizures are sudden, paroxysmal episodes of neurological dysfunction with or without impairment of consciousness, which may be epileptic (*i.e.* due to abnormal synchronous electrical activity within the brain, either focally or generally) or non-epileptic in origin ("pseudoseizures", non-epileptic attack disorder). The two varieties may co-exist. Seizure morphology may be helpful in establishing aetiology and/or focus of onset.

- *Epileptic*:

> Idiopathic generalised: tonic-clonic ("grand mal"); absence attack ("petit mal"); myoclonic epilepsy.
> Partial: simple (no impairment of consciousness), for example jerking of one arm, which may spread sequentially to other body parts (jacksonian march); or complex, in which there is impairment or loss of consciousness: may be associated with specific aura (olfactory, *déjà vu, jamais vu*) and/or automatisms (motor, *e.g.* cursive; or emotional, *e.g.* gelastic, dacrystic); limb posturing (salutatory, fencing posture) and pelvic thrusting may be seen in frontal lobe epilepsy. Secondary generalisation of seizures of partial onset may occur.

Investigation of partial seizures to exclude a symptomatic cause is recommended (MR imaging, EEG). Some are amenbale to surgical intervention. Otherwise, as for idiopathic generalised epilepsies, various anti-epileptic medications are available. Partial seizures may prove more resistant to treatment than generalised seizures.

- *Non-epileptic*:

> Often long lasting, thrashing, pelvic thrusting, carpet burns, eyes closed and resist opening, tongue biting rare, may have urinary incontinence; past history of physical or sexual abuse. Best treated with psychological approaches, or drug treatment of underlying affective disorders; anti-epileptic medications are best avoided.

The differentiation of epileptic from non-epileptic seizures may be difficult; it is sometimes helpful to see a video recording of the attacks, or to undertake in-patient video-telemetry.

Reference
Panayiotopoulos CP. A clinical guide to epileptic syndromes and their treatment: based on the ILAE classifications and practice parameter guidelines. 2nd ed. London: Springer; 2007.

Cross References
Absence; Aura; Automatism; *Déjà vu*; Fencer's posture, Fencing posture; Jacksonian march; *Jamais vu*; Pelvic thrusting; Urinary incontinence

Self-Mutilation
Self-injury to the point of mutilation, especially around the mouth, may be seen in certain neurological conditions, such as Lesch-Nyhan syndrome, Tourette syndrome, and neuroacanthocytosis.

Sensory Ataxia
- see ATAXIA; ROMBERGISM, ROMBERG'S SIGN

Sensory Loss
Sensory examination aims to determine the precise pattern of any sensory complaint, since specific patterns of sensory loss or impairment have localising value. (More details may be found in specific entries.)

Cross References
Balaclava helmet; Dermatomal sensory loss; Dissociated sensory loss; "Glove and stocking" sensory loss; Onion peel, Onion skin; Sacral sparing; Suspended sensory loss

Sensory Tricks
Sensory tricks, also known as *geste antagoniste* or sensory geste, consist of a tactile or proprioceptive stimulus, learned by the patient, which reduces or eliminates a dystonic posture, hence also known as a corrective gesture. For example, touching the chin, face or neck may

overcome cervical dystonia (torticollis), and singing may inhibit blepharospasm. Such tricks may also modify dystonic tremor. They are almost ubiquitous in sufferers of cervical dystonia and have remarkable efficacy. They are said to be absent in psychogenic dystonia.

The neurophysiological mechanisms underpinning sensory tricks are thought to involve a decrease in the abnormal facilitation which leads to dystonia.

Management of dystonic syndromes should include a search for possible sensory tricks.

References
Martino D, Liuzzi D, Macerollo A, Aniello MS, Livrea P, Defazio G. The phenomenology of the geste antagoniste in primary blepharospasm and cervical dystonia. *Mov Disord*. 2010; **25**: 407–12.
Poisson A, Krack P, Thobois S, et al. History of the "geste antagoniste" sign in cervical dystonia. *J Neurol*. 2012; **259**: 1580–4.
Ramos VF, Karp BI, Hallett M. Tricks in dystonia: ordering the complexity. *J Neurol Neurosurg Psychiatry*. 2014; **85**: 987–93.

Cross References
Blepharospasm; Dystonia; Reverse sensory geste; Torticollis

Sequential Paresis
Sequential, or "round the clock", paresis or weakness refers to the sequential development of weakness in one arm, the ipsilateral leg, the contralateral leg, and contralateral arm (*i.e.* hemiparesis, triparesis, tetra- or quadriparesis). This pattern is highly suggestive of a foramen magnum lesion, usually a tumour but sometimes demyelination or other intrinsic inflammatory disorder, sequentially affecting the lamination of corticospinal fibres in the medullary pyramids.

Cross References
Hemiparesis; Paresis; Quadriparesis, Quadriplegia

Setting Sun Sign
The setting sun sign, or sunset sign, consists of tonic downward deviation of the eyes with retraction of the upper eyelids exposing the sclera. There may be downbeating nystagmus. Setting sun sign is a sign of dorsal midbrain compression in children with untreated hydrocephalus.

A similar appearance may also be observed in progressive supranuclear palsy (Steele-Richardson-Olszewski syndrome; Stellwag's sign) and in Parinaud's syndrome, but without the tonic downward deviation.

Cross References
Lid retraction; Nystagmus; Parinaud's syndrome; Stellwag's sign

Shadowing
This describes a neurobehavioural disorder, occasionally seen in patients with dementia, in which the patient follows the spouse or carer around like a shadow.

Cross References
Dementia

Shin-Tapping
This describes a modification of the heel-knee-shin test or heel-shin test in which the heel is tapped repetitively on the shin before sliding it down to the foot, claimed to be a better test of motor co-ordination.

Reference
Fisher CM. An improved test of motor coordination in the lower limbs. *Neurology*. 1961; **11**: 335–6.

Cross References
Ataxia; Cerebellar syndromes; Heel-knee-shin test, Heel-shin test

Sialorrhoea

Sialorrhoea (drooling) is excessive salivation, possibly due to excess flow of saliva but more likely secondary to a reduced frequency of swallowing (*e.g.* in parkinsonian syndromes) or difficulty swallowing (*e.g.* motor neurone disease, developmental perisylvian syndrome). Metallic poisonings (mercury, bismuth, lead) may also produce marked salivation (ptyalism).

If troublesome, options for the treatment of sialorrhoea include hyoscine patches, amitriptyline, carbocisteine, and injections of botulinum toxin into the salivary glands. Anticholinergic agents may cause confusion in Parkinson's disease. In extreme cases, irradiation of the salivary glands has been used.

References

Hobson EV, McGeachan A, Al-Chalabi A, et al. Management of sialorrhoea in motor neuron disease: survey of current UK practice. *Amyotroph Lateral Scler Frontotemporal Degener.* 2013; **14**: 521–7.

Srivanitchapoom P, Pandey S, Hallett M. Drooling in Parkinson's disease: a review. *Parkinsonism Relat Disord.* 2014; **20**: 1109–18.

Tan EK. Botulinum toxin treatment of sialorrhoea: comparing different therapeutic preparations. *Eur J Neurol.* 2006; **13**(Suppl 1): 60–4.

Cross References

Bulbar palsy; Parkinsonism

Sighing

Occasional deep involuntary sighs may occur in multiple system atrophy. Sighing is also a feature, along with yawning, of the early (diencephalic) stage of central herniation of the brainstem with an otherwise normal respiratory pattern. Sudden inspiratory or expiratory sighs are said to be a feature of the hyperkinetic choreiform dysarthria characteristically seen in choreiform disorders such as Huntington's disease.

Reference

Quinn N. Multiple system atrophy. In: Marsden CD, Fahn S, editors. Movement disorders 3. Boston: Butterworth; 1994. pp. 262–81.

Cross References

Blinking; Dysarthria; Yawning

Signe D'applause

- see APPLAUSE SIGN

Signe De L'éventail (Fan Sign)

- see BABINSKI'S SIGN (1); PLANTAR RESPONSE

Signe De Rideau

Signe de rideau, or curtain sign, refers to the motion of the posterior pharyngeal wall toward the intact side, resembling the drawing of a curtain, in unilateral paresis of the superior pharyngeal constrictor muscle, as seen in unilateral vagus (X) nerve palsy.

Signe Du Journal

- see FROMENT'S SIGN

Simian Hand

Simian hand or ape hand has been used to describe the atrophy of the thenar eminence with recession of the metacarpal bones of the thumb to the plane of the other metacarpal bones, as seen in median nerve lesions in the axilla or upper arm.

Cross Reference

Benediction hand

Simian Posture
- see PARKINSONISM

Simultanagnosia
Simultanagnosia is impaired perception of multi-element or multipart visual displays, such that pictures are described in a piecemeal manner. Recognition of single objects is preserved; this is likened to having a fragment or island of clear vision which may shift from region to region. Two types of simultanagnosia are described:

- *Dorsal*:

  An attentional limitation preventing more than one object being seen at a time; although superficially similar to apperceptive visual agnosia, with which it has sometimes been classified, patients with dorsal simultanagnosia can recognise objects quickly and accurately, but unattended objects are not seen. There may be inability to localise stimuli even when they are seen, manifest as visual disorientation. Reading is severely impaired. Patients may grope, as though blind. Dorsal simultanagnosia is associated with bilateral posterior parieto-occipital lesions, and is one feature of Balint's syndrome.

- *Ventral*:

  A limitation in the number of objects which can be recognised in unit time, *i.e.* there is no primary recognition problem in that individual shapes can be recognised. Ventral simultanagnosia is most evident during reading which is severely impaired and empirically this may be the same impairment as seen in pure alexia; otherwise deficits may not be evident, unlike dorsal simultanagnosia. Ventral simultanagnosia may be a form of associative visual agnosia. It is associated with left inferior temporo-occipital cortical lesions.

References
Chechlacz M, Rothstein P, Hansen PC, Riddoch JM, Deb S, Humphreys GW. The neural underpinnings of simultanagnosia: disconnecting the visuospatial attention network. *J Cogn Neurosci*. 2012; **24**: 718–35.
Coslett HB, Saffran E. Simultanagnosia: to see but not two see. *Brain*. 1991; **114**: 1523–45.
Farah MJ. Visual agnosia: disorders of object recognition and what they tell us about normal vision. Cambridge: MIT Press; 1995.
Cross References
Agnosia; Alexia; Balint's syndrome; Visual agnosia; Visual disorientation

Singultus
- see HICCUPS

"Sink Sign"
- see ROMBERG'S SIGN, ROMBERGISM

Skew Deviation
Skew deviation, or the Hertwig-Magendie sign, is a supranuclear vertical misalignment of the visual axes; the final common efferent pathway for eye movements is spared (*cf.* hypertropia, hypotropia, due to ocular motor nerve palsies or extraocular muscle disease). This is thought to reflect damage to otolith-ocular pathways or vestibulo-ocular pathways. There may be concurrent ocular tilt reaction. Bielschowsky's head tilt test is usually negative (*cf.* ocular motor nerve palsies).

Skew deviation has been associated with posterior fossa lesions, from midbrain to medulla. Ipsiversive skew deviation (ipsilateral eye lowermost) has been associated with caudal pontomedullary lesions, whereas contraversive skew (contralateral eye lowermost) occurs with rostral pontomesencephalic lesions, indicating that skew type has localising value.

References

Hernowo A, Eggenberger E. Skew deviation: clinical updates for ophthalmologists. *Curr Opin Ophthalmol*. 2014; **25**: 485–7.

Wong AM. New understanding on the contribution of the central otolithic system to eye movement and skew deviation. *Eye*. 2015; **29**: 153–6.

Cross References

Bielschowsky's sign, Bielschowsky's test; Hypertropia; Hypotropia; Ocular tilt reaction; Tullio phenomenon

Slipping Slipper Sign

This term has been used to describe the inadvertent loss of a shoe (or slipper) whilst walking, occurring in the context of diabetic peripheral neuropathy. In a small study, the sign was not sensitive but had high specificity and positive predictive value for diabetic neuropathy.

Reference

Gayle KA, Tulloch-Reid MK, Wilks RJ, Ferguson TS. The slipping slipper sign: a simple test with high specificity and positive predictive value for peripheral neuropathy among diabetic patients. *Clin Pract*. 2012; **2**: e51.

Smile-Wink Phenomenon

This name has been given to narrowing of the palpebral fissure aggravated by smiling following a contralateral lenticulocapsular infarction. Dysarthria, facial paresis, hemiparesis with or without hemihypoaesthesia, and excessive laughing with or without crying, were common accompanying features in one series.

Reference

Kim JS. Smile-wink phenomenon: aggravated narrowing of palpebral fissure by smiling after lenticulocapsular stroke. *J Neurol*. 2001; **248**: 389–93.

Cross References

Dysarthria; Facial paresis, Facial weakness; Hemiparesis; Hypoaesthesia

Smooth Pursuit

- see PURSUIT

Snarling Facies

- see "MYASTHENIC SNARL"

Sneezing

Sneezing, or ptarmus, or sternutation, is a complex respiratory reflex. Sensory nasal trigeminal afferents run to a putative sneeze centre, localised to the brainstem based on lesions causing loss of sneezing following lateral medullary syndrome and medullary neoplasm. Integration of inputs in this centre reaches a threshold at which point an expiratory phase occurs with exhalation, forced eye closure and contraction of respiratory musculature.

Sneezing may also be triggered by the presence of light: photoptarmosis or the photic sneeze reflex. This may involve not only brainstem but also cortical centres, with increased sensitivity to visual stimuli in the visual cortex and coactivation of somatosensory areas.

References

Fiink JN. Localization of the "sneeze center". *Neurology*. 2001; **56**: 138

Hersch M. Loss of ability to sneeze in lateral medullary syndrome. *Neurology*. 2000; **54**: 520–1.

Langer N, Beeli G, Jancke L. When the sun prickles your nose: an EEG study identifying neural bases of photic sneezing. *PLoS One*. 2010; **5** :e9208.

Cross Reference

Lateral medullary syndrome

Snoring
Reduced muscle tone in the upper airway during sleep leads to increased resistance to the flow of air, and partial obstruction often results in loud snoring. This symptom may be associated with the obstructive sleep apnoea-hypopnoea syndrome (OSAHS), risk factors for which include obesity, alcohol overconsumption, and male sex. OSAHS may be associated with a variety of neurological symptoms including excessive daytime somnolence, episodic loss of consciousness, headache (especially morning), cognitive decline, and increased risk of stroke (snoring may be an independent risk factor for stroke).

References
Huang L, Quinn SJ, Ellis PDM, Ffowcs Williams JE. Biomechanics of snoring. *Endeavour*. 1995; **19**: 96–100.
Jordan AS, McSharryDG, Malhotra A. Adult obstructive sleep apnoea. *Lancet*. 2014; **383**: 736–7.
Lim R, Larner AJ. Obstructive sleep apnoea-hypopnoea syndrome presenting in the neurology clinic: a prospective 5-year study. *Int J Clin Pract*. 2008; **62**: 1886–8.

Cross Reference
Hypersomnolence

Snouting, Snout Reflex
Sometimes used interchangeably with pout reflex, this term should probably be reserved for the puckering or pouting of the lips induced by constant pressure over the philtrum, rather than the phasic response to a tap over the muscle with finger or tendon hammer.

Reference
Rossor M. Snouting, pouting and rooting. *Pract Neurol*. 2001; **1**: 119–21.

Cross References
Frontal release signs; Pout reflex; Primitive reflexes

Somatoparaphrenia
Somatoparaphrenia describes the patient's ascription of hemiplegic limb(s) to another person (*e.g.* the examiner, a family member). This may be a form of asomatognosia, or possibly a confabulation, or a delusional belief.

References
Beato R, Martins W, Nicolato A, Ulhoa TH, Oliveira MM, Avelar IF. Transitory somatoparaphrenia associated with a left frontoparietal meningioma. *J Neurol*. 2010; **257**: 1208–10.
Feinberg TE, Venneri A, Simone AM, Fan Y, Northoff G. The neuroanatomy of asomatognosia and somatoparaphrenia. *J Neurol Neurosurg Psychiatry*. 2010; **81**: 276–81.

Cross References
Anosognosia; Asomatognosia; Autotopagnosia; Confabulation; Delusion

Somatotopagnosia
- see AUTOTOPAGNOSIA

Spasm
The word spasm implies a sudden, involuntary, muscle contraction, which may be painful. Often there is a rapid crescendo over 1–2 s to maximum, followed by a slower decrescendo. For example, flexor spasms in patients with paraplegia due to upper motor neurone lesions are sudden contractions of the flexor musculature, particularly of the legs, either spontaneous or triggered by light touch. Hemifacial spasm is an involuntary contraction of facial musculature. Tonic spasms (paroxysmal dystonia) occur in multiple sclerosis.

Spasm may also refer to a tetanic muscle contraction (tetany), as seen in hypocalcaemic states (*e.g. main d'accoucheur*), tetanus (*e.g.* risus sardonicus), or tonic spasms of various muscles (*e.g.* jaw musculature, trismus) which may be dystonic or spastic in origin. Involuntary movements such as tics may be known as spasms or habit spasms.

Patients may use the word spasm differently, *e.g.* to denote paroxysmal sensory phenomena, or even epileptic seizures. Infantile seizures consisting of brief flexion of the trunk and limbs (emprosthotonos, salaam or jack-knife seizures) may be known as spasms.

Distinction may be drawn between spasms and cramps. The former are of CNS origin, involving groups of neighbouring muscles or becoming generalized, sponatenous, recurrent at regular or irregular intervals, often easily and reproducibly provoked by cutaneous stimulation. Cramps, in contrast, are peripherally generated and involve isolated muscles or parts thereof, and pain is a more prominent feature.

References
Meinck HM. Cramps, spasms, startles and related symptoms. In: Schmitz B, Tettenborn B, Schomer DL, editors. The paroxysmal disorders. Cambridge: Cambridge University Press; 2010. p. 130–44.
Rowland LP. Cramps, spasms, and muscle stiffness. *Rev Neurol (Paris)*. 1985; **141**: 261–73.
Cross References
Contracture; Cramp; Dystonia; Hemifacial spasm; *Main d'accoucheur*; Paraplegia; Quadriparesis, quadriplegia; Risus sardonicus; Seizures; Tic; Tonic spasms; Trismus

Spasmus Nutans
Spasmus nutans is the clinical triad of head nodding, anomalous head postures, and nystagmoid eye movements seen in children aged between about 1 and 8 years of age. This is usually a benign idiopathic condition, but the diagnosis should prompt consideration of an optic pathway tumour.
Reference
Kiblinger GD, Wallace BS, Hines M, Siatkowski RM. Spasmus nutans-like nystagmus is often associated with underlying ocular, intracranial, or systemic abnormalities. *J Neuroophthalmol.* 2007; **27**: 118–22.
Cross Reference
Nystagmus

Spastic Catch
- see SPASTICITY

Spasticity
Spasticity describes an increased resistance to the passive movement of a joint due to abnormally high muscle tone (hypertonus) which varies with the amplitude and speed of displacement of a joint (*cf.* rigidity). The excessive resistance evident at the extremes of joint displacement may suddenly give way, a phenomenon known as clasp-knife (or, confusingly, clasp-knife rigidity). Spasticity may vary in degree from mild, (*e.g.* a spastic catch on supination/pronation of the forearm), to extreme (*e.g.* immobile limbs in fixed flexion with secondary contractures and painful spasms: paraplegia in flexion). Spasticity may need to be differentiated clinically from rigidity and stiffness.

The amount and pattern of spasticity depends on the location of the lesion and tends to be greater with spinal cord than cortical lesions. Scales to quantitate spasticity are available (Ashworth, modified Ashworth, Wartenberg's pendulum test, the Tardieu Scale) but all have shortcomings. Spasticity may also vary in distribution: for lesions above the spinal cord it typically affects the arm flexors and the leg extensors to a greater extent (hemiparetic posture).

Spasticity is a clinical feature of the upper motor neurone syndrome, and may be accompanied by both positive (clonus, hyperreflexia, Babinski's sign, flexor or extensor spasms) and negative phenomena (weakness in a pyramidal distribution, motor underactivity): the latter may be more significant determinants of disability. Pain is often associated.

Slow, laboured speech, with slow voluntary tongue movements, may be referred to as spastic dysarthria, which may occur in the context of a pseudobulbar palsy.

The pathogenesis of spasticity has traditionally been ascribed to damage to the corticospinal and/or corticobulbar pathways at any level from cerebral cortex to spinal cord.

However, various lines of evidence (*e.g.* the failure of pyramidotomy to produce spasticity in animals, rare human cases of isolated pyramid infarction causing hyperreflexia and weakness without spasticity) have led to the implication of other motor tracts in the genesis of spasticity, *viz.*:

- the dorsal reticulospinal tract, which lies in the lateral funiculus of the spinal cord and hence is often damaged concurrently with the adjacent lateral corticospinal tract (*e.g.* in MS, which seems to have a predilection for the lateral funiculus); this descending pathway has an inhibitory effect on stretch reflexes which is under cortical control;
- the medial reticulospinal tract and vestibulospinal tracts which are not under cortical control and whose excitatory effects on extensor tone may remain unopposed.

Physiologically, spasticity has been characterized as an exaggeration of the muscle stretch reflexes, with reduced threshold (hyperexcitable α-motor neurones) and abnormal reflex transmission (increased gain), resulting in intermittent or sustained activation of muscles. The role of neurotransmitters (glutamate, glycine, catecholamines, serotonin) in the pathogenesis of spasticity is unclear, but the efficacy of baclofen (a GABA$_B$ agonist) and benzodiazepines suggest impaired GABAergic neurotransmission may contribute, perhaps through a loss of presynaptic inhibition mediated by interneurones or the inhibition of glutamate release.

Treatment of severe spasticity, for example in multiple sclerosis, often requires a multidisciplinary approach. Urinary infection, constipation, skin ulceration and pain can all exacerbate spasticity, as may inappropriate posture; appropriate management of these features may ameliorate spasticity. Drugs which may be useful include baclofen, dantrolene (a blocker of muscle excitation-contraction coupling), and tizanidine (α_2-adrenoreceptor agonist). Intrathecal baclofen given via a pump may also be of benefit in selected cases, and for focal spasticity injections of botulinum toxin may be appropriate. For painful immobile spastic legs with reflex spasms and double incontinence, irreversible nerve injury with intrathecal phenol or alcohol may be advocated to relieve symptoms. The place of cannabinoids has yet to be fully determined.

References

Haas J. Pathophysiology, assessment and management of multiple sclerosis spasticity: an update. *Expert Rev Neurother*. 2011; **11**(4 Suppl): 3–8.
Nair KPS, Marsden J. The management of spasticity in adults. *BMJ*. 2014; **349**: g4737.
Sheean G. Neurophysiology of spasticity. In: Barnes MP, Johnson GR, editors. Upper motor neurone syndrome and spasticity. Clinical management and neurophysiology. 2nd ed. Cambridge: Cambridge University Press; 2008. p. 9–63.

Cross References

Babinski's sign (1); Clasp-knife phenomenon; Clonus; Contracture; Dysarthria; Hyperreflexia; Hypertonia, Hypertonus; Paraplegia; Pseudobulbar palsy; Reflexes; Spasm; Tonic spasms; Upper motor neurone (UMN) syndrome; Wartenberg's pendulum test; Weakness

Speech Apraxia

Speech apraxia refers to a disorder of communication characterized by slow speech tempo ("groping for words"), impaired articulation of speech sounds, and dysprosody. More errors occur with increasing articulatory complexity (*e.g.* consonant clusters: bdk, bdk, bdk; *vs.* single consonants: b, d, k), and there is reduced articulatory agility. Automatic or reactive speech (*e.g.* expletives, clichés) is without error. This, or a very similar, constellation of features has also been known on occasion as cortical dysarthria, aphemia, or phonetic disintegration. There may be associated orofacial apraxia. The syndrome is thought to reflect disturbances of planning articulatory and phonatory functions.

Speech apraxia has been associated with inferior frontal dominant (left) hemisphere damage in the region of the lower motor cortex or frontal operculum; it has been claimed that involvement of the anterior insula is specific for speech apraxia.

When speech apraxia occurs in isolation, there is relatively intact language function and no dysgraphia. However, it is most often encountered as one feature of the syndrome of progressive non-fluent aphasia (the agrammatic variant of primary progressive aphasia) which may sometimes evolve to corticobasal degeneration.

References
Botha H, Duffy JR, Whitwell JL, et al. Classification and clinicoradiologic features of primary progressive aphasia (PPA) and apraxia of speech. *Cortex.* 2015; **69**: 220–36.
Dronkers NF. A new brain region for coordinating speech articulation. *Nature.* 1996; **384**: 159–61.

Cross References
Aphasia; Aphemia; Apraxia; Orofacial dyspraxia

Spinal Mass Reflex
The spinal mass reflex is involuntary flexion of the trunk in a comatose patient, such that they appear to be attempting to sit up ("rising from the dead").

Cross References
Coma; Lazarus sign; Spinal movements in brainstem death

Spinal Movements in Brainstem Death
Various reflex movements may be observed in patients with brainstem death, due to the absence of descending control of spinal cord neuronal networks. These spinal movements include:

- Flexor or extensor plantar responses
- Abdominal and cremasteric reflexes
- Tonic-neck reflexes
- Isolated jerks of the upper extremities
- Unilateral extension-pronation movements
- Asymmetric opisthotonic posturing of the trunk
- Undulating toe flexion sign
- Myoclonus
- Lazarus sign
- Head rotation
- Respiratory-like movements
- Quadriceps contraction
- Eye opening response
- Leg movements mimicking periodic leg movement
- Facial myokymia
- Spinal mass reflex

These movements do not necessarily invalidate a diagnosis of brainstem death.

Reference
Saposnik G, Basile VS, Young GB. Movements in brain death: a systematic review. *Can J Neurol Sci.* 2009; **36**: 154–60.

Cross References
Abdominal reflexes; Cremasteric reflex; Lazarus sign; Myoclonus; Myokymia; Opisthotonos; Plantar response

Spoonerisms
This term is used for a speech production disorder characterized by the transposition of consonants, so named for the mannerism affecting the speech of Reverend WA Spooner (1844–1930), sometime Warden of New College, Oxford. If not done deliberately, perhaps for the amusement of others, it presumably reflects a left hemisphere dysfunction in the appropriate sequencing of phonemes.

Reference
Mackay DG. Spoonerisms: the structure of errors in the serial order of speech. *Neuropsychologia*. 1970; **8**: 323–50.

Spurling's Sign
Spurling's sign may be used in the diagnosis of compressive cervical radiculopathy. It is judged present if there is increased arm pain (brachalgia) following neck rotation and flexion to the side of the pain (Spurling's neck compression test). A variant of this foraminal compression test involves rotation, side bend and slight extension of the neck with the application of axial pressure to the head.
Reference
Cook C, Cleland J, Huijbregts P. Creation and critique of studies of diagnostic accuracy: use of the STARD and QUADAS methodological quality assessment tools. *J Man Manip Ther*. 2007; **15**: 93–102 [at 95,98,100,101].
Cross Reference
Radiculopathy

Square-Wave Jerks
Square-wave jerks are small saccades which interrupt fixation, moving the eye away from the primary position and then returning. This instability of ocular fixation is a disorder of saccadic eye movements in which there is a saccadic interval (of about 200 ms; *cf.* ocular flutter, opsoclonus). Very frequent square-wave jerks may be termed square-wave oscillations. Very obvious square-wave jerks (amplitude > 7°) are termed macro-square-wave jerks.

Square-wave jerks are often best appreciated on ophthalmoscopy. Their name derives from the appearance they produce on electro-oculographic recordings.

Although square-wave jerks may be normal in elderly individuals, they may be indicative of disease of the cerebellum or brainstem, *e.g.* Huntington's disease, Parkinson's disease, progressive supranuclear palsy, cerebellar degeneration including multiple system atrophy. They have been reported to have close to 100% sensitivity for the diagnosis of PSP.
Reference
Otero-Millan J, Schneider R, Leigh RJ, Macknik SL, Martinez-Conde S. Saccades during attempted fixation in parkinsonian disorders and recessive ataxia: from microsaccades to square-wave jerks. *PLoS One*. 2013; **8**(3): e58535.
Cross References
Nystagmus; Ocular flutter; Opsoclonus; Saccades; Saccadic intrusion, Saccadic pursuit

Square-Wave Oscillations
- see SQUARE-WAVE JERKS

Squint
- see HETEROTROPIA

Stapedius Reflex
- see HYPERACUSIS

Stellwag's Sign
Stellwag's sign is a widening of the palpebral fissure due to upper eyelid retraction. Along with a reduced blink rate, this creates a very typical staring, "astonished", facies. The clinical phenomena of Stellwag's sign overlap with those labelled as the setting sun or sunset sign. Stellwag's sign is seen in progressive supranuclear palsy, and in dysthyroid eye disease.
Cross References
Blinking; Lid lag; Lid retraction; Setting sun sign

Steppage, Stepping Gait
Steppage or stepping gait occurs with a lower motor neurone type of foot drop ("floppy" foot drop), *e.g.* due to a common peroneal nerve palsy, or peripheral neuropathies. Because of the weakness of foot dorsiflexion (weak tibialis anterior) there is compensatory overaction of hip and knee flexors during the swing phase of walking to ensure the foot clears the ground (hence "high-stepping gait"). In the strike phase, there is a characteristic slapping down of the foot, again a consequence of weak ankle dorsiflexion. Proprioceptive loss, as in dorsal column spinal disease, may also lead to a gait characterized by high lifting of the feet, and also stomping (stamping with a heavily accented rhythm) or slapping of the foot onto the floor in the strike phase.

The pattern of gait with upper motor neurone foot drop ("stiff" foot drop), *e.g.* due to a corticospinal tract lesion, is quite different, with the foot being dragged, sometimes with circumduction of the leg. This may leads to falls as a consequence of tripping over the foot, especially on uneven ground or up-hill gradients, and a characteristic pattern of wear on the point of the shoe.

Cross References
Foot drop; Lower motor neurone (LMN) syndrome; Proprioception; Rombergism, Romberg's sign; Upper motor neurone (UMN) syndrome

Stereoanaesthesia
- see ASTEREOGNOSIS

Stereohypaesthesia
- see ASTEREOGNOSIS

Stereotyped Aphasia
- see RECURRENT UTTERANCES

Stereotypy
Stereotypies, or adventitious movements, may be defined as regular repeated movements, which are voluntary but not apparently goal-directed, and which may be carried out in a uniform pattern for long periods of time (*cf.* tic). Whole areas of the body may be involved by stereotypies and hence this movement is more complex than a tic. Examples include patting, tapping, rubbing, clasping, wringing, digit sucking, body or head rocking or banging, grimacing, smelling, licking, spitting, and mouthing of objects.

Stereotypies are common in patients with learning disability, autism, and schizophrenia. Very characteristic manual stereotypies (washing, rubbing movements: "hand washing") may be seen in Rett's disease. The term has also been used to describe movements associated with chronic neuroleptic use; indeed adult-onset stereotypy is highly suggestive of prior exposure to dopamine receptor blocking drugs. Stereotypies are also common in frontotemporal lobar degeneration syndromes, associated with a greater proportion of striatal volume loss to cortical volume loss than in those patients without stereotypies.

The recurrent utterances of global aphasia are sometimes known as verbal stereotypies or stereotyped aphasia. Reiterated words or syllables are produced by patients with profound non-fluent aphasia (*e.g.* Broca's original case, Leborgne, who could only repeat "tan, tan, tan", by which name he was known).

References
Jankovic J. Stereotypies. In: Marsden CD, Fahn S, editors. Movement disorders 3. Boston: Butterworth; 1994. p. 503–17.
Josephs KA, Whitwell JL, Jack CR Jr. Anatomic correlates of stereotypies in frontotemporal lobar degeneration. *Neurobiol Aging*. 2008; **29**: 1859–63
Lees AJ. Tics and related disorders. Edinburgh: Churchill Livingstone; 1985.
Cross References
Aphasia; Broca's aphasia; Recurrent utterances; Tic

Sternocleidomastoid Test

It has been reported that apparent weakness of the sternocleidomastoid muscle is common (80%) in functional hemiparesis, usually ipsilateral to the hemiparesis, whereas it is rare in hemiparesis of vascular origin (11%), presumably because of the bilateral innervation of the muscle.

Reference

Diukova GM, Stolajrova AV, Vein AM. Sternocleidomastoid (SCM) muscle test in patients with hysterical and organic paresis. *J Neurol Sci*. 2001; **187**(Suppl 1): S108.

Cross References

Functional weakness and sensory disturbance; Hemiparesis

Stethoscope Loudness Imbalance Test

- see HYPERACUSIS

Stewart-Holmes Sign

- see REBOUND PHENOMENON

Stiffness

Stiffness of muscles occurs as a feature of all pyramidal and extrapyramidal disorders (as spasticity and rigidity, respectively), but the term stiffness is usually reserved in clinical practice for disorders in which stiffness is the principal symptom due to continuous motor unit activity within muscles. There may be associated muscle pain (cramp). Stiffness may be primarily of muscular origin (myotonia) or of neural origin (myokymia, neuromyotonia). Accompanying signs may prove helpful in diagnosis, such as slow muscle relaxation (myotonia), percussion irritability of muscle (myoedema), and spontaneous and exertional muscle spasms. Hyperlordotic posture is typical of stiff man/stiff person syndrome (SPS). Late and missed diagnosis of SPS is well recognised, with functional disorders sometimes entering the differential diagnosis.

Stiffness must be differentiated from both rigidity and spasticity. Recognised causes of stiffness include:

- Stiff man/stiff person syndrome.
- Stiff limb syndrome.
- Progressive encephalomyelitis with rigidity +/− myoclonus.
- Neuromyotonia (Isaac's syndrome; armadillo syndrome; peripheral nerve hyperexcitability).
- Schwartz-Jampel syndrome (chondrodystrophic myotonia).
- Tetanus.
- Strychnine poisoning.

SPS is probably of autoimmune pathogenesis since it is strongly associated with insulin-dependent diabetes mellitus and the presence of antibodies to glutamic acid decarboxylase (anti-GAD antibodies), the rate-limiting enzyme in the synthetic pathway of GABA. Cases with antibodies to the $GABA_A$ receptor-associated protein and the glycine-alpha1 receptor are also reported, as are anti-amphiphysin antibodes in paraneoplastic cases associated with breast cancer. Intravenous immunoglobulin therapy may be of symptomatic benefit. Spontaneous remissions are unlikely, but long term survival is reported.

References

Baizabal-Carvallo JF, Jankovic J. Stiff-person syndrome: insights into a complex autoimmune disorder. *J Neurol Neurosurg Psychiatry*. 2015; **86**: 840–8.

Duddy ME, Baker MR. Stiff person syndrome. *Front Neurol Neurosci*. 2009; **26**: 147–65.

Cross References

Myokymia; Myotonia; Neuromyotonia; Paramyotonia; Rigidity; Spasticity

"Stops Walking When Talking"
First observed in patients with dementia who were unable to continue walking when a conversation was initiated, the "stops walking when talking" test or sign is a predictor of increased falls risk in older persons. It is essentially a dual-task testing paradigm, which reflects the interaction between gait and cognition.
References
Beauchet O, Annweiler C, Dubost V, et al. Stops walking when talking: a predictor of falls in older adults? *Eur J Neurol.* 2009; **16**: 786–95.
Lundin-Olsson L, Nyberg L, Gustafson Y. "Stops walking when talking" as a predictor of falls in elderly people. *Lancet.* 1997; **349**: 617.

"Stork Legs"
A name given to describe the disproportionate wasting of the lower legs, a pattern characteristic of hereditary motor and sensory neuropathies (Charcot-Marie-Tooth diseases), which may be evident even before the development of gait disorder with foot drop and steppage gait.
Cross References
Foot drop; Steppage, Stepping gait; Wasting

"Stork Manoeuvre"
The patient is asked to stand on one leg, with arms folded across chest, and the eyes open. Absence of wobble or falling is said to exclude a significant disorder of balance, or pyramidal lower limb weakness.

Strabismus
- see HETEROPHORIA; HETEROTROPIA

Straight Leg Raising
- see LASÈGUE'S SIGN

"Straight Thumb Sign"
Median nerve lesions in the forearm cause weakness of flexor pollicis longus, which normally flexes the distal phalanx of the thumb. Hence the thumb remains straight when the patient attempts to grasp something or make a fist. The "pinch sign" may also be present.
Reference
Cherington M. Anterior interosseous nerve syndrome straight thumb sign. *Neurology.* 1977; **27**: 800–1.
Cross Reference
"Pinch sign"

Striatal Hand
Striatal hand refers to an abnormal hand posture characterized by flexion of the metacarpophalangeal joints, extension of the proximal interphalangeal joints, flexion of the distal interphalangeal joints, and ulnar hand deviation, which causes altered dexterity, pain, and disfigurement. It is said to be 100% specific for Parkinson's disease.
References
Ashour R, Tintner R, Jankovic J. Striatal deformities of the hand and foot in Parkinson's disease. *Lancet Neurol.* 2005; **4**: 423–31.
Spagnolo F, Fichera M, Bucello S, et al. Striatal hand in Parkinson's disease: the re-evaluation of an old clinical sign. *J Neurol.* 2014; **261**: 117–20.

Striatal Toe
Striatal toe refers to the spontaneous tonic extension of the hallux which is seen in dystonic syndromes, and as a feature of extrapyramidal disorders, such as dopa-responsive dystonia. Striatal toe may be confused with Babinski's sign (extensor plantar response) and

pseudo-Babinski's sign (= "phasic striatal toe"), the principal difference being that both the latter are elicited by stimulation whereas the former is a sponatenous tonic response. It is found in advanced Parkinson's disease, and has been reported in association with an isolated lentiform nucleus infarct.

References
Ashour R, Tintner R, Jankovic J. Striatal deformities of the hand and foot in Parkinson's disease. *Lancet Neurol.* 2005; **4**: 423–31.
Kumar S, Reddy CR, Prabhakar S. Striatal toe. *Ann Indian Acad Neurol.* 2013; **16**: 304–5.

Cross References
Babinski's sign (1); Parkinsonism; Pseudo-Babinski's sign

String Sign
The string sign has been advocated as a way of testing visual field integrity in patients whose cooperation cannot be easily gained, by asking them to point quickly to the centre of a piece of string held horizontally in the examiner's hands. If visual fields are full, the patient will point to the approximate centre; if there is a left field defect, pointing will be to the right of centre, and vice versa for a right field defect. Altitudinal field defects may be similarly identified by holding the string vertically.

Reference
Ross RT. How to examine the nervous system. 4th ed. Totawa: Humana Press; 2006. p. 16.

Cross Reference
Visual field defects

Stupor
Stupor is a state of altered consciousness characterized by deep sleep or unresponsiveness, in which patients are susceptible to arousal only by vigorous and/or repeated stimuli, with lapse back into unresponsiveness when the stimulus stops. Stupor denotes a less severe impairment of conscious level than coma, but worse than obtundation (torpor). It is suggestive of diffuse cerebral dysfunction, *e.g.* drug-induced.

Reference
Posner JB, Saper CB, Schiff ND, Plum F. Plum and Posner's diagnosis of stupor and coma, 4th ed. Oxford: Oxford University Press; 2007.

Cross References
Coma; Delirium; Encephalopathy; Obtundation

Stutter, Stuttering
Stutter, one of the reiterative speech disorders, is usually a developmental problem, but may be acquired in aphasia with unilateral or bilateral hemisphere lesions (*e.g.* vascular damage, trauma, Alzheimer's disease, Parkinson's disease, progressive supranuclear palsy).

Unlike developmental stutter, acquired stutter may be evident throughout sentences, rather than just at the beginning. Furthermore, developmental stutter tends to occur more with plosives (phonemes where the flow of air is temporarily blocked and suddenly released, as in 'p', 'b'), whereas acquired stutter is said to affect all speech sounds fairly equally.

Onset of stutter after brain infarction (*e.g.* of the anterior corpus callosum) or traumatic injury is reported, as is cessation of developmental stutter following bilateral thalamic infarction in adult life. The basal ganglia likely play an important role in stutter pathogenesis, related to abnormal cueing for the initiation and termination of articulatory movements.

References
Craig-McQuaide A, Akram H, Zrinzo L, Tripoliti E. A review of brain circuitries involved in stuttering. *Front Hum Neurosci.* 2014; **8**: 884.
Lundgren K, Helm-Estabrooks N, Klein R. Stuttering following acquired brain damage: a review of the literature. *J Neurolinguistics.* 2010; **23**: 447–54.

Cross References
Aphasia; Echolalia; Palilalia

Sucking Reflex
Contact of an object with the lips will evoke sucking movements in an infant. The reflex may
re-emerge in patients with dementia.
Cross References
Akinetic mutism; Dementia; Frontal release signs

Summerskill's Sign
- see LID RETRACTION

"Sundowning"
"Sundowning", or sundown syndrome, is increased confusion, agitation or disorientation in
the late afternoon, evening, and night-time, which may be seen in patients with delirium, and
sometimes in dementia. In dementia, there may be complete reversal of sleep schedule with
daytime somnolence and nocturnal wakefulness. Diagnostic criteria to define the phenomenon do not currently exist.

   Although this syndrome may relate to worsening of visual cues with increasing darkness,
it may also occur in well-lit environments. A disorder of circadian rhythms is a possible physiological correlate of "sundowning": EEG recordings in delirious patients may suggest this.

   Suggested management for dementia patients with sundowning includes use of structured
activities at the relevant times (enforcement of external Zeitgebers), and increased staffing or avail-
ability of family members. Sedative medications, such as antipsychotics, are probably best avoided.
References
Bliwise DL. What is sundowning? *J Am Geriatr Soc*. 1994; **42**: 1009–11.
Gnanasekaran G. "Sundowning" as a biological phenomenon: current understandings and
future directions: an update. *Aging Clin Exp Res*. 2015; Aug 5 [Epub ahead of print].
Cross References
Delirium; Dementia

Sunset Sign
- see SETTING SUN SIGN

Suppression
- see EXTINCTION

Supranuclear Gaze Palsy
A supranuclear gaze palsy results from pathology located above the cranial nerve nuclei supplying the extraocular muscles. Voluntary gaze is impaired while the integrity of the oculomotor nuclei and infranuclear connections may be demonstrated by the preservation of:

- Vestibulo-ocular reflexes (VOR): overcoming the ophthalmoplegia, at least in the early stages
  (*e.g.* the supranuclear gaze palsy in the vertical plane in progressive supranuclear palsy).
- Oculocephalic reflex (doll's head, doll's eye manoeuvre).
- Bell's phenomenon.

   Supranuclear gaze palsies may be:

- *Horizontal*:
      Hemisphere (frontal) lesion: eyes deviated to the side of the lesion, or in the case of
      an irritative (*e.g.* epileptic) focus away from the side of the lesion.
      Paramedian pontine reticular formation: eyes deviated to contralateral side.

- *Vertical*:
      Brainstem compression/distortion.

Dorsal upper midbrain (*e.g.* rostral interstitial nucleus of the median longitudinal fasciculus; pineal lesion causing Parinaud's syndrome).

Skew deviation.

Recognised causes of supranuclear gaze palsy include:

- Progressive supranuclear palsy (PSP; Steele-Richardson-Olszewski syndrome).
- Creutzfeldt-Jakob disease.
- Corticobasal degeneration.
- Progressive subcortical gliosis of Neumann.
- Adult-onset Niemann-Pick disease.
- Gaucher's disease.

Reference
Lees AJ. The Steele-Richardson-Olszewski syndrome (progressive supranuclear palsy). In: Marsden CD, Fahn S, editors. Movement disorders 2. London: Butterworth; 1987. p. 272–87.
Cross References
Gaze palsy; Parinaud's syndrome; Parkinsonism; Prevost's sign; Skew deviation; Vestibulo-ocular reflexes

Surface Dyslexia
- see ALEXIA

Suspended Sensory Loss
Sensory loss or impairment involving the trunk and proximal limbs may be described as suspended, or in a "cape-like", "bathing suit", "vest-like", or cuirasse distribution. This may reflect intrinsic or intramedulary spinal cord pathology, in which case other signs of myelopathy may be present, including dissociated sensory loss, but it can also occur in peripheral neuropathic disease such as acute porphyria.
Cross References
Dissociated sensory loss; Myelopathy

"Swan Neck"
This term has been applied to thinning of the neck musculature, for example in myotonic dystrophy type 1.

Swearing
Swearing is not, *in sensu strictu*, a part of language, serving merely to add force of emotion to the expression of ideas; hence it is within the same category as loudness of tone, or violence of gesticulation. As for other prosodic elements of speech, it may be mediated by the non-dominant hemisphere. Swearing may be a feature of Tourette syndrome, and ictal swearing is also described.
Reference
Van Lancker D, Cummings JL. Expletives; neurolinguistic and neurobehavioral perspectives on swearing. *Brain Res Brain Res Rev*. 1999; **31**: 83–104.
Cross References
Coprolalia; Klazomania

Sweat Level
A definable sweat level, below which sweating is absent, is an autonomic change which may be observed below the level of a spinal cord compression.

Swinging Flashlight Sign

The swinging flashlight sign or test, originally described by Levitan in 1959, compares the direct and consensual pupillary light reflexes in one eye; the speed of swing is found by trial and error. Normally the responses are equal but in the presence of an afferent conduction defect an inequality is manifest as pupillary dilatation. The test is known to be unreliable in the presence of bilateral afferent defects of light conduction. Subjective appreciation of light intensity, or light brightness comparison, is a subjective version of this test.

References

Broadway DC. How to test for a relative afferent pupillary defect (RAPD). *Community Eye Health*. 2012; **25**: 58–9.

Thompson HS, Corbett JJ. Swinging flashlight test. *Neurology*. 1989; **39**: 154–6.

Cross References

Marcus Gunn pupil, Marcus Gunn sign; Pupilary reflexes; Relative afferent pupillary defect (RAPD)

Syllogomania

Syllogomania is excessive hoarding behavior, often contributing to domestic squalor, as seen in Diogenes syndrome.

Synaesthesia

Synaesthesia is a perceptual experience in one sensory modality following stimulation of another sensory modality. The most commonly encountered example is colour-word synaesthesia ("coloured hearing" or chromaesthesia), experiencing a visual colour sensation on hearing a particular word. Characteristics ascribed to synaesthetic experience include its involuntary or automatic nature, consistency, generic or categorical and affect-laden quality.

There may be concurrent excellent memory (hypermnesia), sometimes of a photographic nature (eidetic memory). Synaesthetes may demonstrate allochiria and finger agnosia.

Neuropsychologically synaesthesia has been conceptualized as a break down of modularity. Functional imaging studies of colour-word synaesthetes show activation of visual associative areas of cortex (but not primary visual cortex), as well as perisylvian language areas, when listening to words which evoke the experience of colour.

Symptomatic synaesthesia is rare but has been described with epileptic seizures of temporal lobe origin and with drug use (LSD).

Synaesthesia occurs in a small percentage of the normal population. Known synaesthetes include the composers Messiaen and Scriabin, the artist Kandinsky, and the author Nabokov.

References

Baron-Cohen S, Harrison JE, editors. Synaesthesia: classic and contemporary readings. Oxford: Blackwell; 1997.

Cytowic RE, Eagleman DM. Wednesday is indigo blue. Discovering the brain of synesthesia. Cambridge: MIT Press; 2011.

Dann KT. Bright colors falsely seen: synaesthesia and the search for transcendental knowledge. New Haven and London: Yale University Press; 1998.

Larner AJ. A possible account of synaesthesia dating from the seventeenth century. *J Hist Neurosci*. 2006; **15**: 245–9.

Ward J. The frog who croaked blue. Synesthesia and the mixing of the senses. London: Routledge; 2008.

Cross References

Allochiria; Auditory-visual synesthesia; Finger agnosia; Phosphene

Synkinesia, Synkinesis

The term synkinesis may be used in different ways:

- It may refer to involuntary movements which accompany or are associated with certain voluntary movements (*mitbewegungen*, motor overflow). These may be physiological, for example the swinging of the arms when walking. Alternatively, such associated phenomena may be pathological, *e.g.* the involuntary contraction of orbicularis oculi when opening the mouth (the Marin-Amat syndrome: inverse Marcus Gunn phenomenon), acquired after lower motor neurone facial (VII) nerve palsies and presumed to reflect aberrant reinnervation. Aberrant nerve regeneration is common to a number of synkinetic phenomena, such as elevation of a ptotic eyelid on swallowing (Ewart phenomenon) and upper eyelid elevation or retraction on attempted downgaze (pseudo-von Graefe's sign). Crocodile tears, or lacrimation when salivating, due to aberrant reinnervation following a lower motor neurone facial nerve palsy, may also fall under this rubric, although there is no movement *per se* (autonomic synkinesis), likewise gustatory sweating. Abnormal synkinesis may be useful in assessing whether weakness is organic or functional (*cf.* Hoover's sign).

- Synkinesis may also be used to refer to the aggravation of limb rigidity detected when performing movements in the opposite limb (*e.g.* clenching and relaxing the fist), also known as activated rigidity or Froment's sign.

Cross References
Crocodile tears; Ewart phenomenon; Froment's sign; Gustatory sweating; Hoover's sign; Jaw winking; Pseudo-von Graefe's sign; Rigidity

T

"Table Top" Sign

The "table top" sign describes the inability to place the hand flat on a level surface, recognised causes of which include ulnar neuropathy (*main en griffe*), Dupuytren's contracture, diabetic cheiroarthropathy, and camptodactyly.

Cross References

Camptodactyly; "Prayer sign"

Tachylalia

Tachylalia is increased speech velocity. This has been reported in patients with cerebrotendinous xanthomatosis, particularly in the 20–40 year age group.

Reference

Verrips A, Van Engelen B, de Swart B, et al. Increased speech rate (tachylalia) in cerebrotendinous xanthomatosis: a new sign. *J Med Speech-Lang Pathol*. 1998; **6**: 161–4.

Tachyphemia

Tachyphemia is repetition of a word or phrase with increasing rapidity and decreasing volume; it may be encountered as a feature of the speech disorders in parkinsonian syndromes.

Cross Reference

Parkinsonism

Tactile Agnosia

Tactile agnosia is a selective impairment of object recognition by touch despite (relatively) preserved somaesthetic perception. This is a unilateral disorder resulting from lesions of the contralateral inferior parietal cortex. Braille alexia may be a form of tactile agnosia, either associative or apperceptive.

References

Larner AJ. Braille alexia: an apperceptive tactile agnosia? *J Neurol Neurosurg Psychiatry*. 2007; **78**: 907–8.

Veronelli L, Ginex V, Dinacci D, Sappa SF, Corbo M. Pure associative tactile agnosia for the left hand: clinical and anatomo-functional correlations. *Cortex*. 2014; **58**: 206–16.

Cross Reference

Agnosia

Tadpole Pupils

Pupillary dilatation restricted to one segment may cause peaked elongation of the pupil, a shape likened to a tadpole's pupil. This has been recorded in Horner's syndrome, migraine, and Holmes-Adie pupil.

References

Koay KL, Plant G, Wearne MJ. Tadpole pupil. *Eye (Lond)*. 2004; **18**: 93–4.

Thompson HS, Zackon DH, Czarnecki JSC. Tadpole-shaped pupils caused by segmental spasm of the iris dilator muscle. *Am J Ophthalmol*. 1983; **96**: 467–477.

Talantropia

- see NYSTAGMUS

© Springer International Publishing Switzerland 2016
A.J. Larner, *A Dictionary of Neurological Signs*,
DOI 10.1007/978-3-319-29821-4_20

Tandem Walking
Tandem walking, or heel-toe walking, also known as the dynamic Romberg's test, is the ability to walk along a straight line placing one foot directly in front of the other, heel to toe, which may be likened to walking along a tightrope.

In ataxic disorders the ability to tandem walk is impaired, whether this is cerebellar (midline cerebellum, in which axial coordination is most affected) or sensory (loss of proprioception) in origin. Such patients tend to compensate for their incoordination by developing a broad based gait. A timed tandem walk has been advocated as an early marker of motor and cerebellar impairment in ambulatory patients with multiple sclerosis.
Reference
Stellmann JP, Vettorazzi E, Poettgen J, Heesen C. A 3 meter Timed Tandem Walk is an early marker of motor and cerebellar impairment in fully ambulatory MS patients. *J Neurol Sci.* 2014; **346**: 99–106.
Cross References
Ataxia; Cerebellar syndromes; Proprioception; Rombergism, Romberg's sign

Tasikinesia
Tasikinesia is forced walking as a consequence of an inner feeling of restlessness or jitteriness as encountered in akathisia. A neuroleptic-induced tasikinesia has been described.
References
Chokroverty S. Differential diagnosis of restless legs syndrome. In: Hening WA, Allen RP, Chokroverty S, Earley CJ, editors. Restless Legs Syndrome. Philadelphia: Saunders Elsevier; 2009. p. 111.
Freed ED. Neuroleptic-induced tasikinesia. *Med J Aust.* 1981; **2**: 517.
Cross Reference
Akathisia

Tay's Sign
- see CHERRY RED SPOT AT THE MACULA

Teichopsia
Meaning literally "town-wall vision", this term was coined by Airy in 1870 to describe the "bastioned form of transient hemiopsia [*sic*]" which he experienced as part of his own migraine attacks, and illustrated in his paper on the subject.
Reference
Airy H. On a distinct form of transient hemiopsia. *Philos Trans R Soc Lond.* 1870; **160**: 247–64.
Cross Reference
Fortification spectra

Telegraphic Speech
- see AGRAMMATISM

Teliopsia
Teliopsia or telopsia is a visual illusion in which the image is altered in position; the term may also be used to refer to the image appearing abnormally distant (*cf.* porropsia).
Cross References
Illusion; Metamorphopsia; Peliopsia; Porropsia

Temporal Crescent Syndrome
The temporal crescent, or "half moon", syndrome is a monocular visual field defect due to a contralateral anterior parieto-occipital sulcus lesion where the most nasal retinal fibres have an unpaired cortical representation. This is the only retro-chiasmal lesion to produce a

non-homonymous field defect. On testing to confrontation, there is a crescent-shaped restriction in the temporal field contralateral to the lesion, the ipsilateral field is normal.
Reference
Ali K. The temporal crescent syndrome. *Pract Neurol.* 2015; **15**: 53–5.
Cross Reference
Visual field defects

Temporal Desaturation
Temporal desaturation refers to impaired perception of red targets confined to the temporal visual hemifield. This may be the earliest indication of a developing temporal field defect, as in a bitemporal hemianopia due to a chiasmal lesion, or a monocular temporal field defect (junctional scotoma of Traquair) due to a distal ipsilateral optic nerve lesion.
Cross References
Hemianopia; Scotoma

Temporal Pallor
Pallor of the temporal portion of the optic nerve head may follow atrophy of the macular fibre bundle in the retina, since the macular fibres for central vision enter the temporal nerve head. This may be associated with impairment of central vision.
Cross Reference
Optic atrophy

Terson Syndrome
Terson syndrome referes to vitreous haemorrhage in association with any form of intracranial or subarachnoid haemorrhage. Patients with subarachnoid haemorrhage and Terson syndrome may have a worse prognosis.
Reference
Seif GI, Teichman JC, Reddy K, Martin C, Rodriguez AR. Incidence, morbidity, and mortality of Terson syndrome in Hamilton, Ontario. *Can J Neurol Sci.* 2014; **41**: 572–6.

Tetanus, Tetany
- see EMPROSTHOTONOS; *MAIN D'ACCOUCHEUR*; RISUS SARDONICUS; SPASM

Tetraparesis, Tetraplegia
- see QUADRIPARESIS, QUADRIPLEGIA

Threat Reflex
- see BLINK REFLEX

Thumb Reflex
The thumb reflex is a distal muscle stretch reflex which consists of flexion of the distal phalanx of the thumb when the tendon of flexor pollicis longus is tapped in the distal forearm held in the supinated position. It has been reported that, unlike more proximal reflexes, the thumb reflex is preserved in Guillain-Barré syndrome.
Reference
Naik KR, Saroja AO, Mahajan M. Intact thumb reflex in areflexic Guillain-Barré syndrome: a novel phenomenon. *Ann Indian Acad Neurol.* 2014; **17**: 199–201.
Cross Reference
Reflexes

Thumb Rolling Test
The thumb rolling test is a variant of the forearm rolling test for the detection of subtle upper motor neurone lesions, by rotating the thumbs around one another ("twiddling").

Reference
Nowak DA. The thumb rolling test: a novel variant of the forearm rolling test. *Can J Neurol Sci*. 2011; **38**: 129–32.
Cross References
Bed cycling test; Forearm and finger rolling; Upper motor neurone (UMN) syndrome

Tibialis Anterior Response
The tibialis anterior response or idiomuscular response describes the response to direct muscle percussion of the anterior tibialis muscle. In patients with bilateral lower limb weakness, brisk ankle dorsiflexion on percussion of tibialis anterior is said to be both sensitive and specific for acute inflammatory demyelinating polyneuropathy, whereas an inversion response was both sensitive and specific for an upper motor neurone lesion.
Reference
Lehn AC, Dionisio S, Airey CA, Brown H, Blum S, Henderson R. The tibialis anterior response revisited. *J Neurol*. 2014; **261**: 1340–3.
Cross Reference
Upper motor neurone (UMN) syndrome

Tic
A tic is an abrupt, jerky, repetitive movement involving discrete muscle groups, hence a less complex movement than a stereotypy. Vocal (phonic) tics are also described. Tics vary in intensity, lack rhythmicity, and are relatively easy to imitate. They may temporarily be voluntarily suppressed (perhaps accounting for their previous designation as "habit spasms") but this is usually accompanied by a growing inner tension or restlessness, only relieved by the performance of the movement. Indeed tic may be defined as a wilful capitulation to a premonitory involuntary inner urge, which sufferers may characterize as an itch or not feeling right (somatic hypersensitivity).

The pathophysiology of tics is uncertain. The belief that Tourette syndrome was a disorder of the basal ganglia has now been superseded by evidence of dysfunction within the cingulate and orbitofrontal cortex, perhaps related to excessive endorphin release. The aetiological differential diagnosis of tic includes:

* Idiopathic.
* Tourette syndrome.
* Tics related to structural brain damage.
* Drug-induced tics.
* Tics triggered by streptococcal infection.

Treatment of tics is most usually with dopamine antagonists (haloperidol, sulpiride, aripiprazole) and opioid antagonists (naltrexone); clonidine (central α_2 adrenergic receptor antagonist) and tetrabenazine (dopamine-depleting agent) have also been reported to be beneficial on occasion. Botulinum toxin injections and deep brain stimulation have also been tried.

The word tic has also been used to describe the paroxysmal, lancinating pains of trigeminal neuralgia (tic douloureux).
References
Bestha DP, Jeevarakshagan S, Madaan V. Management of tics and Tourette's disorder: an update. *Expert Opin Pharmacother*. 2010; **11**: 1813–22.
Lees AJ. Tics and related disorders. Edinburgh: Churchill Livingstone; 1985.
Martino D, Madhusudan N, Zis P, Cavanna AE. An introduction to the clinical phenomenology of Tourette syndrome. *Int Rev Neurobiol*. 2013; **112**: 1–33.
Yael D, Vinner E, Bar-Gad I. Pathophysiology of tic disorders. *Mov Disord*. 2015; **30**: 1171–8.
Cross References
Klazomania; Stereotypy

Tic Convulsif

Tic convulsif is a name that has been given to the combination of trigeminal neuralgia (tic douloureux) with hemifacial spasm. Both may be characterised as neurovascular compression syndromes.

Reference

Maurice-Williams RS. Tic convulsif: the association of trigeminal neuralgia and hemifacial spasm. *Postgrad Med J*. 1973; **49**: 742–5.

Cross Reference

Hemifacial spasm

"Tie Sign"

- see VISUAL DISORIENTATION

Tilted Disc

Tilted optic disc is a benign anomaly, causing the discs (it is usually bilateral) to look oval or lopsided, with a bitemporal superior visual field defect which does not respect the vertical midline.

Reference

Williams A. The tilted disc syndrome. *Pract Neurol*. 2005; **5**: 54–5.

Cross References

Bitemporal hemianopia; Visual field defects

Tilt Illusion

- see ENVIRONMENTAL TILT

Tinel's Sign (Hoffmann-Tinel Sign)

Tinel's sign (or Hoffmann-Tinel sign) is present when tingling (paraesthesia) is experienced when tapping lightly with a finger or a tendon hammer over a compressed or regenerating peripheral nerve. The tingling (Tinel's "sign of formication") is present in the cutaneous distribution of the damaged nerve ("peripheral reference").

Although originally described in the context of peripheral nerve regeneration after injury, Tinel's sign may also be helpful in diagnosing focal entrapment neuropathy such as carpal tunnel syndrome. However, it is a "soft" sign; like other provocative tests for carpal tunnel syndrome (*e.g.* Phalen's sign) it is not as reliable for diagnostic purposes as electromyography (EMG). Its specificity has been reported to range between 23 and 60% and sensitivity between 64 and 87%.

A "motor Tinel sign" has been described, consisting of motor EMG activity and jerking of muscles evoked by manipulation of an entrapped nerve trunk.

The neurophysiological basis of Tinel's sign is presumed to be the lower threshold of regenerating or injured (demyelinated) nerves to mechanical stimuli, which permits ectopic generation of orthodromic action potentials, as in Lhermitte's sign.

References

D'Arcy CA, McGee S. Does this patient have carpal tunnel syndrome? *JAMA*. 2000; **283**: 3110–7.

Hi ACF, Wong S, Griffith J. Carpal tunnel syndrome. *Pract Neurol*. 2005; **5**: 210–7.

Montagna P. Motor Tinel sign: a new localising sign in entrapment neuropathy. *Muscle Nerve*. 1994; **17**: 1493–4.

Pietrzak K, Grzybowski A, Kaczmarczyk J. Jules Tinel (1879–1952). *J Neurol*. 2016; **263**. (In press).

Cross References

Closed fist sign; Durkan's compression test; "Flick sign"; Hand elevation test; Lhermitte's sign; Phalen's sign; Pressure provocation test; Scratch collapse test

Tinnitus

Tinnitus is the perception of elementary non-environmental sound or noise in the ear. This is most usually a subjective phenomenon (*i.e.* heard only by the sufferer), occurring in the absence of acoustic stimulation. It may occur in conjunction with either conductive or sensorineural hearing loss. However, in about one-fifth of sufferers, tinnitus is objective (*i.e.* heard also by an observer). This may result from:

- vascular causes: *e.g.* arteriovenous malformation, fistula; carotid or vertebrobasilar bruit.
- mechanical causes: *e.g.* palatal myoclonus (ear click).

The common causes of subjective tinnitus are:

- middle/inner ear disease: cochlear hydrops (Ménière's disease), presbycusis, acoustic tumour.
- pulsatile: normal heartbeat, glomus jugulare tumour, raised intracranial pressure, cervical/intracranial aneurysm, arteriovenous malformation.

Cross References
Hallucination; Palatal myoclonus

"Tip-of-the-Tongue" Phenomenon
- see CIRCUMLOCUTION

Titubation
- see HEAD TREMOR

Todd's Paralysis, Todd's Paresis

Todd's paralysis (or Todd's paresis) is a transient localised weakness (usually hemiparesis), lasting seconds to minutes (exceptionally 24–48 h), observed following a focal motor epileptic seizure or Jacksonian seizure originating in the central motor strip, or febrile convulsion, a phenomenon first described by Robert Bentley Todd (1809–1860) in 1854. The pattern and duration of post-ictal signs is quite heterogeneous. Aphasia is also described. A postictal "paralytic" conjugate ocular deviation may be observed after adversive seizures. Todd's paresis is of localising value, being contralateral to the epileptogenic hemisphere.

The differential diagnosis of transient postictal hemiparesis includes stroke, hemiplegic migraine, and, in children, alternating hemiplegia.

References
Binder DK. A history of Todd and his paralysis. *Neurosurgery*. 2004; **54**: 480–6.
Kellinghaus C, Kotagal P. Lateralizing value of Todd's palsy in patients with epilepsy. *Neurology*. 2004; **62**: 289–91.
Rolak LA, Rutecki P, Ashizawa T, Harati Y. Clinical features of Todd's post-epileptic paralysis. *J Neurol Neurosurg Psychiatry*. 1992; **55**: 63–4.
Cross References
Hemiparesis; Seizures

Toe Walking

Toe walking, or cock walking, is walking on the balls of the toes, with the heel off the floor. A tendency to walk on the toes may be a feature of hereditary spastic paraplegia, and the presenting feature of idiopathic torsion dystonia in childhood.
Cross References
Dystonia; Paraplegia

Tongue Biting
Tongue biting is one feature of a seizure. In a generalised tonic-clonic epileptic seizure the side or sides of the tongue are typically bitten: a specific but not very sensitive sign. In a non-epileptic seizures the tip of the tongue may be more likely to be bitten.
Reference
Benbadis SR, Wolgamuth BR, Goren H, Brener S, Fouad-Tarazi F. Value of tongue biting in the diagnosis of seizures. *Arch Intern Med.* 1995; **155**: 2346–9.
Cross Reference
Seizure

Tonic Spasms
Painful tonic spasms occur in multiple sclerosis, especially with lesions of the posterior limb of the internal capsule or cerebral peduncle, perhaps due to ephaptic activation, or following putaminal infarction. Similar phenomena were also seen in tetanus.
References
Merchut MP, Brumlik J. Painful tonic spasms caused by putaminal infarction. *Stroke.* 1986; **17**: 1319–21.
Spissu A, Cannas A, Ferrigno P, Pelaghi AE, Spissu M. Anatomic correlates of painful tonic spasms in multiple sclerosis. *Mov Disord.* 1999; **14**: 331–5.
Cross Reference
Spasm

Topographagnosia
Topographagnosia or topographical disorientation describes the loss of the ability to make a correct representation of the surrounding environment, such that patients may become lost in previously familiar surroundings (sometimes known as "landmark agnosia"), including their own home. This form of visual agnosia is dissociable from prosopagnosia, and is often associated with non-dominant hemisphere occipito-temporal lesions.
Cross Reference
Agnosia; Prosopagnosia; Visual agnosia

Torpor
- see OBTUNDATION

Torticollis
Torticollis (also known as wryneck, cervical dystonia, nuchal dystonia, spasmodic torticollis) is a movement disorder characterized by involuntary contraction of neck musculature, involving especially sternocleidomastoid, trapezius, and splenius capitis. In the majority of cases (>50%) this produces head rotation, but laterocollis, retrocollis, tremulous ("no-no") and complex (*i.e.* variable) forms are seen; antecollis is unusual. Contractions are usually unilateral, may be associated with local pain. As with other types of dystonia, the movements may be relieved by a sensory trick (*geste antagoniste*). Recognised causes of torticollis include:

- Idiopathic (the majority).
- Secondary to acquired cervical spine abnormalities, trauma.
- Cervical spinal tumour.
- Tardive effect of neuroleptics.

The treatment of choice is botulinum toxin injections into the affected muscles. Injections benefit up to 70–80% of patients, but need to be repeated every 3 months or so.

Reference
Comella CL. Cervical dystonia. In: Warner TT, Bressman SB, editors. Clinical diagnosis and management of dystonia. Abingdon: Informa; 2007. p. 73–80.
Cross References
Antecollis; Dystonia; Laterocollis; Retrocollis; Sensory tricks

Tortopia
- see ENVIRONMENTAL TILT

Tourettism
- see TIC

Transcortical Aphasias
Transcortical aphasias may be categorised as either motor or sensory.

- *Transcortical motor aphasia (TCMA)*:

  There is a dissociation between preserved repetition (*cf.* conduction aphasia) and impaired fluency, manifest as delayed initiation, even mutism, impaired lexical selection, and reduced capacity to generate unconstrained syntactic forms. TCMA is associated with pathology (usually infarction) in the supplementary motor area, superior to Broca's area (left lateral frontal cortex) or in subcortical structures including white matter projections and dorsal caudate nucleus; it has clinical similarities with Broca's aphasia.
- *Transcortical sensory aphasia (TCSA)*:

  There is dissociation between preserved repetition (*cf.* conduction aphasia) and impairments of spoken and written language comprehension without phonemic paraphasia. TCSA is associated with pathology (usually infarction) in the ventral and ventrolateral temporal lobe involving the fusiform gyrus and the inferior temporal gyrus, and posterior convexity lesions involving the posterior middle temporal gyrus and the temporo-occipital junction. It has similarities with Wernicke's aphasia.

Some authorities prefer to label these conditions as "extrasylvian aphasic syndromes", to distinguish them from the perisylvian aphasic syndromes (Broca, Wernicke, conduction); moreover, these syndromes are not "transcortical" in any literal sense.

Dynamic aphasia may be a lesser version of TCMA, in which there are no paraphasias and minimal anomia, preserved repetition and automatic speech, but reduced spontaneous speech. This may be associated with lesions of dorsolateral prefrontal cortex ("frontal aphasia") in the context of frontal lobar degeneration. There may be incorporational echolalia, when the patient uses the examiner's question to help form an answer.
References
Alexander MP. Transcortical motor aphasia: a disorder of language production. In: D'Esposito M, editors. Neurological foundations of cognitive neuroscience. Cambridge: MIT Press; 2003. p. 165–74.
Boatman D, Gordon B, Hart J, Selnes O, Miglioretti D, Lenz F. Transcortical sensory aphasia: revisited and revised. *Brain*. 2000; **123**: 1634–42.
Cross References
Aphasia; Broca's aphasia; Conduction aphasia; Dynamic aphasia; Echolalia; Paraphasia; Wernicke's aphasia

Transverse Smile
- see "MYASTHENIC SNARL"

Tremblement Affirmatif, Tremblement Negatif
- see HEAD TREMOR

Tremor
Tremor is an involuntary movement, roughly rhythmic and sinusoidal, although some tremors (*e.g.* dystonic) are irregular in amplitude and periodicity. Tremors may be classified clinically:

- *Rest tremor*:

    is present when a limb is supported against gravity and there is no voluntary muscle activation, *e.g.* the 3.5–7 Hz "pill rolling" hand tremor of Parkinson's disease; midbrain/rubral tremor.
- *Action tremor*:

    is present during any voluntary muscle contraction.
    Various subtypes of action tremor are recognised:

- *Postural tremor*:

    this is present during voluntary maintenance of a posture opposed by gravity, *e.g.* arm tremor of essential tremor; 6 Hz postural tremor sometimes seen in Parkinson's disease ("re-emergent tremor"), which may predate emergence of akinesia/rigidity/ rest tremor; modest postural tremor of cerebellar disease; some drug-induced tremors (including alcohol withdrawal, delirium tremens); tremor of IgM paraprotein-aemic neuropathy; wing-beating tremor of Wilson's disease.
- *Kinetic tremor*:

    present with movement, often with an exacerbation at the end of a goal-directed movement (intention tremor), *e.g.* cerebellar/midbrain tremor (3–5 Hz).
- *Task-specific tremor*:

    evident only during the performance of a highly-skilled activity, *e.g.* primary writing tremor.
- *Isometric tremor*:

    present when voluntary muscle contraction is opposed by a stationary object, *e.g.* primary orthostatic tremor (14–18 Hz).
- *Psychogenic tremors*:

    these are difficult to classify, with changing characteristics; the frequency with which such tremors are observed varies greatly between different clinics; the co-activation sign (increase in tremor amplitude with peripheral loading) is said to be typical of psychogenic tremor. The entrainment test may be helpful in identifying psychogenic tremor.

Diagnosis of tremor is usually clinical. EMG may be useful for determining tremor frequency, but is only diagnostic in primary orthostatic tremor.

Various treatments are available for tremor, with variable efficacy. Essential tremor often responds to alcohol, and this is a reasonable treatment (previous anxieties that such a recommendation would lead to alcoholism seem unjustified); alternatives include propranolol, topiramate, primidone, alprazolam, flunarizine, and nicardipine. In Parkinson's disease, tremor is less reliably responsive to levodopa preparations than akinesia and rigidity; anticholinergics such as benzhexol may be more helpful but may cause confusion. Primary orthostatic tremor has been reported to respond to gabapentin, clonazepam, primidone, and levodopa. Cerebellar tremor is often treated with isoniazid, but seldom with marked benefit, likewise carbamazepine, clonazepam, ondansetron, limb weights. Stereotactic neurosurgery may be an option in some patients who are significantly disabled with tremor.

References
Bain PG, Findley LJ. Assessing Tremor Severity. London: Smith-Gordon; 1993.
Bhatia KP, Schneider SA. Psychogenic tremor and related disorders. *J Neurol*. 2007; **254**: 569–74.
Fasano A, Bove F, Lang AE. The treatment of dystonic tremor: a systematic review. *J Neurol Neurosurg Psychiatry*. 2014; **85**: 759–69.
Govert F, Deuschl G. Tremor entities and their classification: an update. *Curr Opin Neurol*. 2015; **28**: 393–9.
Cross References
Asterixis; Co-activation sign; Entrainment test; Head tremor; Holmes' tremor; Knee tremor; Palatal tremor; Parkinsonism; Vocal tremor, Voice tremor; Wing-beating tremor

Trendelenburg's Sign
Trendelenburg's sign is tilting of the pelvis toward the side of the unaffected raised leg in a unilateral superior gluteal nerve lesion.

Trick Manoeuvres
- see SENSORY TRICKS, TORTICOLLIS

Triparesis
- see SEQUENTIAL PARESIS

Triplopia
Triplopia is seeing triple, a rare complaint, which may be due to oculomotor (III) nerve palsy, internuclear ophthalmoplegia and abducens (VI) nerve palsy. It may result from an unusual interpretation of abnormal eye movements
Reference
Keane JR. Triplopia: thirteen patients from a neurology inpatient service. *Arch Neurol*. 2006; **63**: 388–9.
Cross References
Abducens (VI) nerve palsy; Diplopia; Internuclear ophthalmoplegia (INO); Oculomotor (III) nerve palsy

Trismus
Trismus is an inability to open the jaw due to tonic spasm or contracture of the masticatory muscles, principally masseter and temporalis, effecting forced jaw closure ("lockjaw"). Recognised neurological causes and associations of trismus include:

- Dystonia of the jaw muscles (*e.g.* drug-induced dystonic reaction).
- Generalised tonic-clonic epileptic seizure.
- Neuromuscular diseases: polymyositis, tetanus, nemaline myopathy, trauma to the muscles of mastication, rabies, strychnine poisoning.
- Metabolic disorders: Gaucher's disease (type II).
- Central disorders: brainstem encephalopathy, multiple sclerosis, pseudobulbar palsy, stroke, traumatic brain injury.

It may also occur after jaw fractures, with infection in the pterygomandibular space, and following treatment of head and neck cancers.
Reference
Lai MM, Howard RS. Pseudobulbar palsy associated with trismus. *Postgrad Med J*. 1994; **70**: 823–4.
Cross References
Dystonia; Pseudobulbar palsy; Spasm; Tonic spasms

Trombone Tongue
Trombone tongue, or flycatcher tongue, refers to an irregular involuntary darting of the tongue in and out of the mouth when the patient is requested to keep the tongue protruded. This sign may be seen in choreiform movement disorders such as Huntington's disease and neuroacanthocytosis, and in tardive dyskinesia.

The term has also been used to describe repetitive protrusion-intrusion tongue movements in a patient with medullary compression at the craniovertebral junction.

Reference
Lee CH, Casey AT, Allibone JB, Chelvarajah R. Trombone tongue: a new clinical sign for significant medullary compression at the craniovertebral junction. Case report. *J Neurosurg. Spine*. 2006; **5**: 550–3.

Cross References
Chorea, Choreoathetosis; Impersistence; Milkmaid's grip

Trömner's Sign
Trömner's sign is flexion of the thumb and index finger in response to tapping or flicking the volar surface of the distal phalanx of the middle finger, held partially flexed between the examiner's finger and thumb. This is an alternative method to Hoffmann's sign ("snapping" the distal phalanx) to elicit the finger flexor response. As in the latter, it is suggestive of a corticospinal tract (upper motor neurone) lesion above C5 or C6 segments, especially if unilateral, although it may be observed in some normal individuals.

Reference
Chang CW, Chang KY, Lin SM. Quantification of the Trömner signs: a sensitive marker for cervical spondylotic myelopathy. *Eur Spine J*. 2011; **20**: 923–7.

Cross References
Hoffmann's sign; Upper motor neurone (UMN) syndrome

Trousseau's Sign
Trousseau described the signs and symptoms of tetany, including anaesthesia, paraesthesia, the *main d'accoucheur* posture, as well as noting that the latter could be reproduced by applying a bandage or inflating a cuff around the arm so as to impede circulation; the latter is now known as Trousseau's sign, and indicates latent tetany.

Trousseau also noted the concurrence of venous thrombosis and migrating thrombophlebitis with malignant disease, also referred to as Trousseau's sign or Trousseau's syndrome; this may present with cerebral venous thrombosis.

References
Pearce JMS. Armand Trousseau, physician and neurologist. In: Fragments of neurological history. London: Imperial College Press; 2003. p. 528–47.
Rehman HU, Wunder S. Trousseau's sign in hypocalcemia. *CMAJ*. 2011; **183**: E498.

Cross References
Achromatopsia; Chvostek's sign; *Main d'accoucheur*

Troxler Effect
The Troxler effect, first described in 1804, is a physiological sensory habituation phenomenon: a visual stimulus in peripheral vision fades and disappears following a few seconds of steady visual fixation, as conscious perception "fills in" the background, perhaps due to the closure of a thalamic sensory gating mechanism.

Tullio Phenomenon
The Tullio phenomenon is the experience of vestibular symptoms and signs (vertigo, nystagmus, oscillopsia, postural imbalance, ocular tilt reaction, +/− skew deviation) on exposure to high intensity acoustic stimuli. These sound-induced signs are presumed to reflect hyperexcitability of the normal vestibular response to sound, causing pathological stimulation of the

semicircular canals and/or otoliths. This unusual phenomenon may be associated with peri-lymph leaks or a defect in the capsule forming the roof of the anterior semicircular canal (superior semicircular canal dehiscence). The sound sensitivity is probably at the level of the receptors rather than the vestibular nerve.

Reference
Kaski D, Davies R, Luxon L, Bronstein AM, Rudge P. The Tullio phenomenon: a neurologically neglected presentation. *J Neurol*. 2012; **259**: 4–21.

Cross References
Nystagmus; Ocular tilt reaction; Oscillopsia; Skew deviation; Vertigo

"Tunnel Vision"
A complaint of "tunnel vision" may indicate constriction of the visual field. This may be observed with enlargement of the blind spot and papilloedema as a consequence of raised intracranial pressure or with a compressive optic neuropathy.

The normal visual field enlarges the further away from the eye a visual target used to map the field is held, a simple consequence of the optics of light, hence there is in fact physiological "funnel vision". In non-organic visual impairment, in contrast, the visual field stays the same size with more distant targets, so-called tunnel vision or tubular vision.

A tunnel vision phenomenon has also been described as part of the aura of seizures of anteromedial temporal and occipitotemporal origin. A closing in of vision may be described as a feature of presyncope.

Cross References
Aura; Blind spot; Hemianopia; Papilloedema; Visual field defects

Two-Point Discrimination
Two-point discrimination is the ability to discriminate two adjacent point stimuli (*e.g.* applied using a pair of calipers, or a two-point discriminator or aesthesiometer) as two rather than one. The minimum detectable distance between the points (acuity) is smaller on the skin of the finger tips (*i.e.* greater acuity) than, say, the skin on the back of the trunk. There is an age-dependent increase in two-point discrimination values.

Impairments of two-point discrimination may occur with peripheral neuropathies, such as diabetic polyneuropathy, and in dorsal column spinal cord lesions, in which proprioception (and possibly vibration) is also impaired. Cortical parietal lobe lesions may produce a cortical sensory syndrome of astereognosis, agraphaesthesia, and impaired two-point discrimination.

Reference
Van Nes SI, Faber CG, Hamers RM, et al. Revising two-point discrimination assessment in normal aging and in patients with polyneuropathies. *J Neurol Neurosurg Psychiatry*. 2008; **79**: 832–4.

Cross References
Age-related signs; Astereognosis; Graphaesthesia; Proprioception; Vibration

U

Uhthoff's Phenomenon

Uhthoff's phenomenon or symptom is the worsening of visual acuity ("amblyopia" in Uhthoff's 1890 description) with exercise in optic neuritis, reflecting the temperature sensitivity of demyelinated axons (*i.e.* reduced safety factor for faithful transmission of action potentials). The term has subsequently been applied to symptoms related to exercise and/or temperature in other demyelinated pathways. It has also been described in the context of other optic nerve diseases, including Leber's hereditary optic neuropathy, sarcoidosis and tumour.

Evidence suggesting that Uhthoff's phenomenon is associated with an increased incidence of recurrent optic neuritis, and may be a prognostic indicator for the development of multiple sclerosis, has been presented.

Uhthoff's phenomenon is often persistent after an episode of optic neuritis; recovery usually occurs within eight weeks. In those with Uhthoff's phenomenon, other non-visual heat-related phenomena are more common.

An inverse Uhthoff sign, improved vision with warming, has been described.

References

Fraser CL, Davagnanam I, Radon M, Plant GT. The time course and phenotype of Uhthoff phenomenon following optic neuritis. *Mult Scler*. 2012; **18**: 1042–4.

Grzybowski A, Pieniazek M, Justynska A. Wilhelm Uhthoff (1853–1927). *J Neurol*. 2015; **262**: 243–4.

Guthrie TC, Nelson DA. Influence of temperature changes on multiple sclerosis: critical review of mechanisms and research potential. *J Neurol Sci*. 1995; **129**: 1–8.

Uhthoff W. Untersuchungen uber die bei der multiplen Herdsklerose vorkommenden Augenstorungen. *Archiv für Psychiatrie und Nervenkrankheit*. 1890; **21**: 55–106. 303–410.

Cross References

Lhermitte's sign; Phosphene

Unterberger's Sign

Unterberger's sign, or Unterberger's stepping test, is said to examine the integrity of vestibulospinal connections and attempts to define the side of a vestibular lesion. The patient is asked to march on the spot with the eyes closed (*i.e.* proprioceptive and visual cues are removed) and the extent of rotation is recorded. It is said that the patient will rotate towards the side of a unilateral vestibular lesion (Unterburger's sign). However, few data on test validity have been published; one study reported that the test was not very useful, particularly in chronic, progressive, or partially compensated vestibular lesions.

Reference

Hickey SA, Ford GR, Buckley JG, Fitzgerald O'Connor AF. Unterberger stepping test: a useful indicator of peripheral vestibular dysfunction?. *J Laryngol Otol*. 1990; **104**: 599–602.

Cross References

Proprioception; Vertigo

Upbeat Nystagmus

- see NYSTAGMUS

© Springer International Publishing Switzerland 2016
A.J. Larner, *A Dictionary of Neurological Signs*,
DOI 10.1007/978-3-319-29821-4_21

"Upgoing Thumb Sign"
Hachinski noted that patients with corticospinal tract involvement of the upper limb display an "upgoing thumb sign" when asked to extend their arms with palms facing each other, a sign which he thought had similar significance to an upgoing toe (Babinski's sign) with corticospinal tract involvement of the lower limb. The exact status of this sign remains to be examined.
References
Hachinski V. The upgoing thumb sign. *Arch Neurol.* 1992; **49**: 346.
Van Gijn J. The Babinski sign: a centenary. Utrecht: Universiteit Utrecht; 1996. p. 83–4.
Cross References
Babinski's sign (1); Plantar response

Upper Motor Neurone (UMN) Syndrome
An upper motor neurone (UMN) syndrome constitutes a constellation of motor signs resulting from damage to upper motor neurone pathways, *i.e.* proximal to the anterior horn cell. These may be termed "pyramidal signs", constituting a "pyramidal syndrome", but since there are several descending motor pathways (*e.g.* corticospinal, reticulospinal, vestibulospinal), of which the pyramidal or corticospinal pathway is just one, "upper motor neurone syndrome" is preferable. "Long tract signs" may be a more accurate, if less precise, term, often used interchangeably with "pyramidal signs".

The syndrome may be variable in its clinical features but common elements, following the standard order of neurological examination of the motor system, include:

● *Appearance*:

usually normal, but there may be muscle wasting in chronic UMN syndromes, although this is usually not as evident as in lower motor neurone (LMN) syndromes; contractures may be evident in chronically spastic limbs.

● *Tone*:

hypertonus, with spasticity, clasp-knife phenomenon, and sustained clonus.

● *Power*:

weakness, often in a so-called pyramidal distribution (*i.e.* affecting extensors more than flexors in the upper limb, and flexors more than extensors in the lower limb); despite its clinical utility, the term pyramidal is, however, a misnomer (see Weakness).

● *Co-ordination*:

depending on the degree of weakness, it may not be possible to comment on the integrity of co-ordination in UMN syndromes; in a pure UMN syndrome co-ordination will be normal, but syndromes with both ataxia and UMN features do occur (*e.g.* spinocerebellar syndromes, ataxic hemiparesis syndromes). Loss of dexterity is part of the syndrome.

● *Reflexes*:

limb hyperreflexia, sometimes with additional reflexes indicative of corticospinal tract involvement (Hoffmann's sign, Trömner's sign, crossed adductor reflex); Babinski's sign (extensor plantar response); cutaneous reflexes (abdominal, cremasteric) are lost.

The most reliable ("hardest") signs of UMN syndrome are increased tone, clonus, and upgoing plantar responses. The most subtle (*i.e.* earliest) sign of UMN involvement is debated but may be pronator drift, or impaired forearm/finger/thumb rolling.

The clinical phenomena comprising the upper motor neurone syndrome may be classified as "positive" and "negative" depending on whether they reflect increased or decreased activity in neural pathways:

- *Positive*:

    Exaggerated stretch/tendon reflexes, flexor spasms.

    Clonus.

    Autonomic hyperreflexia.

    Contractures.

- *Negative*:

    Muscle weakness, pronator drift.

    Loss of dexterity

These features help to differentiate UMN from LMN syndromes, although clinically the distinction is not always easy to make: a "pyramidal" pattern of weakness may occur in LMN syndromes (*e.g.* Guillain-Barré syndrome) and acute UMN syndromes may transiently cause flaccidity and areflexia (*e.g.* "spinal shock").

Reference

Barnes MP, Johnson GR, editors. Upper motor neurone syndrome and spasticity. Clinical management and neurophysiology. 2nd ed. Cambridge: Cambridge University Press; 2008.

Cross References

Abdominal reflexes; Ataxic hemiparesis; Babinski's sign (1); Bed cycling test; Clasp-knife phenomenon; Clonus; Contracture; Cremasteric reflex; Forearm and finger rolling; Hoffmann's sign; Hyperreflexia; Hypertonia, Hypertonus; Lower motor neurone (LMN) syndrome; Pronator drift; Pseudobulabr palsy; Spasticity; Thumb rolling test; Trömner's sign; "Upgoing thumb sign"; Weakness

Urgency
- see URINARY INCONTINENCE

Urinary Incontinence

Urinary incontinence may result from neurological, as well as urological, disease. Neurological pathways subserving the appropriate control of micturition encompass the medial frontal lobes, a micturition centre in the dorsal tegmentum of the pons, spinal cord pathways, Onuf's nucleus in the spinal cord segments S2-S4, the cauda equina, and the pudendal nerves. Thus the anatomical differential diagnosis of neurological incontinence is broad. Moreover incontinence may be due to inappropriate bladder emptying or a consequence of loss of awareness of bladder fullness with secondary overflow.

Features of the history and/or examination may give useful pointers as to localisation. Incontinence of neurological origin is often accompanied by other neurological signs, especially if associated with spinal cord pathology (see Myelopathy). The pontine micturition centre lies close to the medial longitudinal fasciculus and local disease may cause an internuclear ophthalmoplegia. However, other signs may be absent in disease of the frontal lobe or cauda equina. Causes of urinary incontinence include:

- Idiopathic generalised epilepsy with tonic-clonic seizures; however, the differential diagnosis of "loss of consciousness with incontinence" also encompasses syncopal attacks with or without secondary anoxic convulsions, non-epileptic attacks, and hyperekplexia.
- Frontal lobe lesions: frontal lobe dementia; normal pressure hydrocephalus.

- Spinal cord pathways: urge incontinence of multiple sclerosis; loss of awareness of bladder fullness with retention of urine and overflow in tabes dorsalis.
- Sacral spinal cord injury; degeneration of the sacral anterior horn cells in Onuf's nucleus (multiple system atrophy).
- Cauda equina syndrome; tethered cord syndrome (associated with spinal dysraphism).
- Pelvic floor injury.

Neurogenic incontinence may be associated with urgency, which results from associated abrupt increases in detrusor pressure (detrusor hyperreflexia); this may be helped by anticholinergic medication (*e.g.* oxybutinin, tolterodine). In addition there may be incomplete bladder emptying, which is usually asymptomatic, due to detrusor sphincter dyssynergia; for post-micturition residual volumes of greater than 100 ml (assessed by in-out catheterisation or ultrasonography), this is best treated by clean intermittent self-catheterisation.

References
Fowler CJ. Investigaion of the neurogenic bladder. In: Hughes RAC, editor. Neurological Investigations. London: BMJ Publishing; 1997. p. 397–414.
Garg BP. Approach to the patient with bladder, bowel, or sexual dysfunction and other autonomic disorders. In: Biller J, editor. Practical neurology. 2nd ed. Philadelphia: Lippincott Williams & Wilkins; 2002. p. 366–76.

Cross References
Cauda equina syndrome; Dementia; Frontal lobe syndromes; Hyperekplexia; Internuclear ophthalmoplegia (INO); Myelopathy; Seizures; Urinary retention

Urinary Retention

Although urinary retention is often urological in origin (*e.g.* prostatic hypertrophy) or a side effect of drugs (*e.g.* with anticholinergic activity), it may have neurological causes. It may be a sign of acute spinal cord compression, with or without other signs in the lower limbs, or of acute cauda equina compression, for example with a central L1 disc herniation. Sometimes the level of the pathology is several segments above that expected on the basis of the neurological signs ("false localizing signs"). Loss of awareness of bladder fullness may lead to retention of urine with overflow.

A syndrome of urinary retention in young women has been described, associated with myotonic-like activity on sphincter EMG; this condition, known as Fowler's syndrome, may be associated with polycystic ovary disease and is best treated with clean intermittent self-catheterisation.

References
Aning JJ, Horsnell J, Gilbert HW, Kinder RB. Management of acute urinary retention. *Br J Hosp Med*. 2007; **68**: 408–11.
Osman NI, Chapple CR. Fowler's syndrome – a cause of unexplained urinary retention in young women? *Nat Rev Urol*. 2014; **11**: 87–98.

Cross References
Cauda equina syndrome; "False localising signs"; Myelopathy; Paraplegia; Radiculopathy; Urinary incontinence

Useless Hand of Oppenheim

The deafferented hand or arm is functionally useless, and manifests involuntary movements due to severe proprioceptive loss. This was first described in multiple sclerosis by Oppenheim in 1911, and reflects plaques in the dorsal root entry zone of the relevant spinal cord segment(s).

References
Coleman RJ, Russon L, Blanshard K, Currie S. Useless hand of Oppenheim – magnetic resonance imaging findings. *Postgrad Med J*. 1993; **69**: 149–50.
Oppenheim H. Discussion on the different types of multiple sclerosis. *BMJ*. 1911; **2**: 729–33.

Cross References
Proprioception; Pseudoathetosis; Pseudochoreoathetosis

Utilization Behaviour

Utilization behaviour describes a disturbed response to external stimuli, a component of the environmental dependency syndrome, in which seeing an object implies that it should be used. Two forms of utilization behaviour are described:

- *Induced*:

    when an item is given to the patient, or their attention is directed to it, *e.g.* handing them a pair of spectacles which they put on, followed by a second pair, which are put on over the first pair.

- *Incidental* or *Spontaneous*:

    when the patient uses an object in their environment without their attention being specifically directed towards it.

Another element of the environmental dependency syndrome which coexists with utilization behaviour is imitation behaviour (*e.g.* echolalia, echopraxia). Primitive reflexes and hypermetamorphosis may also be observed.

Utilization behaviour is associated with lesions of the frontal lobe, affecting the inferior medial area bilaterally. It has also been reported following paramedian thalamic infarction. One study found utilization behavior to be relatively common (by history) in frontotemporal dementia but it was not seen in Alzheimer's disease (as for imitation behaviour).

References

Ghosh A, Dutt A, Bhargava P, Snowden J. Environmental dependency behaviours in frontotemporal dementia: have we been underrating them? *J Neurol*. 2013; **260**: 861–8.

Lhermitte F. Human autonomy and the frontal lobes. Part II. Patient behaviour in complex and social situations: the "environmental dependency syndrome". *Ann Neurol*. 1986; **19**: 335–43.

Lhermitte F, Pillon B, Serdaru M. Human autonomy and the frontal lobes. Part I: imitation and utilization behaviour: a neuropsychological study of 75 patients. *Ann Neurol*. 1986; **19**: 326–34.

Schott JM, Rossor MN. The grasp and other primitive reflexes. *J Neurol Neurosurg Psychiatry*. 2003; **74**: 558–60.

Cross References

Automatic writing behaviour; Echolalia; Echopraxia; Frontal lobe syndromes; Hypermetamorphosis; Imitation behaviour; Primitive reflexes

V

Valsalva Manoeuvre

The Valsalva manoeuvre is a simple test of autonomically-mediated cardiovascular reflexes, comprising forced expiration against resistance ("straining"), followed by release of the resistance and completion of expiration. The first phase produces impaired cardiac filling due to impaired venous return as a consequence of elevated intrathoracic pressure, with a consequent fall in cardiac output and blood pressure which induces peripheral vasoconstriction (via sympathetic pathways) to maintain blood pressure. The second phase produces a transient overshoot in blood pressure as the restored cardiac output is ejected into a constricted circulation, followed by reflex slowing of heart rate (via parasympathetic pathways).

In autonomic (sympathetic) dysfunction, reflex vasoconstriction, blood pressure overshoot and bradycardia do not occur. The latter may be conveniently assessed by measuring R-R intervals in a prolonged ECG recording, an R-R interval ratio between the straining and release phases of less than 1.1 suggesting impaired baroreceptor response.

Cross Reference
Orthostatic hypotension

Vegetative States

Vegetative states are characterized by wakefulness with absent awareness. It is a state in which there is preserved capacity for spontaneous or stimulus-induced arousal, evidenced by the presence of sleep-wake cycles and a range of reflexive and spontaneous behaviours. However, there is complete absence of behavioural evidence for self- or environmental awareness. The term originated because of the preservation of vegetative (autonomic, respiratory) functions due to intact brainstem centres despite the loss of cognitive function due to neocortical damage (hence no awareness, response, or speech). Primitive postural and reflex limb movements may also be observed. It may also be known as the unresponsive wakefulness syndrome or the apallic syndrome.

Vegetative states may be seen after extensive ischaemic-hypoxic brain injury, for example following resuscitation after prolonged cardiac arrest, and need to be distinguished from coma, minimally conscious state, akinetic mutism, and the locked-in syndrome.

Persistent vegetative state (PVS) is defined by persistence of this state for >12 months (UK) or >6 months (USA) after brain trauma, or >6 months (UK) or >3 months (USA) following brain anoxia. The prognosis of PVS is poor, but occasional reports of very late recovery have appeared.

Experimental studies initially interpreted as showing evidence of retained capacity for covert cognition in patients with persistent vegetative state have been challenged.

References
Jennett B. The vegetative state. Medical facts, ethical and legal dilemmas. Cambridge: Cambridge University Press; 2002.
Jennett B, Plum F. Persistent vegetative state after brain damage. A syndrome in search of a name. *Lancet*. 1972; 1: 734–7.
Nachev P, Hacker PM. Covert cognition in the persistent vegetative state. *Prog Neurobiol*. 2010; **91**: 68–76.
Royal College of Physicians. Prolonged disorders of consciousness: national clinical guidelines. London: Royal College of Physicians; 2013. p. 3, 12.

Cross References
Akinetic mutism; Coma; Locked-in syndrome; Minimally conscious state

© Springer International Publishing Switzerland 2016
A.J. Larner, *A Dictionary of Neurological Signs*,
DOI 10.1007/978-3-319-29821-4_22   329

Venous Pulsation
- see RETINAL VENOUS PULSATION

Vernet's Syndrome
- see JUGULAR FORAMEN SYNDROME

Vertigo

Vertigo describes an illusion of movement, a sense of rotation or of tilt, causing a feeling of imbalance or dysequilibrium. It is a subtype of "dizziness', to be distinguished from the light-headedness of general medical conditions (vasovagal attacks, presyncope, cardiac dysrhythmias). Vertigo is often triggered by head movement and there may be associated autonomic features (sweating, pallor, nausea, vomiting). Vertigo may be horizontal, vertical or rotatory.

Pathophysiologically, vertigo reflects an asymmetry of signalling anywhere in the central or peripheral vestibular pathways. Clinically it may be possible to draw a distinction between central and peripheral lesions. In peripheral lesions there may be concurrent hearing loss and tinnitus, reflecting involvement of the vestibulocochlear (VIII) nerve. With central lesions there may be concurrent facial weakness (VII) and ipsilateral ataxia, suggesting a cerebello-pontine angle lesion, or diplopia, bulbar dysfunction and long tract signs suggesting an intrinsic brainstem lesion.

Peripheral vertigo tends to compensate rapidly and completely with disappearance of nystagmus after a few days, whereas central lesions compensate slowly and nystagmus persists. The clinical pattern of vertigo may gives clues as to underlying diagnosis:

Vertigo	Peripheral	Central
Acute	Labyrinthitis	
Prolonged, spontaneous	Otomastoiditis Vestibular neur(on)itis Labyrinthine concussion Isolated labyrinthine infarct Vestibular nerve section Drug-induced	Brainstem/cerebellum haemorrhage/infarct/ demyelination
Recurrent, episodic	Migraine Menière's disease (endolymphatic hydrops) Autoimmune inner ear disease (isolated, systemic) Perilymph fistula Epilepsy (rare)	Vertebrobasilar ischaemia (with associated features)
Positional	Benign paroxysmal positional vertigo (BPPV)	Fourth ventricle lesions: multiple sclerosis, Chiari malformation, brainstem/cerebellar tumours Spinocerebellar atrophy
Chronic	Vestibular decompensation/ failure	Neurological disorder Psychogenic

All patients with vertigo should have a Hallpike manoeuvre performed during the examination. Head impulse test may also be helpful to differentiate acute cerebellar strokes from vestibular neuritis.

Specific treatments are available for certain of these conditions. A brief course of a vestibular sedative (cinnarizine, Serc) is appropriate in the acute phase, but exercises to "rehabilitate" the semicircular canals should be begun as soon as possible in peripheral causes. In BPPV, most patients respond to the Epley manoeuvre to reposition the otoconia which are thought to cause the condition (canalolithiasis). Brandt-Daroff exercises are an alternative. Cawthorne-Cooksey exercises are helpful in vestibular decompensation or failure.

References

Bronstein AM, Lempert T. Dizziness: a practical approach to diagnosis and management. Cambridge: Cambridge University Press; 2007.

Cha YH. Migraine-associated vertigo: diagnosis and treatment. *Semin Neurol.* 2010; **30**: 167–74.

Chawla N, Olshaker JS. Diagnosis and management of dizziness and vertigo. *Med Clin N Am.* 2006; **90**: 291–304.

Macleod D, McAuley D. Vertigo: clinical assessment and diagnosis. *Br J Hosp Med.* 2008; **69**: 330–4.

Cross References

Ataxia; Caloric testing; Facial paresis, Facial weakness; Hallpike maneouvre, Hallpike test; Head impulse test; Hennebert's sign; Illusion; Nystagmus; Vestibulo-ocular reflexes

Vestibulo-Ocular Reflexes

The vestibulo-ocular reflexes (VOR) are a physiological mechanism to generate eye rotations that compensate for head movements, especially during locomotion, so stabilizing the retinal image on the fovea. VORs depend upon the integrity of the connections between the semicircular canals of the vestibular system (afferent limb of reflex arc) and oculomotor nuclei in the brainstem (efferent limb). Loss of vestibular function, as in acute bilateral vestibular failure, causes gaze instability due to loss of VORs, causing the symptom of oscillopsia when the head moves. As well as vestibular input, compensatory eye rotations may also be generated in response to visual information (pursuit-optokinetic eye movements) and neck proprioceptive information; anticipatory eye movements may also help stabilize the retinal image.

VORs are also useful in assessing whether ophthalmoplegia results from a supranuclear or infranuclear disorder, since in the former the restriction of eye movement may be overcome, at least in the early stages, by the intact VOR, *e.g.* the supranuclear gaze palsy in the vertical plane in progressive supranuclear palsy.

VORs are difficult to assess in conscious patients because of concurrent pursuit-optokinetic eye movements, and because rotation of the head through large angles in conscious patients leads to interruption of VORs by vestibular nystagmus in the opposite direction (optokinetic nystagmus). The head impulse test may be used to test VORs in conscious patients, for example those with vertigo in whom vestibular failure is suspected. VOR may also be assessed using a slow (0.5–1.0 Hz) doll's head manoeuvre whilst directly observing the eyes ("catch up" saccades may be seen in the absence of VOR), or by measuring visual acuity (dynamic visual acuity, or illegible E test; dropping two to three lines on visual acuity with head movement *vs.* normal if VOR impaired), and by ophthalmoscopy (optic disc moves with head if VOR abnormal).

In unconscious patients, slow phase of the VORs may be tested by rotating the head and looking for contraversive conjugate eye movements (oculocephalic responses, doll's head eye movements) or by caloric testing. VORs are lost in brainstem death.

Another important element of VOR assessment is suppression or cancellation of VOR by the pursuit system during combined head and eye tracking. VOR suppression may be tested by asking the patient to fixate on their thumbs with arms held outstretched whilst rotating at the trunk or sitting in a swivel chair. VOR suppression can also be assessed during caloric testing: when the nystagmus ceases with fixation, removal of the fixation point (*e.g.* with Frenzel's glasses) will lead to recurrence of nystagmus in normals but not in those with reduced or absent VOR suppression. VOR suppression is impaired (presence of nystagmus even with slow head movements) in cerebellar and brainstem disease.

References
Bronstein AM. Vestibular reflexes and positional manoeuvres. *J Neurol Neurosurg Psychiatry*. 2003; **74**: 289–93.
Leigh RJ, Brandt T. A reevaluation of the vestibulo-ocular reflex: new ideas of its purpose, properties, neural substrate, and disorders. *Neurology*. 1993; **43**: 1288–95.
Cross References
Caloric testing; Coma; Doll's eye manoeuvre, Doll's head manoeuvre; Hallpike maneouvre, Hallpike test; Head impulse test; Ocular tilt reaction; Oculocephalic response; Oscillopsia; Supranuclear gaze palsy; Vertigo

Vibration
Vibratory sensibility (pallesthesia) represents a temporal modulation of tactile sense. On this ground, some would argue that the elevation of vibration to a "sensory modality" is not justified. Vibratory sensibility is easily tested using a tuning fork (128 Hz). This assesses the integrity of rapidly adapting mechanoreceptors (Pacinian corpuscles) and their peripheral and central connections; the former consist of large afferent fibres, the latter of ascending projections in both the dorsal and lateral columns. The classification of both vibration and proprioception as "posterior column signs", sharing spinal cord and brainstem pathways, is common in neurological parlance (and textbooks) but questioned by some. Instances of dissociation of vibratory sensibility and proprioception are well recognised, for instance the former is usually more impaired with intramedullary myelopathies.

Decrease in sensitivity of vibratory perception (increased perceptual threshold) is the most prominent age-related finding on sensory examination, thought to reflect distal degeneration of sensory axons.

References
Calne DB, Pallis CA. Vibratory sense: a critical review. *Brain*. 1966; **89**: 723–46.
Gilman S. Joint position sense and vibration sense. *J Neurol Neurosurg Psychiatry*. 2002; **73**: 473–7.
Wickremaratchi MM, Llewellyn JG. Effects of ageing on touch. *Postgrad Med J*. 2006; **82**: 301–4.
Cross References
Age-related signs; Myelopathy; Proprioception; Two-point discrimination

Visual Agnosia
Visual agnosia describes a disorder of visual object recognition. The term derives from Freud (1891), but it was Lissauer (1890), speaking of *seelenblindheit* (psychic blindness), who suggested the categorization into two types:

- *Apperceptive visual agnosia*:

    A defect of higher order visual perception leading to impaired shape recognition, manifested as difficulty copying shapes or matching shapes, despite preserved primary visual capacities, including visual acuity and fields (adequate to achieve recognition), brightness discrimination, colour vision and motion perception (indeed motion may facilitate shape perception; see Riddoch's phenomenon). Reading is performed with great difficulty, with a "slavish" tracing of letters which is easily derailed by any irrelevant lines; such patients may appear blind.

- *Associative visual agnosia*:

    An impairment of visual object recognition thought not to be due to a perceptual deficit, since copying shapes of unrecognised objects is good. The scope of this impairment may vary, some patients being limited to a failure to recognise faces (prosopagnosia) or visually presented words (pure alexia, pure word blindness).

These terms continue to be used, although some authors (*e.g.* Critchley) have taken the view that there is always some qualitative or quantitative disorder of sight (*i.e.* there is always a perceptual, as opposed to a gnostic, disorder), and hence that to isolate subtypes is a "vain pursuit".

Visually agnosic patients can recognise objects presented to other sensory modalities. Clinically, apperceptive visual agnosia may be said to lie between cortical blindness and associative visual agnosia.

Apperceptive visual agnosia results from diffuse posterior brain damage; associative visual agnosia has been reported with lesions in a variety of locations, usually ventral temporal and occipital regions, usually bilateral but occasionally unilateral. Pathological causes include cerebrovascular disease, tumour, degenerative dementia (visual agnosia may on occasion be the presenting feature of Alzheimer's disease, the so-called visual variant, or posterior cortical atrophy), and carbon monoxide poisoning. A related syndrome which has on occasion been labelled as apperceptive visual agnosia is simultanagnosia, particularly the dorsal variant in which there is inability to recognise more than one object at a time. Associative visual agnosia has sometimes been confused with optic aphasia.

References
Critchley M. The citadel of the senses and other essays. New York: Raven Press; 1986. p. 87, 236.
Farah MJ. Visual agnosia: disorders of object recognition and what they tell us about normal vision. Cambridge: MIT Press; 1995.
Riddoch MJ, Humphreys GW. Visual agnosia. *Neurol Clin.* 2003; **21**: 501–20.
Cross References
Agnosia; Alexia; Cortical blindness; Optic aphasia; Prosopagnosia; Riddoch's phenomenon; Simultanagnosia; Topographagnosia; Visual disorientation; Visual form agnosia

Visual Disorientation
Visual disorientation refers to the inability to perceive more than a fragment of the visual field at any one time; it is sometimes characterized as a shifting fragment or an island of clear vision. There may be difficulty fixating static visual stimuli and impaired visual pursuit eye movements.

Visual disorientation may be demonstrated by sitting directly opposite the patient and asking them, whilst looking at the bridge of the examiner's nose, to reach for the examiner's hand held up in the peripheral field of vision. Once contact is made with the hand, the examiner holds up the other hand in a different part of the field of vision. Individuals with visual disorientation will find it hard to see the hand and will grope for it, sometimes mistakenly grasping the examiner's clothing ("tie sign") or face.

Visual disorientation is secondary to, and an inevitable consequence of, the attentional disorder of dorsal simultanagnosia, in which the inability to attend two separate loci leads to impaired localization. It may be a feature of Alzheimer's disease; indeed, sometimes it may be the presenting feature, but there are usually signs of more generalized cognitive problems (*e.g.* impairment of episodic memory). Visual disorientation may be localizing to the non-dominant hemisphere.

References
Brain WR. Visual disorientation with special reference to lesions of the right cerebral hemisphere. *Brain.* 1941; **64**: 244–72.
Farah MJ. Visual agnosia: disorders of object recognition and what they tell us about normal vision. Cambridge: MIT Press; 1995.
Cross References
Simultanagnosia; Visual agnosia

Visual Extinction
Visual extinction is the failure to respond to a novel or meaningful visual stimulus on one side when a homologous stimulus is given simultaneously to the contralateral side (*i.e.* double simultaneous stimulation), despite the ability to perceive each stimulus when presented singly.
Cross References
Extinction; Neglect

Visual Field Defects
Visual fields may be mapped clinically by confrontation testing. Various methods are available to do this, including use of a small (5 mm) red pin (ubiquitous badge of office of neurologists of yore), a waggling finger, or a red laser pointer and a wall. Peripheral fields are tested by moving the target in from the periphery, and the patient is asked to indicate when the colour red/moving finger becomes detectable, not when they first see the pinhead/finger. The central field may be mapped using the same target presented statically to points within the central field. All these methods are insensitive, requiring a cooperative patient who can maintain fixation. Nevertheless, visual field defects may be detectable and so prompt further investigation as to cause.

The exact pattern of visual field loss may have localising value due to the retinotopic arrangement of fibres in the visual pathways: any unilateral area of restricted loss implies a pre-chiasmatic lesion (choroid, retina, optic nerve), although lesions of the anterior calcarine cortex can produce a contralateral monocular temporal crescent. Bilateral homonymous scotomata are post-chiasmal in origin; bilateral heteronymous scotomata may be seen with chiasmal lesions. Topographically, typical visual field defects are:

- Retina: monocular visual loss, altitudinal field defects; central or centrocaecal scotoma, arcuate scotoma, annular or ring scotoma.
- Optic nerve: central or centrocaecal scotoma, arcuate scotoma; junctional scotoma of Traquair.
- Optic chiasm: bitemporal hemianopia; junctional scotoma.
- Optic tract: homonymous hemianopia, usually incongruous.
- Lateral genciulate nucleus: homonymous hemianopia, usually incongruous.
- Optic radiations: homonymous hemianopia, usually congruous; quadrantanopia.
- Visual cortex: homonymous hemianopia, usually congruous; quadrantanopia; cortical blindness.

References
Cooper SA, Metcalfe RA. How to do it: assess and interpret the visual fields at the bedside. *Pract Neurol*. 2009; **9**: 324–34.
Kerr NM, Chew SS, Eady EK, Gamble GD, Danesh-Meyer HV. Diagnostic accuracy of confrontation visual field tests. *Neurology*. 2010; **74**: 1184–90.
Schiefer U. Visual field defects: essentials for neurologists. *J Neurol*. 2003; **250**: 407–11.
Stark R. Clinical testing of visual fields using a laser pointer and a wall. *Pract Neurol*. 2013; **13**: 258–9.
Cross References
Altitudinal field defect; Annular scotoma; Arcuate scotoma; Hemianopia; Junctional scotoma, Junctional scotoma of Traquair; Macula sparing, Macula splitting; Quadrantanopia; Scotoma; Temporal crescent syndrome; Tilted disc

Visual Form Agnosia
This name has been given to an unusual and highly selective visual perceptual deficit, characterised by loss of the ability to identify shape and form, although colour and surface detail can still be appreciated, but with striking preservation of visuomotor control (*i.e.* a pattern of deficits inverse to those seen in optic ataxia). This syndrome of loss of shape recognition but

with preserved vision to guide actions may reflect selective damage to the ventral ("what") stream of visual processing in the lateral occipital area, whilst the dorsal ("where") stream remains intact, yet the workings of the latter are not available to consciousness.

References

Bridge H, Thomas OM, Minini L, Cavina-Pratesi C, Milner AD, Parker AJ. Structural and functional changes across the visual cortex of a patient with visual form agnosia. *J Neurosci.* 2013; **33**: 12779–91.

Goodale MA, Milner AD. Sight unseen. An exploration of conscious and unconscious vision. Oxford, Oxford University Press; 2003.

Cross References

Agnosia; Optic ataxia; Visual agnosia

Visual Grasp Reflex

- see SACCADES

Visual Perseveration

Visual perseveration may refer to more than one (unusual) subjective visual experience:

- Hallucinatory and recurring appearance of an object after its removal: palinopsia (*q.v.*);
- Visual perseveration *in sensu strictu*, when a disappearing visual stimulus does not fade from view; no recurrence as in palinopsia;
- Visual stimulus sensed over an unduly extensive area of environmental space, also known as visuospatial perseveration or illusory visual spread; rare; no temporal factor, the effect disappears when the stimulus is removed.

References

Critchley M. The divine banquet of the brain and other essays. New York: Raven Press; 1979. p. 149–55.

Larner AJ. Illusory visual spread or visuospatial perseveration. *Adv Clin Neurosci Rehabil.* 2009; **9**(5): 14.

Cross References

Palinopsia; Perseveration

Visual Snow

Visual snow describes persistent positive visual symptoms characterised as tiny white dots throughout the visual field, likened to the noise of an analogue television screen. It may often be comorbid with migraine, and other visual phenomena such as palinopsia and nyctalopia. The pathophysiology remains to be explained.

References

Bessero AC, Plant GT. Should "visual snow" and persistence of after-images be recognised as a new visual syndrome? *J Neurol Neurosurg Psychiatry.* 2014; **85**: 1057–8.

Schankin CJ, Maniyar FH, Digre KB, Goadsby PJ. "Visual snow" – a disorder distinct from persistent migraine aura. *Brain.* 2014; **137**: 1419–28.

Cross References

Nyctalopia; Palinopsia

Visuopalpebral Reflex

- see BLINK REFLEX

Vocal Tremor, Voice Tremor

Vocal or voice tremor is a shaking, quivering, or quavering of the voice. It may be heard in:

- Essential tremor
- Cerebellar disorders
- Spasmodic dysphonia/laryngeal dystonia

- Parkinson's disease
- Motor neurone disease.

The pathophysiology is uncertain but may relate to rhythmic contractions of the crico-thyroid and rectus abdominis muscles.

Cross References
Dysphonia; Tremor

Von Graefe's Sign
Von Graefe's sign, or Graefe's sign, is the retarded descent of the upper eyelid during movement of the eye from the primary position to downgaze; the lid "follows" the eye. This may be termed "lid lag", although some authorities reserve this term for a static situation in which the lid is higher than the globe on downgaze. Von Graefe's sign may be seen in thyroid ophthalmopathy.

Cross References
Lid lag; Pseudo-von Graefe's sign

Vorbereiden
- see GANSER PHENOMENON, GANSER SYNDROME

VOR Suppression
- see VESTIBULO-OCULAR REFLEXES

Vulpian's Sign
- see PREVOST'S SIGN

W

Waddling Gait
Weakness of the proximal leg and hip girdle muscles, most often of myopathic origin, impairs the stability of the pelvis on the trunk during walking, leading to exaggerated rotation with each step, an appearance likened to the waddling of a duck. In addition, the hips may be slightly flexed and lumbar lordosis exaggerated. Neurogenic causes include spinal muscular atrophy and Guillain-Barré syndrome.
Cross Reference
Myopathy

"Waiter's Tip" Posture
Lesions of the upper trunk of the brachial plexus (Erb-Duchenne type) produce weakness and sensory loss in the distribution of C5 and C6 roots, typically with the arm hanging at the side, internally rotated at the shoulder with the elbow extended and the forearm pronated: the so-called "waiter's tip" posture, also sometimes known as the "porter's tip" or "policeman's tip".
Cross References
Plexopathy; Radiculopathy

Wallenberg's Syndrome
- see LATERAL MEDULLARY SYNDROME

Wall-Eyed
- see EXOTROPIA; INTERNUCLEAR OPHTHALMOPLEGIA (INO)

Warm-Up Phenomenon
The warm-up phenomenon describes the easing of muscle stiffness (*i.e.* normalized function) with repeated contraction or movement which is reported by many patients with myotonic syndromes such as myotonia congenita (Thomsen's disease, Becker's disease), in contrast to the situation in paramyotonia. This may be a reflection of the biophysical properties of the skeletal muscle voltage-gated sodium channel Nav 1.4 (gene name SCN4A), deficient conductance through which plays a role in some myotonic disorders.
Reference
Lossin C. Nav 1.4 slow-inactivation: is it a player in the warm-up phenomenon of myotonic disorders? *Muscle Nerve*. 2013; **47**: 483–7.
Cross References
Myotonia; Paramyotonia

Wartenberg's Pendulum Test
Wartenberg's pendulum test was originally developed to assess muscle tone in patients with Parkinson's disease, but it can be used to assess not only rigidity but also spasticity. In Wartenberg's original description (1951) the patient's leg, hanging freely from the knee, was lifted to the horizontal and then released to swing freely under the action of gravity. The swing pattern may be modified by reflex muscle activity (quadriceps stretch reflex). Other similar tests to assess tone include passive swinging of the wrist or elbow joint; or, with the patient standing, the examiner holds the shoulders and gently shakes backwards and forwards, the two sides out of phase. Normally the passive arm swing induced by this movement

will be out of phase with the trunk movements, but in rigidity the limbs and trunk tend to move *en bloc*.

Reference
Wartenberg R. Pendulousness of the legs as a diagnostic test. *Neurology*. 1951; **1**: 18–24.
Cross References
Parkinsonism; Rigidity; "Rolex" sign; Spasticity

Wartenberg's Sign (1)
In ulnar neuropathy, Wartenberg's sign refers to the slightly greater abduction of the fifth digit on the affected side, due to paralysis of the adducting palmar interosseous muscle and unopposed action of the radial-innervated extensor muscles (digiti minimi, digitorum communis).
Cross Reference
Froment's sign

Wartenberg's Sign (2)
- see CORNEOMANDIBULAR REFLEX

Wasting
Wasting refers to a thinning of the musculature, also known as atrophy or, if it is neurogenic, amyotrophy. Wasting may be a consequence of disorders of:

- muscle (myopathies, dystrophies).
- peripheral nerve (more so in axonal than demyelinating peripheral neuropathies).
- anterior horn cells (*e.g.,* motor neurone disease).

Wasting may occur in chronic upper motor neurone syndromes (*e.g.,* chronic hemiplegia) but is not as evident as in lower motor neurone syndromes where wasting may appear subacutely (over a few weeks).

Wasting may also be seen in general medical disorders associated with a profound catabolic state, *e.g.,* cancer cachexia, uncontrolled heart failure, liver cirrhosis, renal failure.
Cross References
Amyotrophy; Atrophy; Lower motor neurone (LMN) syndrome; Upper motor neurone (UMN) syndrome

Weakness
Weakness is an objective loss of muscle strength. This is conveniently quantified or rated using the MRC grading system:

- 5 = normal power
- 4 = active movement against gravity and resistance
- 3 = active movement against gravity
- 2 = active movement with gravity eliminated
- 1 = flicker or trace of contraction
- = no contraction (paralysis).

However, though ordinal, this is not a linear scale. Grade 4 is often subdivided by clinicians into 4−, 4, and 4+ (or even 5−) according to the increasing degree of resistance which the examiner must apply to overcome active contraction. Testing records only the best forced maximal contraction. Testing should not develop into an unseemly trial of strength between patient and examiner.

It is also important to assess what effort the patient is making to comply with the testing. Terms such as "apparent weakness" or "pseudoparesis" may be shorthand for lack of patient effort. Sudden "giving way" of muscle contraction may be an indicator of this. Non-uniform resistance may also be due to pain (algesic pseudoparesis). Accepting these difficulties, it should be acknowledged that the grading of weakness, like all clinical observations, is subject to some degree of observer bias.

The specific pattern of muscle weakness may suggest its anatomical origin (as for sensory loss). So-called "pyramidal weakness" (*i.e.,* affecting upper limb extensors more than flexors, and lower limb flexors more than extensors), suggests an upper motor neurone lesion (corticospinal pathways). However, there is no evidence that pure lesions of the pyramidal tracts produce this picture: pyramidotomy in the monkey results in a deficit in fine finger movements, but without weakness. Moreover, a similar pattern of weakness may be observed in lower motor neurone disorders such as Guillain-Barré syndrome. Coexistent wasting suggests muscle weakness is of lower motor neurone origin, especially if acute, although wasting may occur in long-standing upper motor neurone lesions. Weakness with minimal or no muscle wasting may be non-organic, but may be seen in conditions such as multifocal motor neuropathy with conduction block.

Reference
Aids to the examination of the peripheral nervous system. London: HMSO; 1976.

Cross References
Collapsing weakness; Hyperreflexia; Lower motor neurone (LMN) syndrome; Sensory loss; Upper motor neurone (UMN) syndrome; Wasting

Weber's Test
Weber's test is one of the tuning fork tests, which may be used to confirm a conductive component in unilateral or asymmetric hearing loss. The vibrating tuning fork (512 Hz preferred) is put on the middle of the forehead and the patient asked in which ear it is heard; this depends entirely upon bone conduction (BC). Hence the sound localises to the side of a conductive hearing loss (where bone conduction is greater than air conduction, BC > AC), and away from the side of a sensorineural hearing loss.

Reference
Miyamoto RT, Wynne MK. Approach to the patient with hearing loss. In: Biller J, editor. Practical neurology. 2nd ed. Philadelphia: Lippincott Williams & Wilkins; 2002. p. 206–26.

Cross Reference
Rinne's test

Wernicke's Aphasia
Wernicke's aphasia is the classical "receptive aphasia", in distinction to the "expressive aphasia" of Broca, although this terminology is problematic since there are concurrent "expressive" problems in Wernicke's aphasia (and "receptive" problems in Broca's aphasia). Other terms sometimes used for Wernicke-type aphasia are sensory aphasia or posterior aphasia.

Considering each of the features suggested for the clinical classification of aphasias (see Aphasia), Wernicke's aphasia is characterized by:

- *Fluency*: fluent speech with phonemic and semantic paraphasias and paragrammatism (inappropriate use of syntax); "empty speech" with few verbs and nouns; prosody usually preserved; at worst, flowing speech (logorrhoea) devoid of semantic meaning (jargon aphasia, semantic aphasia); automatic speech is often better preserved than spontaneous, *e.g.,* counting, days of week, overlearned phrases ("I'm fine").
- *Comprehension*: impaired auditory comprehension (*sine qua non*; "word deafness"); impaired reading comprehension probably also required (not specifically discussed by Wernicke).
- *Repetition*: impaired.
- *Naming*: severely impaired (anomia) and not aided by cueing (*cf.* Broca's aphasia).
- *Reading*: usually impaired, with numerous paralexic errors, and impaired reading comprehension (*cf.* pure word deafness).
- *Writing*: similarly affected.

There may be associated anxiety, with or without agitation and paranoia, and concurrent auditory agnosia. Because of a loss of self-monitoring of speech output, patients are often not aware of the impairment, and behavioural disturbance is sometimes misdiagnosed as "acute confusional state" and even referral or admission to psychiatric hospital may occur, particularly if there is no or minimal accompanying hemiparesis. The differential diagnosis of Wernicke's aphasia includes delirium and schizophasia.

The neuroanatomical substrate of Wernicke's aphasia has been a subject of debate. Wernicke placed it in the posterior two-thirds of the superior temporal gyrus and planum temporale (Brodmann area 22), but more recent neuroradiological studies (structural and functional imaging) suggest that this area may be more associated with the generation of paraphasia whereas more ventral areas of temporal lobe and angular gyrus (Brodmann areas 37, 39 and 40) may be associated with disturbance of comprehension. A correlation exists between the size of the lesion and the extent of the aphasia. A similar clinical picture may occur with infarcts of the head of the left caudate nucleus and left thalamic nuclei.

References

Binder JR. Wernicke aphasia: a disorder of central language processing. In: D'Esposito M, editor. Neurological foundations of cognitive neuroscience. Cambridge: MIT Press; 2003. p. 175–238.

Pillmann F. Carl Wernicke (1848–1905). *J Neurol*. 2003; **250**: 1390–1.

Robson H, Grube M, Lambon Ralph MA, Griffiths TD, Sage K. Fundamental deficits of auditory perception in Wernicke's aphasia. *Cortex*. 2013; **49**: 1808–22.

Wise RJS, Scott SK, Blank SC, Mummery CJ, Murphy K, Warburton EA. Separate neural subsystems within "Wernicke's area". *Brain*. 2001; **124**: 83–95.

Cross References

Agnosia; Agraphia; Alexia; Anomia; Aphasia; Broca's aphasia; Jargon aphasia; Logorrhoea; Paraphasia; Pure word deafness; Schizophasia; Transcortical aphasias

"Wheelchair Sign"

The so-called "wheelchair sign" describes patients with parkinsonism who start to use a wheelchair because of mobility problems early in the course of their disease, usually because of repeated falls. Early falls are a typical feature of progressive supranuclear palsy (Steele-Richardson-Olszewski syndrome), but not idiopathic Parkinson's disease or other parkinsonian syndromes.

Cross References

Parkinsonism; "Rocket sign"

Wilbrand's Sign

This name has sometimes been used to describe tracing the shape of letters with a finger to aid recognition in patients with pure alexia.

Reference

Allsion RS. The senile brain. A clinical study. London: Edward Arnold; 1962. p. 163.

Cross Reference

Alexia

Wing-Beating Tremor

Wing-beating tremor is absent at rest but develops when the arms are abducted, hence this is a postural tremor, of low-frequency and high amplitude, with flexed elbows and palms facing downwards. It is said to be typical of Wilson's disease (hepatolenticular degeneration) although can be seen with other conditions affecting the dentatorubrothalamic pathway (superior cerebellar peduncle), such as multiple sclerosis, stroke, or tumour.

Reference

Mahajan R, Zachariah U. Images in clinical medicine: Wing-beating tremor. *N Engl J Med*. 2014; **371**: e1.

Cross Reference

Tremor

Winging of the Scapula

Winging of the scapula, or scapula alata, is a failure to hold the medial border of the scapula against the rib cage when pushing forward with the hands. It is most easily observed by asking the patient to push or press against a wall or the examiner's hand whilst observing the scapula which lifts away from the posterior chest wall.

Winging of the scapula may be a consequence of weakness of the serratus anterior muscle, usually due to a neuropathy of the long thoracic nerve of Bell, but sometimes as a consequence of brachial plexus injury or cervical root (C7) injury. It may also be of myopathic origin, as in facioscapulohumeral muscular dystrophy.

Weakness of trapezius, particularly the middle trapezius muscle, may also cause winging of the upper part of the scapula, more prominent on abduction of the arm, when the superior angle of the scapula moves farther from the midline. Hence spinal accessory (XI) nerve palsy enters the differential diagnosis of scapular winging.

Witzelsucht

Witzelsucht, or the joking malady, refers to excessive and inappropriate facetiousness or jocularity, a term coined in the 1890s for one of the personality changes observed following frontal (especially orbitofrontal) lobe injury. This phenomenon may overlap with those described as moria or emotional lability. It may be seen in frontotemporal dementia.

Reference
Mendez MF. Moria and Witzelsucht from frontotemporal dementia. *J Neuropsychiatry Clin Neurosci*. 2005; **17**: 429–30.

Cross References
Emotionalism, Emotional lability; Frontal lobe syndromes; Moria

Woltman's Sign

Woltman's sign denotes slow-relaxing, or "hung-up", tendon reflexes. These are most commonly seen in the context of untreated hypothyroidism (myxoedema), but have also been recorded in other situations, including treatment with β-blockers, diabetes mellitus, and complete heart block. The phenomenon is sometimes labelled "pseudomyotonia" because of its superficial resemblance to the slow muscle relaxation of myotonia, but myotonic discharges are not seen on neurophysiological testing.

Chorea may result in apparently "hung-up" reflexes, perhaps due to a choreiform jerk after muscle relaxation.

The mechanisms underlying Woltman's sign are uncertain: changes in basal metabolic rate and in muscle fibre types (selective loss of fast twitch fibres) have been suggested.

References
Burkholder DB, Klaas JP, Kumar N, Boes CJ. The origin of Woltman's sign of myxedema. *J Clin Neurosci*. 2013; **20**: 1204–6.

Larner AJ. Normalisation of slow-relaxing tendon reflexes (Woltman's sign) after cardiac pacing for complete heart block. *Br J Clin Pract*. 1995; **49**: 331–2.

Todman D. Henry Woltman (1889–1964): pioneering American neurologist. *J Med Biogr*. 2008; **16**: 162–6.

Cross References
Chorea, Choreoathetosis; Myotonia; Pseudomyotonia

Word Blindness
- see ALEXIA

Word Deafness
- see PURE WORD DEAFNESS

"Wrestler's Sign"
This name has sometimes been applied to the excessive effort in irrelevant muscle groups accompanied by prominent non-verbal signs of effort such as grunting in patients with apparent ("functional") weakness. It may coexist with intermittent voluntary effort, collapsing weakness, co-contraction of agonist and antagonist muscles and inconsistency in clinical examination (*e.g.,* inability to lift leg from couch when recumbent, despite preserved ability to stand up and walk).
Cross References
Collapsing weakness; Functional weakness and sensory disturbance

Wrist Drop
Wrist drop describes a hand hanging in flexion due to weakness of wrist extension. This results from radial nerve palsy, located either in the axilla or the spiral groove of the humerus ("Saturday night palsy", although other nerves may also be compressed by hanging the arm over a chair, *e.g.,* ulnar, median). Distal radial nerve lesions affecting branches of the posterior interosseous branch may produce more circumscribed deformity, such as weak extension of metacarpophalangeal joints ("finger drop", "thumb drop").
Cross Reference
Neuropathy

Writer's Cramp
Writer's cramp, also known as graphospasm, *la crampe des écrivains,* or scrivener's palsy, is a focal dystonia involving the hand and/or arm muscles, causing abnormal posturing of the hand when writing; it is the most common of the task-specific dystonias (these were once known as "craft palsies"). When attempting to write, patients may find they are involuntarily gripping the pen harder, and there may also be involuntary movement at the wrist or in the arm. A tremor may also develop, not to be confused with primary writing tremor in which there is no dystonia. Handwriting becomes illegible. Attempts to use the contralateral hand may be made, but this too may become affected with time ("mirror dystonia"). The problem may be exclusive to writing (simple writer's cramp) but some people develop difficulties with other activities as well (*e.g.,* shaving; dystonic writer's cramp), reflecting a dystonia of the hand or arm. Muscle fatigue may make writing more legible. Familial forms may be associated with mutations in the epsilon sarcoglycan gene (DYT11). There may be an association between writer's cramp and carpal tunnel syndrome.

There is some neurophysiological evidence that the condition is due to abnormalities within the spinal cord segmental motor programmes and muscle spindle afferent input to them.

Writer's cramp may be amenable to treatment with local botulinum toxin injections into the hand or arm muscles responsible for the involuntary movement. Other strategies which may be used include writing with a different pen grip (*e.g.,* whole hand grip), using a fat-bodied pen, or using a word processor.
References
Jhunjhunwala K, Lenka A, Pal PK. A clinical profile of 125 patients with writer's cramp. *Eur Neurol.* 2015; **73**: 316–20.
Sheehy MP, Marsden CD. Writer's cramp – a focal dystonia. *Brain.* 1982; **105**: 461–80.
Cross References
Dystonia; Fatigue; Tremor

Wrong-Way Eyes
- see PREVOST'S SIGN

Wry Neck
- see TORTICOLLIS

X

Xanthopsia

Xanthopsia is a visual disturbance characterized by excessive perception of yellow colours (literally "yellow vision"). It may be associated with the use of various drugs including digoxin (especially if levels are toxic), thiazides (especially chlorothiazide), sulphonamides, and barbiturates. The mechanism is uncertain, but one possibility is that this is a partial form of achromatopsia, affecting one colour more than others. It has been suggested that the artist Vincent van Gogh (1853–1890) may have suffered from xanthopsia as a consequence of digitalis toxicity, accounting for the bright yellows in many of his later canvases, although documentary evidence is lacking.

References

Arnold WN, Loftus LS. Xanthopsia and van Gogh's yellow palette. *Eye (Lond)*. 1991; **5**: 503–10.

Critchley M. Acquired anomalies of colour perception of central origin. *Brain*. 1965; **88**: 711–24.

Cross References

Achromatopsia; "Monochromatopsia"

Xerophthalmia, Xerostomia

Xerophthalmia, dryness of the eyes, and xerostomia, dryness of the mouth, due to impaired secretion from the lacrimal glands and the salivary glands respectively, often occur together (sicca syndrome). This may reflect autonomic dysfunction, as for example in Lambert Eaton myasthenic syndrome, or be due to autoimmune disorders such as Sjögren's syndrome. Other causes of xerostomia include medications with anticholinergic properties (*e.g.,* amitriptyline), dehydration, diabetes, and radiotherapy for head and neck cancer. Xerophthalmia may result from vitamin A deficiency.

Reference

Visvanathan V, Nix P. Managing the patient presenting with xerostomia: a review. *Int J Clin Pract*. 2010; **64**: 404–7.

Cross References

Facilitation; Orthostatic hypotension

© Springer International Publishing Switzerland 2016
A.J. Larner, *A Dictionary of Neurological Signs*,
DOI 10.1007/978-3-319-29821-4_24

Y

Yawning

Yawning is an arousal reflex thought to be generated in the brainstem reticular formation to counteract brain hypoxia; it may precede vasovagal syncope.

Excessive or pathological yawning (chasm) is compulsive, repetitive yawning not triggered by physiological stimuli such as fatigue or boredom. Known associations of excessive yawning or salvos of yawning include:

- Presyncope.
- Hypoglycaemia.
- Drugs: SSRIs, imipramine, valproate, dopamine agonists.
- Migraine prodrome.
- Temporal lobe epileptic seizures.
- Encephalitis.
- Multiple sclerosis.
- Tumours of the 4th ventricle, frontal lobes.
- Electroconvulsive therapy.
- Post-thalamotomy.
- Neuroleptic withdrawal.
- Parkinson's disease, progressive supranuclear palsy, restless legs syndrome.
- Pseudobulbar palsy of motor neurone disease.

Although the mechanisms are uncertain, yawning may represent a disturbance of dopaminergic neurotransmission. Levodopa may help.

Reference

Walusinski O, editor. The mystery of yawning in physiology and disease. Basel: Karger; 2010.

Cross References

Parakinesia, Parakinesis; Parkinsonism; Sighing

Yips

Yips is the name given to a task-specific focal dystonia seen in golfers, especially associated with the action of putting or chipping.

References

Adler CH, Crews D, Hentz JG, Smith AM, Caviness JN. Abnormal co-contraction in yips-affected but not unaffected golfers: evidence for focal dystonia. *Neurology*. 2005; **64**: 1813–4.

Dhungana S, Jankovic J. Yips and other movement disorders in golfers. *Mov Disord*. 2013; **28**: 576–81.

Cross Reference

Dystonia

Yo-Yo-Ing

Yo-yo-ing is the name given to a form of dyskinesia experienced by patients with idiopathic Parkinson's disease who have been treated for several years with levodopa preparations, in which there are sudden and unpredictable swings between hypokinesia/akinesia ("off" state; freezing) and severe hyperkinesia ("on" state), sometimes known as the "on-off

© Springer International Publishing Switzerland 2016
A.J. Larner, *A Dictionary of Neurological Signs*,
DOI 10.1007/978-3-319-29821-4_25

phenomenon". Yo-yo-ing is difficult to treat: approaches include levodopa dose fraction-ation, improved drug absorption, or use of dopaminergic agonists with concurrent reduction in levodopa dosage.

Reference
Marsden CD, Parkes JD. "On-off" effects in patients with Parkinson's disease on chronic levodopa therapy. *Lancet*. 1976; **1**: 292–6.

Cross References
Akinesia; Dyskinesia; Hypokinesia

Z

Zeitraffer Phenomenon

The *zeitraffer* phenomenon describes altered perception of the speed of moving objects. It has sometimes been described as part of the aura of migraine, in which the speed of moving objects appears to increase, even the vehicle in which the patient is driving. It may share certain characteristics with akinetopsia, the loss of visual ability to perceive motion.

References

Critchley M. The citadel of the senses and other essays. New York: Raven Press; 1986. p. 202.
Klein R, Mayer-Gross W. The clinical examination of patients with organic cerebral disease. London: Cassell; 1957. p. 36.

Cross Reference

Akinetopsia

Zooagnosia

The term zooagnosia has been used to describe a difficulty in recognising animal faces. This may be observed as a component of prosopagnosia. In one case, this deficit seemed to persist despite improvement in human face recognition, suggesting the possibility of separate systems for animal and human face recognition; however, the evidence is not compelling. In a patient with developmental prosopagnosia seen by the author, there was no subjective awareness that animals such as dogs might have faces.

References

Assal G, Favre C, Anderes J. Nonrecogntion of familiar animals by a farmer: zooagnosia or prosopagnosia for animals. *Rev Neurol (Paris)*. 1984; **140**: 580–4.
Larner AJ, Downes JJ, Hanley JR, Tsivilis D, Doran M. Developmental prosopagnosia: a clinical and neuropsychological study. *J Neurol*. 2003; **250**(Suppl 2): II156. (abstract P591).

Cross References

Agnosia; Prosopagnosia

Zoom Effect

The zoom effect describes a metamorphopsia occurring as a migraine aura in which images increase and decrease in size sequentially.

Cross Reference

Metamorphopsia

© Springer International Publishing Switzerland 2016
A.J. Larner, *A Dictionary of Neurological Signs*,
DOI 10.1007/978-3-319-29821-4_26